T0192615

Fieldwork Educator's Guide to

Guide to

Level II

Fieldwork

Fieldwork Educator's Guide to Level II Fieldwork

Editors

Elizabeth D. DeIuliis, OTD, MOT, OTR/L, CLA
Clinical Associate Professor
John G. Rangos Sr. School of Health Sciences
Department of Occupational Therapy
Duquesne University
Pittsburgh, Pennsylvania

Debra Hanson, PhD, OTR/L, FAOTA
Professor
St. Gianna School of Health Sciences
Department of Occupational Therapy
University of Mary
Bismarck/Fargo, North Dakota

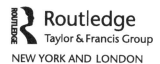

Routledge
Taylor & Francis Group

NEW YORK AND LONDON

First published in 2023 by SLACK Incorporated

Published in 2024 by Routledge
605 Third Avenue, New York, NY 10158

and by Routledge
4 Park Square, Milton Park, Abingdon, Oxon, OX14 4RN

Routledge is an imprint of the Taylor & Francis Group, an informa business

© 2023 Taylor & Francis Group

Cover: Tinhouse Design

Library of Congress

LCCN: 2022045837

ISBN: 9781630919658 (pbk)
ISBN: 9781003524175 (ebk)

DOI: 10.4324/9781003524175

DEDICATION

We would like to dedicate this book and Level I to academic fieldwork coordinators, who are often serving in this essential role within occupational education without a lot of training and resources, but serve with ingenuity, dedication, and resourcefulness.

We would also be remiss without a formal dedication to fieldwork educators who essentially volunteer their time, expertise, and energy, which makes a significant contribution to occupational therapy student learning and the future of the profession.

CONTENTS

ABOUT THE EDITORS

Elizabeth D. DeIuliis, OTD, MOT, OTR/L, CLA, is a clinical associate professor at Duquesne University, which maintains dually accredited occupational therapy programs at the master's-level and the entry-level occupational therapy doctorate level in Pittsburgh, Pennsylvania. Dr. DeIuliis served as the AFWC at Duquesne University for more than 11 years and assumed the role of program director in 2021. Dr. DeIuliis received a bachelor's degree in Health Sciences and a master's degree in Occupational Therapy from Duquesne University. She completed a Post-Professional Occupational Therapy Doctorate Program at Chatham University. Dr. DeIuliis also earned the credential Academic Leader via successful completion of the AOTA's Academic Leadership Institute in 2018. Dr. DeIuliis has had various leadership roles within academia and the occupational therapy profession, such as serving on the Board of Directors within the Pennsylvania Occupational Therapy Association and as a subject matter expert and volunteer within the National Board for Certification in Occupational Therapy. She has published several textbooks, numerous peer-reviewed publications, and has presented at state, national, and international conferences on topics related to fieldwork education, doctorate capstone, professionalism, interprofessional education, and teaching methodologies.

Debra Hanson, PhD, OTR/L, FAOTA, is currently a professor at the University of Mary, which maintains dually accredited doctoral programs at Bismarck, North Dakota and Fargo, North Dakota campuses, and an affiliated doctoral program in Billings, Montana. Dr. Hanson previously served as faculty and academic fieldwork coordinator (AFWC) at the University of North Dakota in Grand Forks, North Dakota for more than 30 years, transitioning to the University of Mary, Fargo, North Dakota campus in 2019. Dr. Hanson completed her bachelor's degrees in Occupational Therapy (1980) and Psychology (1979) and a master's degree in Counseling (1990), all at the University of North Dakota, and a PhD in Adult Education in 2009 from North Dakota State University in Fargo, North Dakota. Dr. Hanson served as the American Occupational Therapy Association (AOTA) Commission on Education AFWC representative from 2010 to 2013 and was recognized in 2014 as a Fellow in the AOTA related to her leadership in fieldwork education. She has served as a content expert and reviewer on the topic of fieldwork education for various academic journals and coordinated the Fieldwork Issues column for *OT Practice* from 2010 to 2017. She has published several book chapters and numerous peer-reviewed publications and has presented at state, national, and international conferences on topics related to fieldwork education, student clinical reasoning development, evolution of occupational therapy practice, professional identity, considerations for rural practice, spirituality, and integration of occupational therapy theory in practice and various teaching methods.

CONTRIBUTING AUTHORS

Julie A. Bednarski, OTD, MHS, OTR (Chapter 3)
Clinical Associate Professor
Program Director
Department of Occupational Therapy
School of Health and Human Sciences
Indiana University
Indianapolis, Indiana

Ann B. Cook, EdD, OTD, OTR/L, CPAM
(Chapter 13)
Associate Professor
Program Director
Department of Occupational Therapy
College of Health, Engineering and Science
Slippery Rock University
Slippery Rock, Pennsylvania

Anna Domina, OTD, OTR/L (Chapter 9)
Associate Professor and Vice Chair of
Education and Clinical Practice
Capstone Coordinator
Department of Occupational Therapy
Creighton University
Omaha, Nebraska

Cherie Graves, PhD, OTR/L (Chapter 6)
Assistant Professor and Academic
Fieldwork Coordinator
University of North Dakota
Grand Forks, North Dakota

Caryn Reichlin Johnson, MS, OTR/L, FAOTA
(Chapter 10)
Associate Professor and
Academic Fieldwork Coordinator (Retired)
Department of Occupational Therapy
College of Rehabilitation Sciences
Thomas Jefferson University
Philadelphia, Pennsylvania

Angela Lampe, OTD, OTR/L (Chapter 9)
Associate Professor and Director
Post-Professional Occupational
Therapy Doctoral Program
Department of Occupational Therapy
School of Pharmacy and Health Professions
Creighton University
Omaha, Nebraska

Patricia Laverdure, OTD, OTR/L, BCP, CLA,
FAOTA (Chapter 11)
Assistant Professor and Program Director
Department of Occupational Therapy
School of Rehabilitation Sciences
College of Health Sciences
Old Dominion University
Norfolk, Virginia

Elizabeth LeQuieu, PhD, OTR/L, CLA
(Chapter 7)
Assistant Professor
Associate Dean of Academics
Academic Fieldwork Coordinator and
Doctoral Capstone Coordinator
School of Occupational Therapy
Arkansas Colleges of Health Education
Fort Smith, Arkansas

Amy Mattila, PhD, OTR/L (Chapter 7)
Assistant Professor and Department Chair
Department of Occupational Therapy
Duquesne University
Pittsburgh, Pennsylvania

Ranelle Nissen, PhD, OTR/L (Chapter 5)
Associate Professor and Department Chair
Department of Occupational Therapy
School of Health Sciences
University of South Dakota
Vermillion, South Dakota

Hannah Oldenburg, EdD, OTR/L, BCPR
(Chapter 6)
Assistant Professor and Academic
Fieldwork Coordinator
St. Catherine University
St. Paul, Minnesota
Mayo Clinic
Rochester, Minnesota

Rebecca Ozelie, DHS, OTR/L, BCPR (Chapter 4)
Associate Professor and Program Director
(Former Academic Fieldwork Coordinator)
Department of Occupational Therapy
College of Health Sciences
Rush University
Chicago, Illinois

Alexandria Raymond, OTD, OTR/L (Chapter 8)
Department of Occupational Therapy
John G. Rangos Sr. School of Health Sciences
Duquesne University
Pittsburgh, Pennsylvania

Michael Roberts, OTD, OT/L (Chapter 2)
Associate Professor and Program Director
Master's of Science Occupational Therapy
Program
Regis College
Weston, Massachusetts

Rebecca L. Simon, EdD, OTR/L, FAOTA
(Chapter 9)
Associate Professor and Academic
Fieldwork Coordinator
Occupational Therapy Doctorate Program
College of Health and Wellness
Johnson & Wales University
Providence, Rhode Island

Bridget Trivinia, OTD, MS, OTR/L (Chapter 10)
Education and Development Coordinator
Children's Hospital of Pennsylvania
Philadelphia, Pennsylvania

Jayson Zeigler, DHSc, MS, OTR (Chapter 12)
Clinical Assistant Professor and
Academic Fieldwork Coordinator
Indiana University
Indianapolis, Indiana

PREFACE

An intended outcome after reading this book is to consciously link the philosophy of occupational therapy to the philosophy of education. There are clear synergies that exist between occupational therapy and teaching and learning best practices that might not be fully grasped by practitioners that serve in essential roles such as fieldwork educators (FWeds).

As occupational therapy practitioners, we are trained to become experts in understanding fit between people, occupations, and environments. We understand the significance of adaptation and person-centered philosophies. We study how to be astute observers and to perform activity analyses and grade tasks and demands to influence performance. We place value in ensuring a just-right challenge. These essential ingredients also make up a good teacher, instructor, or educator. As paradigms in health care and clinical practice transform and change, so does the landscape of education. We need to adapt. Although fieldwork education has existed in occupational therapy for nearly 100 years, there are limited resources that exclusively focus on best practice and skill development specific to the FWed role and, more importantly, how best to promote student learning in fieldwork.

New models for clinical learning have emerged in the occupational therapy profession and in the broader arena of health care education. Today's learners and current health professional students have changed, and generational differences in learning need consideration. One should not have a one-size-fits-all or cookie-cutter approach as a FWed. While ensuring your fieldwork student can manage a full caseload, keep up with the documentation quota, and perform safe handling techniques are certainly essential aspects of entry-level performance across various practice settings, this book challenges FWeds to shift their mindset to facilitating skill acquisition (learning) and to adjusting the teaching approach to match the learning needs and developmental level of the student. *The nuts and bolts of the matter is that there is a skill of teaching skills, and more specifically a skill to teach clinical skills.*

This book is designed to complement *Fieldwork Educator's Guide to Level I Fieldwork*. Although the books can be utilized separately, they are designed to be used sequentially and in tandem to holistically develop service competency as FWed in both Level I and II fieldwork experiences. Both of these books align with the American Occupational Therapy Association's (AOTA) Vision 2025, which provides a distinct call for the profession to *inform*, *educate*, and *activate* occupational therapy practitioners (AOTA, 2017). Fieldwork education by tradition has been integral to occupational therapy education and central to our profession. This book is designed to *inform* and *educate* occupational therapy practitioners on best practice teaching and learning approaches in order to enhance their effectiveness and identity as FWeds. Finally, it is the hope of the contributing authors that this book *activates* practitioners to link arms with and serve alongside occupational therapy educators and academic fieldwork coordinators as partners in fieldwork education to propel the occupational therapy profession forward together. As former academic fieldwork coordinators, we can confidently say that we cannot do what we do without the dedication and commitment of our FWeds.

Quality Fieldwork Is Key to Quality Occupational Therapists

This book is intended to build upon Level I's model of providing a comprehensive resource to guide the FWed with a specific focus on Level II fieldwork. In occupational therapy, fieldwork is organized by levels to include an introductory-competence level (Level I), and progressive-entry level (Level II), to develop the generalist occupational therapy practitioner (Accreditation Council for Occupational Therapy Education [ACOTE], 2018). As a desired outcome of Level II fieldwork is preparation for entry-level practice, the role and expectations of the Level II FWed are not exclusive to only being an instructor or evaluator of student performance, but also act as a facilitator of professionalism, mentor, resource curator, and clinical reasoning guide. Evolving contextual factors, such as the current and future generation of occupational therapy students, new accreditation

Figure I-1. Purpose of the book.

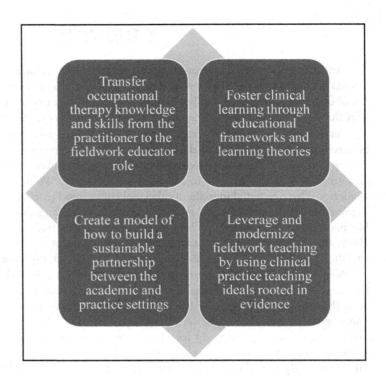

requirements impacting the preparation in the classroom, and the dynamic nature of health care require Level II FWeds to have a widening skill set compared to the past. This book is the first of its kind to serve as a practical working guide for all Level II fieldwork types and for situating pedagogy of learning in Level II fieldwork. As editors, our overall ambitions can be summarized in Figure I-1.

We are so grateful to have partnered with an all-star cast of contributing authors to actualize a big, hairy, audacious, goal that has been on our vision boards as AFWCs for some time. One of the remarkable aspects of the book sequence is the wealth of knowledge and experience behind the contributing authors. Across both books, the authors have a combined sum of more than 463 years of experience as occupational therapy practitioners, and a combined sum of more than 150 years of experience as AFWCs. The authors represent occupational therapy programs at different degree levels and from different geographical regions across the United States, as represented in Figure I-2.

Our authors have directly supervised or placed thousands of occupational therapy fieldwork students throughout their careers. They are recognized leaders in their field, as evidenced by their attainment of service leadership within the AOTA, ACOTE, National Board of Certification in Occupational Therapy (NBCOT), and state occupational therapy organizations. The contributing authors have served on AOTA AFWC-Capstone Coordinator Research Committees and task forces, served as trainers in the AOTA Fieldwork Educator Certificate Workshop, engaged as mentors and mentees in AOTAs Academic Education Special Interest Section new AFWC mentorship program, been a representative on the Roster of Accreditation Evaluation Committee, and appointed as committee members on AOTA's Commission of Education. We are so thankful to have garnered occupational therapy scholars and leaders that epitomize bona fide experts in occupational therapy fieldwork education to share their wisdom and guidance.

Frequently in occupational therapy literature, fieldwork is referred to as a bridge. Each chapter in this book is intentionally designed to serve as building block in order to create a robust infrastructure (a bridge) to connect the occupational therapy classroom to practice.

A bridge, by definition, requires support, span, and foundation to be functional and ultimately serve its purpose. Fieldwork is intended to serve as the conduit between the classroom and the

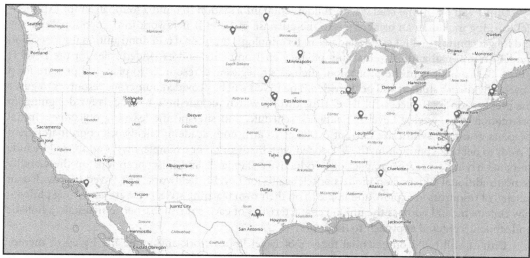
Figure I-2. Geographical locations of contributing authors.

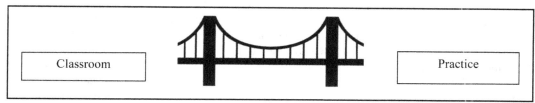
Figure I-3. Fieldwork as a bridge metaphor schematic.

clinic (Figure I-3), yet often FWeds are underprepared or unsure of how to be effective in this role. Sometimes this bridge, this infrastructure, is not sound nor stable, lacks connection, and, therefore, does not provide a solid learning experience for the occupational therapy student. As clinicians, occupational therapists are expected to be lifelong learners and engage in continued competency to support their individual clinical practice and the future of the occupational therapy profession. Practitioners that are called to serve as FWeds should embody this same professional responsibility to enhance their performance and skill set as FWeds. This is referred to as *service competency*; engaging in learning and training to develop a specific level of knowledge and skill. Each chapter in this book contributes to a comprehensive blueprint on how to develop service competency as a FWed. This next section will provide a general overview of the book as a whole and the unique features of each chapter.

Book at a Glance

A distinct aspect of this book is the showcasing of best practice teaching and learning approaches that allow the FWed to view themselves as an authentic educator. This is coupled with a similar emphasis on integrating best practice ideals of the occupational therapy profession, which include person-centeredness, inclusivity, ethics and professionalism, and occupation-based practice. Using these best practice ideals as a foundation not only enhances the professional identity of the FWed, but also the occupational therapy profession as a whole. As experts in the field, the authors thoughtfully respond to common pitfalls and challenges prevalent in Level II fieldwork today and outline a framework of action steps to address them. Vision 2025 calls upon the occupational therapy profession to be solutions-oriented, influential, effective, and responsive (AOTA, 2017). Each chapter in this book serves as an essential stepping stone to realize Vision 2025.

Unit I will orient the reader with fundamental information to build a foundation for experiential learning including an orientation to the purpose of Level II fieldwork in occupational therapy and how it contrasts with Level I, updates in terminology, traditional and nontraditional supervision models, traditional and role-emerging practice environments, and expanded roles for the Level II FWed. Best practices in the profession, such as strategies and resources to plan and prepare for a Level II fieldwork student will be provided. The FWed will be provided numerous resources to guide the preparation for a successful Level II fieldwork, which include how-to models for designing an orientation plan, weekly Level II fieldwork schedule, and site-specific learning objectives. Initial chapters also help synthesize current evidence to arm both academic fieldwork coordinators and FWeds to debunk common myths associated with fieldwork. For example, myths addressed include students having a negative impact on productivity standards and misconceptions on the viability of nontraditional supervision models or telehealth for Level II fieldwork. The FWed is provided an arsenal of resources to explore and home in on their own teaching style, cultivate a teaching philosophy statement, and address the unique characteristics of each student learner to maintain a holistic and student-centered approach to fieldwork.

Unit II will build on essential themes of Level II fieldwork and guide the FWed to mentor occupational therapy students in such areas as occupation-based, client-centered, evidence-based practice, and ethics, which are important pillars of the AOTA Vision 2025 for the profession. Best practices to spark and nurture clinical reasoning throughout the Level II fieldwork experience will also be examined. Based upon the vast experience and knowledge of the authors, frequently asked questions by FWeds and novice academic fieldwork coordinators are addressed via authentic case scenarios. Common situations illustrated include supporting students with disabilities, navigating student learning accommodations, remediating fieldwork performance problems, scaffolding clinical learning for the high-performing student, resolving intergenerational mishaps, and more. Exemplar templates to guide remediation (learning contracts) and progressive independence of the occupational therapy student will also be included.

Unit III will foster deep reflection and explore the evaluation of learning and performance during Level II fieldwork. FWeds will be empowered to consider the true value of fieldwork and link up to trends in value-based health care. The FWed will be challenged to think about evaluation as more than just a form that is completed at midterm and final. Competencies expected for student learning will be linked back to the experiential learning frameworks utilized to design the learning experience. Strategies to guide FWed self-assessment to improve proficiency in the FWed role will be provided. Lastly, as many occupational therapy programs offer an entry-level doctorate degree, the final chapter will clarify the distinct elements of the Level II fieldwork and the doctoral capstone and differentiate the roles of the Level II FWed and doctoral capstone site mentor. In addition, the reader will find helpful strategies to encourage the critical thinking and problem-solving abilities of students as they transition from Level II fieldwork to the doctoral capstone.

As occupational therapists, we know that learning occurs through doing, which is the quintessential methodology behind experiential learning such as fieldwork education. Readers are encouraged to *do* and *reflect* throughout the book. Each chapter provides opportunities for reflection, meaningful resources, and learning activities that empower the reader to translate key knowledge and skills learned to their own practice site or experience.

In Closing

Though the primary intended audience is practitioners as FWeds, these books will be meaningful to other stakeholders. For instance, occupational therapy doctoral students that are interested in exploring education as a focus area for the doctoral capstone (ACOTE, 2018) will benefit from the pedagogical groundwork and frameworks of learning threaded throughout the book sequence. To that end, serving as a FWed is often an opportunity for practitioners to test the waters as an educator within the occupational therapy classroom, serving as lab assistants, adjunct instructors, part-time instructors, or, ultimately, pursuing a full-time faculty role in academia. Those practitioners that are hypothesizing a potential career move from the clinic to higher-education will find value in learning how to connect the dots between their capacity and skill sets as a FWed to pedagogical guideposts that can be used to foster teaching and adult learning in the didactic classroom. Finally, academic fieldwork coordinators will also benefit from learning best practice teaching and learning strategies to strengthen the skill set of their own network of FWeds and to develop innovative and unique fieldwork experiences in their program. Essentially, we have provided a blueprint for academic fieldwork coordinators to design, implement, and manage fieldwork programs in diverse settings and with diverse instructional methods.

This book uniquely puts together learning frameworks, educational theories, and clinical instructional techniques within and outside of occupational therapy to uniquely equip FWeds for the future of fieldwork education. In addition to infusing these new practices into everyday fieldwork practice, it is hoped that FWeds and academic fieldwork coordinators feel inspired to continue to innovate and expand upon these fieldwork education pedagogies. What is next in the realm of occupational therapy fieldwork education? We challenge our readers to question, hypothesize, trial, reflect, learn from, and then repeat.

What we are most curious about, is what questions you have about your own fieldwork practice? For instance, have you ever wondered …

- *Is what I am doing with my students working?*
- *What is my students' experience with particular teaching approaches I use? Are they effective?*
- *Do students appreciate having site-specific learning objectives and a weekly schedule? In what ways does it help them?*
- *How did trialing a different supervision model work in my setting?*
- *Doe my students like to have weekly check-ins to discuss performance and feedback?*
- *How do diverse feedback models impact my students' learning and performance?*
- *In what ways do fieldwork students create value to my clients, work site, and my own professional development?*
- *Are the comments I provide during midterm and final evaluations meaningful to the student's growth and development?*
- *What are the most effective techniques to develop clinical reasoning in Level II fieldwork?*

Questions likes these are important ones to have and even more important to act upon and to study. Did you know that the scholarship surrounding fieldwork education in the United States falls behind other countries (Roberts et al., 2015)? Examining and expanding instructional methods and educator-development resources are critical research priorities set forth by the Occupational Therapy Research Agenda, designed to propel the occupational therapy profession forward (AOTA, 2016). Armed with a stronger pedagogical foundation and deeper appreciation for the FWed role, FWeds and academic fieldwork coordinators truly have the power to transform the future of the occupational therapy profession. Quality fieldwork is key to quality occupational therapists.

We are truly grateful for your commitment to expand and intensify your knowledge and skill set as a FWed. We hope you enjoy the books!

Warm regards,
Liz and Deb

References

Accreditation Council for Occupational Therapy Education. (2018). Standards and interpretative guide [PDF]. https://www.aota.org/~/media/Corporate/Files/EducationCareers/Accredit/StandardsReview/2018-ACOTE-Standards-Interpretive-Guide.pdf

American Occupational Therapy Association. (2017). Vision 2025. *American Journal of Occupational Therapy, 71*(3), 7103420010p7103420011-7103420010p7103420011. https://doi.org/10.5014/ajot.2017.713002

American Occupational Therapy Association. (2018). Occupational therapy education research agenda–revised. *American Journal of Occupational Therapy, 72*(Suppl. 2), 7212420070p1-7212420070p5. https://doi.org/10.5014/ajot.2018.72S218

Roberts, M. E., Hooper, B. E., Wood, W. H., & King, R. M. (2014). An international systematic mapping of fieldwork education in occupational therapy. *Canadian Journal of Occupational Therapy, 82*(2), 106-118. https://doi.org/10.1177/0008417414552187

Unit I

Getting Ready for a Level II Fieldwork Student

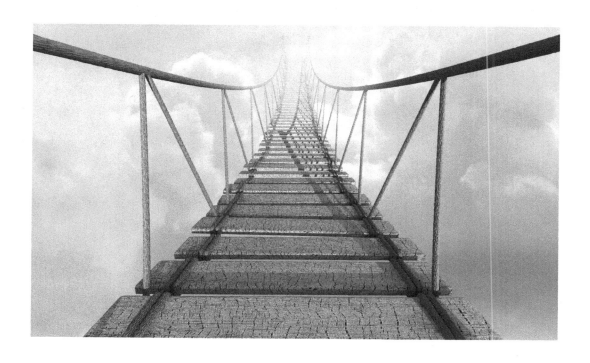

1

Overview of Level II Fieldwork

Elizabeth D. DeIuliis, OTD, MOT, OTR/L, CLA
and Debra Hanson, PhD, OTR/L, FAOTA

Historically, the occupational therapy profession has branded experiential learning for student-generalists as *fieldwork education*. Fieldwork education is often described in the literature via a metaphor of a bridge, which symbolizes a structure that provides a vital connection between theoretical didactic classroom instruction to real-world clinical practice and is argued as the most integral piece of the occupational therapy education process. Fieldwork is integrated with occupational therapy coursework to nurture the development of clinical knowledge and technical skills, as well as the core values and attitudes expected by the profession. Therefore, the role of the fieldwork educator (FWed) is essential not just to the development of individual student practitioners but the overall functioning and future of the occupational therapy profession.

Experiential learning is a required training component among various professions. Disciplines may utilize various terms to describe this required curricular component, such as apprenticeship, clinical education, practicum, residencies, externships, or internships. What is not common within health professional education is an intentional, progressive, step-wise approach, with initial, introductory experiential experiences, followed by a more immersive, intensive experience such as the nature of occupational therapy fieldwork education. A review of the educational requirements for physical therapy, nursing, speech-language pathology, physician assistant studies, and even training requirements for teachers and lawyers demonstrate that these other disciplines do not clearly stipulate different levels of experiential learning (American Academy of Physician Associates, 2019; American Speech-Language-Hearing Association, 2018; Commission on Accreditation in

DeIuliis, E. D., & Hanson, D. (Eds.).
Fieldwork Educator's Guide to Level II Fieldwork (pp. 3-28).
© 2023 Taylor & Francis Group.

Physical Therapy Education, 2017; Commission of Collegiate Nursing Education, 2018; Council for the Accreditation of Educator Preparation, 2015). Academic programs within these disciplines may differentiate levels within their individual curricula, but there is not a clear or formally defined process that distinguishes different levels of clinical training by their accreditors and/or professional organizations. Unique to occupational therapy, the desired outcome of this progressive model of fieldwork education is to achieve competency status aligned with entry-level practice expectations in the field.

Service competency is a concept in occupational therapy that includes the need for practitioners to possess a certain skill set and level of experience prior to using an intervention approach or technique (American Occupational Therapy Association [AOTA], 2009). For instance, prior to using an electrotherapeutic modality in clinical practice, a novice-practitioner will want to engage in an appropriate study of the modality, demonstrate a certain level of knowledge, and be supervised by another individual that has expertise with the use of the modality. Establishing service competency in the role of FWed is just as important. However, some occupational therapy practitioners only have their own individual fieldwork experiences as a fieldwork student to guide their attitudes and actions as a FWed. This book is designed to be a blueprint to develop service competency in the Level II FWed role. This first chapter will serve as an introduction to Level II fieldwork, including an overview of the history, an examination of the roles and unique responsibilities of the fieldwork team, and an initial synopsis of the inherent benefits and common myths associated with serving as a Level II FWed.

KEY WORDS

- **Academic fieldwork coordinator (AFWC):** Full-time, core faculty member in an occupational therapy program who is principally responsible for developing, coordinating, organizing, and monitoring the entire fieldwork process, including the oversight of the FWed and the fieldwork student.

- **American Occupational Therapy Association Fieldwork Performance Evaluation of the Level II Fieldwork Student (AOTA FWPE):** A tool designed to measure a student's performance of the occupational therapy process across multiple settings in the context of a Level II fieldwork experience.

- **Clinical coordinator of fieldwork education (CCFW):** The fieldwork site's formal representative and liaison to the academic institution; this individual is responsible for the development, management, and logistic details of fieldwork education at the fieldwork site.

- **Direct supervision:** "Two-way communication that occurs in real-time and offers both audio and visual capabilities to ensure opportunities for timely feedback" (Accreditation Council for Occupational Therapy Education [ACOTE], 2018, p. 54).

- **Fieldwork educator (FWed):** "An individual, typically a clinician, who works collaboratively with the program and is informed of the curriculum and fieldwork program design. This individual supports the fieldwork experience, serves as a role model, and holds the requisite qualifications to provide the student with the opportunity to carry out professional responsibilities during the experiential portion of their education" (ACOTE, 2018, p. 50).

- **Indirect supervision:** Supervision that occurs when the FWed gathers information from the supervisee after performance through a variety of methods, such as electronic, written, telephone communications, or interaction with other colleagues who have interacted with the student.

- **Level I fieldwork:** An introductory fieldwork experience that provides students the opportunity to apply knowledge to practice and to develop an understanding of the needs of clients (ACOTE, 2018).

- **Level II fieldwork:** A 16- or 24-week in-depth learning experience to develop competent, professional, entry-level, generalist occupational therapists who are capable of clinical reasoning and reflective practice, as well as to transmit the values and beliefs that enable ethical practice while providing occupational services to clients across the lifespan (ACOTE, 2018).

- **Student evaluation of fieldwork experience (SEFWE):** A tool through which a fieldwork student can provide feedback to their FWed or site.

- **Supervision:** Intentional intervention by a FWed aimed at helping fieldwork students develop clinical and professional skills; a mutual process involving participation from both the fieldwork students and the FWeds to establish, maintain, promote, or enhance clinical and professional performance.

LEARNING OBJECTIVES

By the end of reading this chapter and completing the learning activities, the reader should be able to:

1. Understand the value and purpose of Level II fieldwork education.
2. Identify members of and the functioning of the fieldwork education team.
3. Compare and contrast the Level I and II FWed role.
4. Identify intrinsic and extrinsic benefits and challenges associated with the Level II FWed role.

THE HISTORY OF LEVEL II FIELDWORK EDUCATION IN THE UNITED STATES

Practical, hands-on training has been required within occupational therapy education for almost 100 years. Table 1-1 provides a historical overview of the evolving regulations that have guided occupational therapy education, with a particular focus on clinical training requirements. Early on in the profession, terms such as practice-work, handiwork, practice training, and clinical training were used to describe required experiential learning for occupational therapy students. It was not until 1973 that the term *fieldwork education* was officially used by the profession, as well as a formal differentiation between Level I and Level II fieldwork. Furthermore, the label used to identify the supervising occupational therapist (or person providing supervision) in the field has also adapted over time. In earlier documents guiding occupational therapy education, the practitioners providing supervision and clinical teaching in the practice setting were referred to as supervisors or clinical trainers. In 1983, the occupational therapy profession was formally introduced to the FWed role. Although this occurred nearly 40 years ago, there continues to be various terms used among the occupational therapy field to identify and describe the FWed. The value and importance of using the FWed name vs. clinical instructor (CI) or preceptor will be discussed later in this chapter. In 1998, the accreditation standards outlined a new requirement to ensure occupational therapy students developed an understanding of the professional responsibility of and the importance of the FWed role. This was an important consideration to add to the training of occupational therapy students, as one day they will serve within this role and play a significant part in the development of the future of the profession. This academic requirement continued to be enforced by ACOTE for the next two, subsequent accreditation documents. However, in the 2018 accreditation standard that went into effect July 1, 2020, this requirement to address the FWed role in the classroom was removed. Although it is not clear why this change occurred,

TABLE 1-1
A HISTORICAL OVERVIEW OF OCCUPATIONAL THERAPY EDUCATION REGULATIONS ON FIELDWORK

DATE	TITLE	SIGNIFICANT CHANGES	SOURCE
1923	*Minimum Standards for Courses of Training in Occupational Therapy*	Minimum of 1080 hours of practice and handiwork, including drawing and design, woodworking, weaving, basketry, metalwork and jewelry, drawing, and design.	AOTA, 1924
1935	*Essentials of an Acceptable School of Occupational Therapy*	First record of being published in the *Journal of the American Medical Association*. Practical work of at least 25 semester hours in design, textiles, wood, metal, leather, plastic arts, and recreation.	AMA, 1935
1943		Requires 36 weeks of hospital practice training in either general, mental, tuberculosis, children's, or orthopedic hospital. No fewer than 30 semester hours of technical instruction in therapeutic activities.	AMA, 1943
1949		64 hours of didactic instruction with a minimum of 25 hours of technical activities in therapeutic activities. No fewer than 9 months (36 weeks) of clinical training in psychiatric, physical disabilities, tuberculosis, pediatrics, general medicine, and surgery.	AMA, 1949
1965	*Essentials of an Accredited Curriculum in Occupational Therapy*	Supervisors of clinical experience should be members of the college faculty with at least 2 years of clinical experience. 6 months of clinical experience under a registered occupational therapist. 3 months in physical dysfunction and 3 months in psychosocial dysfunction. Director of the Curriculum is responsible for selecting clinical experience sites.	AMA & AOTA, 1965

(continued)

TABLE 1-1 (CONTINUED)

A HISTORICAL OVERVIEW OF OCCUPATIONAL THERAPY EDUCATION REGULATIONS ON FIELDWORK

DATE	TITLE	SIGNIFICANT CHANGES	SOURCE
1973	*Essentials and Guidelines of an Accredited Educational Program for the Occupational Therapist*	The first time the term *fieldwork experience* is used and divided by descriptions of Level I and Level II. • Level I: Initial experiences in directed observation and participation in various field settings. • Level II: Supervised fieldwork placement with a focus on application to provide an in-depth experience. Fieldwork experience is an integral part of an educational program.	AMA & AOTA, 1973
1983	*Essentials of an Accredited Educational Program for the Occupational Therapist*	*Fieldwork educator* as a term to describe the supervisor is introduced. Collaboration between academic and fieldwork educators. Level I: Part of didactic courses; not expected to emphasize independent performance. • Supervised by qualified personnel (e.g., teachers, social workers, public health nurses, physical therapists). Level II: At least 3 months of fieldwork is full time with opportunities for supervised entry-level occupational therapist roles. • Supervised by registered occupational therapist who collaborates with academic faculty with a minimum of 1 year of experience. All fieldwork completed no later than 24 months of academic preparation.	AOTA, 1983

(continued)

it provides a valid argument for the overall need of a resource like this text to help contextualize occupational therapy fieldwork education and best practice approaches for students, practitioners, and educators.

VALUE AND PURPOSE OF LEVEL II FIELDWORK

Although the focus of this textbook is on Level II fieldwork, to develop service competency as a FWed it is important to understand the differences between the two levels. One of the differences

		TABLE 1-1 (CONTINUED)	

A HISTORICAL OVERVIEW OF OCCUPATIONAL THERAPY
EDUCATION REGULATIONS ON FIELDWORK

DATE	TITLE	SIGNIFICANT CHANGES	SOURCE
1991	*Essentials and Guidelines for an Accredited Educational Program for the Occupational Therapist*	Fieldwork center must be documented as a formal affiliation. Fieldwork to be conducted in settings equipped to provide an application of principles learned in the classroom. Advising is a collaborative process between faculty and FWed. Level I: Supervised by qualified personnel (e.g., occupational therapists, certified occupational therapy assistants, teachers, social workers, nurses, physical therapists). Level II: Required to promote clinical reasoning and reflective practice. • Minimum of 6 months (940 hours) of Level II fieldwork. • Supervised by certified occupational therapist with a minimum of 1 year of experience in practice setting. Fieldwork provided with various groups across the lifespan with various physical and psychosocial deficits. International fieldwork may be provided under certain circumstances.	AOTA, 1991

(continued)

between Level I and Level II fieldwork is that the accreditation requirements set by ACOTE are more structured for Level II. Where Level I fieldwork accreditation requirements do not provide guidelines regarding length and time, ACOTE states that 16 weeks of Level II fieldwork are required for occupational therapy assistant educational programs and 24 weeks for occupational therapist programs. There is also more structure regarding the supervision requirements and qualifications of those who serve as FWeds to Level II fieldwork students. For example, Level II fieldwork students are required to be supervised by a currently licensed or otherwise regulated occupational therapist, or, for occupational therapy assistant programs, an occupational therapy assistant (under the supervision of an occupational therapist) who has a minimum of 1 year full-time (or the equivalent) practice experience subsequent to initial certification and who is adequately prepared to serve as a FWed. The supervising therapist may be engaged by the fieldwork site or by the educational program. (ACOTE, 2018; Amini & Gupta, 2012). See Table 1-2 for a brief comparison between Level I and Level II fieldwork.

TABLE 1-1 (CONTINUED)

A HISTORICAL OVERVIEW OF OCCUPATIONAL THERAPY EDUCATION REGULATIONS ON FIELDWORK

DATE	TITLE	SIGNIFICANT CHANGES	SOURCE
1998	*Standards for an Accredited Educational Program for the Occupational Therapist* and *Standards for an Accredited Educational Program for the Occupational Therapy Assistant*	ACOTE adopted the *Standards for an Accredited Educational Program for the Occupational Therapist* and *Standards for an Accredited Educational Program for the Occupational Therapy Assistant.* Plan is documented to ensure collaboration between academic and fieldwork representatives with agreed-upon student objectives. Level I: Goal is to provide an introduction to fieldwork to have a basic comfort level of client needs. • Supervised by qualified personnel (e.g., occupational therapists, psychologists, physician assistants, teachers, social workers, nurses, physical therapists). • Experience must be documented. • Formal evaluation of student performance documented. Level II: The goal is to develop generalist entry-level occupational therapy skills. • Completed in minimum of one setting and maximum of four different settings. • Require minimum of 24 weeks full time. • Student must receive 6 hours of occupational therapy supervision per week (direct observation and client interaction). International fieldwork must be supervised by an occupational therapist who graduated from approved World Federation of Occupational Therapy with 1 year of experience. New standard requiring programs to specifically educate students on the ongoing professional responsibility for providing fieldwork education and supervision (B.7.16).	ACOTE, 1998

(continued)

TABLE 1-1 (CONTINUED)

A HISTORICAL OVERVIEW OF OCCUPATIONAL THERAPY EDUCATION REGULATIONS ON FIELDWORK

DATE	TITLE	SIGNIFICANT CHANGES	SOURCE
2006	*ACOTE Standards for an Accredited Educational Program for the Occupational Therapist or Occupational Therapy Assistant*	ACOTE adopted new *Accreditation Standards for Master's-Degree-Level Educational Programs for the Occupational Therapist* and new *Accreditation Standards for Educational Programs for the Occupational Therapy Assistant*. ACOTE adopted *Accreditation Standards for a Doctoral-Degree-Level Educational Program for the Occupational Therapist* Term *academic fieldwork coordinator* is introduced. • Responsible for advocating for links between curriculum and communication to FWed. Level I: No changes from previous standards. Level II: • For a site with no occupational therapy services, the student must be supervised for a minimum of 8 hours/week. • Formal evaluation required using *Fieldwork Performance Evaluation for the Occupational Therapy Student*	ACOTE, 2006
2011	*ACOTE Standards and Interpretive Guide*	AFWC responsible for ensuring at least one fieldwork experience has focused on psychosocial or social factors Level I: No changes from previous standards. Level II: 24 week full time can be completed part-time as long as it is at least 50% of a full-time equivalent at that site.	ACOTE, 2011

(continued)

To summarize, the goal of Level II fieldwork is "to develop competent, entry-level, generalist occupational therapists," to promote clinical reasoning and reflective practice, to transmit the values and beliefs that enable ethical practice, and to develop professionalism and competence in career responsibilities (ACOTE, 2018, p. 41). As the purpose, goal, and value of Level I and Level II fieldwork contrast, the skill set and expectations among the members of the fieldwork education team also differ. This next section will introduce and provide an initial overview of the members of the fieldwork education team.

		TABLE 1-1 (CONTINUED)	
		A HISTORICAL OVERVIEW OF OCCUPATIONAL THERAPY EDUCATION REGULATIONS ON FIELDWORK	
DATE	TITLE	SIGNIFICANT CHANGES	SOURCE
2018	*ACOTE Standards and Interpretive Guide*	Level I: • Requirements can be met through simulated environments, standardized patients, faculty practice, faculty-led site visits, or supervision by a FWed in a practice environment. Level II: • Require minimum of 16 weeks full time. • Supervision is direct and decreases over time as appropriate per setting. No longer a standard requiring programs to teach about the professional responsibility for providing fieldwork education and the criteria of the FWed role.	ACOTE, 2018

THE FIELDWORK EDUCATION TEAM

Occupational therapy generalists are expected to have comprehensive skills and knowledge from a set of core knowledge that is essential for all occupational therapy practitioners (established by ACOTE) and deliver care across a whole spectrum of ages, conditions, and practice settings. The role of an occupational therapy practitioner has long been referred to as multifaceted (Figure 1-1) even at the generalist level and demands a vast set of responsibilities, functions, and performance areas (AOTA, 1993). Although not every occupational therapy student comes into their academic journey with the expectation of becoming a teacher, as practitioners we frequently use elements of teaching and learning in clinical practice. We may teach our clients how to move their body safely via joint protection or ergonomic principles. We may educate family members or caregivers on how to don and doff an orthosis. We instruct other members of the interprofessional team on the value and importance of occupation to physical health, well-being, and quality of life. We train occupational therapy aides or volunteers how to perform routine tasks like set-up and clean-up of treatment spaces to support service delivery. Despite this, practitioners may not consider themselves fully as educators, nor have been exposed to best practices in adult learning theory and teaching and learning principles. Chapter 3 will help FWeds to think like educators and dive deeper into this realm of understanding theory behind adult learning and specific teaching and learning styles.

Figure 1-1 also portrays that the FWed plays a major function in the overall role of the occupational therapist. Along with other members of the fieldwork education team, the FWed is an essential role that helps grow the profession.

TABLE 1-2
OVERVIEW OF LEVEL I VERSUS LEVEL II FIELDWORK

	LEVEL I	LEVEL II
Structure	• No guidelines for length/time, yet all experiences within a curriculum need to be consistent in rigor • Several methods permitted by ACOTE, such as simulated environments, standardized patients, and faculty practice	• 16 weeks (occupational therapy assistant) or 24 weeks (occupational therapist) • Traditional practice setting: Supervised by a registered/licensed occupational therapist who has minimum of 1-year experience • Role-emerging setting: Supervision by a registered/licensed occupational therapist for a minimum of 8 hours per week
Purpose	• Apply knowledge to practice • Understand basic needs of clients • Opportunity for directed observation and participation	• In-depth experience • Develop professionalism • Develop competence in occupational therapist responsibilities • Develop entry-level generalist skills
Goal/ Value	• Introduction • Exposure • Active observation	• Promote clinical reasoning* • Application of evidence-based meaningful occupation, search, administration of occupational therapy • Exposure to variety of settings across the lifespan Strategies of how to develop and build clinical reasoning within Level II fieldwork students can be found in Chapter 7 of this book

*Clinical reasoning was initially recognized as an integral outcome of fieldwork in 1991 (ACOTE, 1991). This is significant as it began a discourse that fieldwork is greater than just a place where technical skills are performed. This was essential to the evolution of the role of the FWed.

Adapted from ACOTE, 2018 and Amini & Gupta, 2012.

There are several members of the fieldwork education team who are instrumental in the preparation, delivery, and evaluation of Level II fieldwork. Understanding one another's roles and responsibilities is an inherent aspect of engaging in collaborative practice, which is essential within fieldwork education (Jung et al., 2008). As fieldwork education functions as a bridge between the classroom and the clinic, the team members overlap between the academic institution and the fieldwork practice setting. This section will provide an overview of the different roles as well as a general description of their responsibilities.

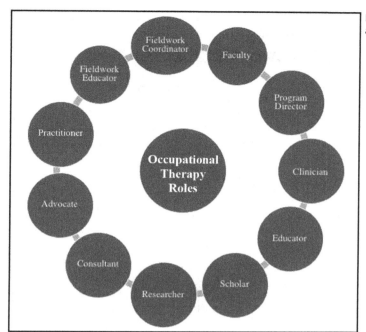

Figure 1-1. Schematic of the roles of an occupational therapy practitioner.

BOX 1-1

FWeds need to be mindful of the current strengths and areas of growth of the current generation of students. The current generation of occupational therapy students has unique viewpoints and needs regarding patterns of learning and knowledge sharing. Chapter 3 will explore adult learning theory and strategies for the FWed to understand themselves as an educator and how to adapt their teaching to meet the needs of the student.

Fieldwork Student

Fieldwork education is a collaborative process. The occupational therapy student plays an active role throughout the progression of fieldwork education. While we have already demonstrated the evolution of terminology and focus of fieldwork over time, it is also important to understand that the needs and expectations of occupational therapy students have also adapted over time. See Box 1-1.

The expectations and goals of Level II fieldwork differ from Level I. Fieldwork students need to be knowledgeable about the desired goal of Level II fieldwork, which includes generalist and entry-level practice. Furthermore, a fieldwork student needs to be aware of the progressive nature of Level II fieldwork, and that increased efficiency and independence are expected in order to assume entry-level practice expectations. Tables 1-3 and 1-4 outline attributes that contribute to or hinder a successful Level II fieldwork experience. A strong foundation of clinical knowledge (hard skills) is very important in the success of a fieldwork student. However, having resilient soft skills or practice-ready skills is just as important (DeIuliis, 2023), if not more important, to meet entry-level practice requirements across practice settings.

TABLE 1-3
EFFECTIVE FIELDWORK STUDENTS

CHARACTERISTICS	STRATEGIES
• Professional	• Build therapeutic relationships
• Ethical	• Demonstrate conflict resolution skills
• Assertive	• Initiate plans
• Accountable	• Seek feedback
• Empathetic	• Take risks
• Flexible	• Ask questions
• Adaptable	• Make eye contact
• Social	• Actively engage
• Hands-on	• Collaborate with others
• Self-aware	• Demonstrate safety and judgment
• Honest	• Accept supervision
• Responsible	• Ask for help when necessary
• Self-directed	• Balance productivity, leisure, and rest
• Strong organization skills	• Demonstrate commitment and dedication to profession
• Strong problem solver	
• Strong communication	

Adapted from Deluliis, E. (2017). Professionalism and fieldwork education. In E. Deluliis (Ed.), *Professionalism across occupational therapy practice* (pp. 201-221). SLACK Incorporated.

Academic Fieldwork Coordinator

ACOTE (2018) defines the AFWC to be a core, full-time faculty member who is responsible for the academic program's compliance with the development, implementation, management, and evaluation of fieldwork education. This faculty member is required to have at least 2 years of occupational therapy clinical experience, hold a necessary degree requirement based on the degrees offered by the institution, and be a licensed/credentialed occupational therapy practitioner (ACOTE, 2018). The position ensures that affiliated fieldwork sites reflect sequence, depth, focus, and scope of curriculum design along with verifying qualifications and preparedness of the FWeds. An essential responsibility of the AFWC is to ensure continuous collaboration among FWeds and students. In addition to the AFWC responsibilities, this individual can also be involved with other faculty responsibilities such as teaching, scholarship, and service expectations (DeIuliis et al., 2021). Some occupational therapy programs may have more than one AFWC depending upon the degrees offered and the scope of the curriculum design. As this faculty member is responsible for the academic program's fieldwork education curricula, understanding the progressive nature of Level II fieldwork and how to mentor FWeds and support fieldwork students is essential.

TABLE 1-4
INEFFECTIVE FIELDWORK STUDENTS

CHARACTERISTICS	STRATEGIES
• Unenthusiastic	• Difficulty relating to other professionals
• Disinterested	• Difficulty responding to feedback
• Outwardly overwhelmed	• Difficulty making decisions
• Resistive	• Hesitates excessively
• Defensive	• Difficulty engaging in the supervisory process
• Not confident	• Lack of insight into personal learning style
• Overly confident	
• Uncomfortable handling patients	• Lack of emotional intelligence
• Poor communication skills	• Reduced flexibility
• Poor organization skills	• Reflects passively
• Limited personal awareness	• Does not ask questions
	• Inability to multitask
	• Does not progress with efficacy or independence
	• Lacks good safety and judgment

Adapted from Deluliis, E. (2017). Professionalism and fieldwork education. In E. Deluliis (Ed.), *Professionalism across occupational therapy practice* (pp. 201-221). SLACK Incorporated.

Clinical Coordinator of Fieldwork

As depicted by AOTA (1993), a FWed may be responsible for a singular occupational therapy fieldwork student or the functioning of an entire fieldwork program at a practice setting. Some practice settings have a site coordinator role, who serves as the overarching liaison between the site and the academic program. This individual may be an occupational therapist by trade, another health profession in the department, or even centralized in the institution's human resource or education department (Hanson & Deluliis, 2015). The clinical coordinator of fieldwork (CCFW) can serve in several leadership capacities designed to promote best practice in fieldwork education, such as handling administrative details (e.g., the affiliation agreement), arranging for staff trainings surrounding fieldwork topics, collaborating with academic programs to develop site-specific learning objectives, mentoring new or novice FWeds, and troubleshooting challenging fieldwork scenarios (many will be discussed in this book) with the FWed and the academic program. The CCFW is not a required role within the fieldwork education team; yet, the role can strengthen a site's overall management of fieldwork education and streamline communication with the academic institution.

Box 1-2

SUPERVISION VERSUS EDUCATION

- *Supervision*: The action, process of supervising; **watching** and direction of activities (oversight, surveillance; Merriam-Webster, n.d.b)
- *Education:* The act or process of education; involves **teaching and learning** (Merriam-Webster, n.d.a)

Fieldwork Educator

As indicated earlier in this chapter, the term *fieldwork educator* is a purposeful title and designation endorsed by the profession of occupational therapy since 1983. While other disciplines may use CI, supervisor, trainer, or preceptor, in occupational therapy, the sanctioned role and descriptor is FWed. According to ACOTE (2018), a FWed is:

> An individual, typically a clinician, who works collaboratively with the program and is informed of the curriculum and fieldwork program design. This individual supports the fieldwork experience, serves as a role model, and holds the requisite qualifications to provide the student with the opportunity to carry out professional responsibilities during the experiential portion of their education. (p. 50)

There are a variety of reasons to support the use of the FWed title. First, fieldwork experiences can take place in a variety of practice settings, not just clinically oriented medical environments. Second, the educator vs. supervisor is chosen language in the role to emphasize the educational nature of the experience. See Box 1-2 for the definitions of education and supervision.

Although academic faculty play a significant role in the delivery of didactic coursework and lay the foundation for clinical knowledge and socialization to professionalism, it can be argued that the occupational therapy student spends more direct time learning from their FWeds (Crist, 2004; Provident et al., 2009; Ryan et al., 2018). Table 1-5 provides an example to break down the time spent with core occupational therapy faculty in a traditional post-baccalaureate program compared to fieldwork. Figure 1-2 provides another illustration to show the quantity of time that an occupational therapy student traditionally spends with the FWed.

Another reason to support the use of the name fieldwork educator is what has been proven in the literature about the significance and importance of embracing and using the language of our discipline (Wilding & Whiteford, 2007). See Box 1-3 for further discussion on the language used in our discipline.

Finally, the FWed role is designed to encompass deeper responsibilities than just instructing and teaching clinical skills. In her 2006 white paper, Dickerson used AOTA's *Standards for Continuing Competence* and transformed the competencies to intentionally describe the FWed. The *Role Competencies for a Fieldwork Educator* document consists of five standards, each with subparts that describe the values, knowledge, skills, and responsibilities expected in fulfilling the role of the FWed: knowledge, critical reasoning, interpersonal skills, performance skills, and ethical reasoning (Table 1-6).

TABLE 1-5
TIME SPENT IN COURSEWORK VERSUS FIELDWORK

		LENGTH OF TERM	QUANTITY	HOURS (LENGTH OF TERM X QUANTITY)	TOTAL HOURS
DIDACTIC COURSEWORK	Campus	225 (15 hours x 15 weeks)	5 semesters	1125	1125
FIELDWORK	Level I fieldwork	3 x 40 hour placements = 120	N/A	120	1080
	Level II fieldwork	480 (40 hours x 12 weeks)	2 rotations	960	

1 semester = 15 weeks ; 1 credit = 1 hour. (Adapted from Musselman, L. [2007]. Achieving AOTA's centennial vision: The role of educators. *Occupational Therapy in Health Care, 21*[1/2], 295-300. https://doi.org/10.1300/j003v21n01_29)

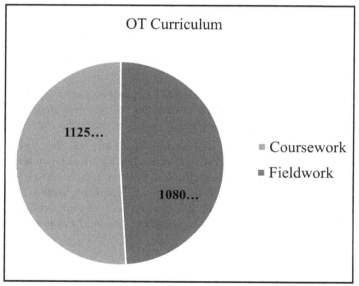

Figure 1-2. Hours in fieldwork vs. coursework.

In 2009, AOTA published the *Specialized Knowledge and Skills of Occupational Therapy Educators of the Future*, which recognized the FWed role as a critical component of the future of occupational therapy education. The desired attributes described in this white paper include a developmental perspective to build competency as a FWed, yet also provide a unique lens to view this role outside of just a supervisor or instructor. AOTA (2009) stretches outside the traditional viewpoint of the FWed toward a more complex understanding of this role as an innovator/visionary, scholar/explorer, leader, integrator, and mentor. More simply put, a FWed **supervises**, **educates**, **mentors**, **guides**, and **evaluates** occupational therapy students.

> **Box 1-3**
>
> Wilding and Whiteford (2007) led an important research study in Australia that revealed how the language we use changes our identity. For more than 100 years, leaders and scholars in occupational therapy have argued that we need to be able to define and describe occupational therapy. The participants in Wilding and Whiteford's (2007) study discuss how they conformed their language to meet the needs of society (i.e., to not be confusing). Despite this call-to-action, there are still many stakeholders who remain unclear in the role and value of occupational therapy. If we want to be better represented and validated on the same level as other allied health professions, we need to not shy away from our language and scope. Using the language endorsed by our discipline is an important strategy to help support professional representation and validate the occupational therapy discipline.
>
> This leads to an important question: Do you use the term FWed or CI/fieldwork supervisor?

- *Supervising:* The core process of overseeing and managing the learning process (i.e., regulating that the fieldwork student is complying with site policies and procedures. (*Does your fieldwork student know what to do if there is a Code Blue called on your unit?*)

- *Educating:* FWeds are responsible for providing knowledge to and teaching fieldwork students skills and techniques. (*Does your fieldwork student know how to implement the* Peabody Developmental Motor Scales, Second Edition *according to the standardized procedures of the tool?*)

- *Mentoring:* FWeds are responsible for fostering personal and professional growth within fieldwork students through role-modeling and taking a personal interest in the student as an occupational being. (*Does your fieldwork student know how to present themselves and speak up appropriately during an interprofessional team meeting?*)

- *Guiding:* FWeds are responsible for facilitating and nurturing the fieldwork process by challenging the student's thinking and encouraging reflective dialogue. (*Does your fieldwork student know how to handle a difficult question from a parent or family member of a client?*)

- *Evaluating:* FWeds create expectations and responsibilities, establish goals and learning objectives for the student, and provide feedback to the AFWC on the student's performance both informally and formally. Resources used to assist in the evaluation process include setting up an orientation schedule, week-by-week site-specific objectives, and implementing weekly formal and informal meetings to provide constructive feedback. (*Do you provide your fieldwork student with frequent constructive feedback [not just during midterm and final evaluations], and also praise their strengths?*)

Attributes of Successful Fieldwork Educators

Due to the broad responsibilities and expectations inherent in the role, being a strong clinician should not be the only deciding factor in pursuing the FWed role. While the specific act of providing hands-on experience is a necessary component, there are other valuable attributes that a FWed should demonstrate in order to provide the student a rich learning experience and role model socialization to the norms of the workplace and the profession (Tables 1-7 and 1-8).

One strategy to better understand if you possess the recommended behaviors and skills to be a FWed is to use the Self-Assessment Tool for the Fieldwork Educator Competency (SAFECOM; AOTA, 2009). The SAFECOM is a tool created by AOTA to help FWeds evaluate their competencies in the FWed role within five categories: administration, evaluation, education, supervision, and professional practice. Each category provides a definition statement as well as measurable

TABLE 1-6
ROLE COMPETENCIES FOR A FIELDWORK EDUCATOR

COMPETENCY	DEFINITION	EXAMPLE
Knowledge	Shall possess understanding and comprehension required for the role they assume.	Be up to date on the rules and regulations regarding student supervision in your practice setting.
Critical reasoning	Use sound reasoning for decision making.	Use clinical education tools that stimulate clinical reasoning for students.
Interpersonal skills	Develop and maintain professional relationships.	Be a role model; project appropriate workplace norms.
Performance skills	Demonstrate skills to competently perform within role.	Codevelop site objectives with occupational therapy program that promotes optimal learning and entry-level practice.
Ethical reasoning	Exhibit awareness of ethical issues.	Recognize important legal aspects of occupational therapy fieldwork, such as the Americans with Disabilities Act and Family Educational Rights and Privacy Act.

Adapted from Dickerson, A. E. (2006). Role competencies for a fieldwork educator. *American Journal of Occupational Therapy, 60*(6), 650-651. http://dx.doi.org/10.5014/ajot.60.6.650

BOX 1-4
"Fieldwork educators are mentors for the students they *supervise*, they *lead by example*, provide *inspiration, challenge students* to think on their feet, *encourage* when the going gets tough, and demonstrate their *commitment to professional excellence and lifelong learning*." (Costa, 2008, p 24)

---

behaviors that emulate that competency. Koski et al. (2013) have demonstrated that the importance and value of these SAFECOM competencies are dependent on the type of Level II fieldwork experience. For example, in their study, students on their first fieldwork experience value supervision, vs. organization, which is more valued during the second, final Level II fieldwork experience (Koski et al., 2013).

Administration

"... develops and/or implements an organized fieldwork program in keeping with legal and professional standards and environmental factors (physical, social, and cultural)" (AOTA, 2009).

This competency includes behaviors and skills that encompass solid interpersonal and communication skills as well good organization and time management abilities. Chapters 4 and 5 will provide various resources to guide the FWed to develop these competencies in administration to create and implement an effective fieldwork program at their practice site.

TABLE 1-7
ATTRIBUTES OF SUCCESSFUL FIELDWORK EDUCATORS

CHARACTERISTICS	STRATEGIES
• Flexible	• Communicate in a clear, specific, consistent manner
• Friendly	• Provide a detailed orientation
• Welcoming	• Provide constructive feedback
• Encouraging	• Provide validation
• Organized	• Provide structured supervision
• Caring	• Provide positive reinforcement
• Empathetic	• Provide variety for patient caseload and other experiences
• Competent	• Demonstrate legal and ethical behavior
• Knowledgeable practitioner	• Demonstrate professional attitudes and actions
• Authoritative	• Demonstrate consistent work behaviors
• Supportive	• Build the student's confidence
• Passionate about the profession	• Model the use of reflection
• Committed to teaching	• Stimulate clinical reasoning
• Interested in the student as an occupational being	• Utilize shared problem solving
• Role model	• Utilize active learning
	• Ask probing or provoking questions: "Tell me why?"
	• Make the student feel like a member of the team
	• Create a positive space for student learning
	• Create a supportive learning environment
	• Create clear and realistic entry-level expectations
	• Adapt teaching style to the needs of the student
	• Match teaching to the student's learning style
	• Maintain a professional relationship with students
	• Act as a facilitator and a guider

Adapted from Deluliis, E. (2017). Professionalism and fieldwork education. In E. Deluliis (Ed.), *Professionalism across occupational therapy practice* (pp. 201-221). SLACK Incorporated.

TABLE 1-8

ATTRIBUTES OF UNSUCCESSFUL FIELDWORK EDUCATORS

CHARACTERISTICS	ACTIONS
• Unprofessional	• Do not actively include the student
• Intimidating	• Do not make the student feel like a part of the team
• Close-minded	• Do not introduce the student to other team members
• A micromanager	
• Not evidence based	• Do not respect the confidentiality of clients
• Not enthusiastic	• Cannot clearly explain complex concepts
• Not supportive	• Do not provide the student a workspace in the clinic
• Burnt out	
• Unapproachable	• Do not provide student-centered learning
• Unethical	• Do not provide sufficient supervision
• Unavailable to teach	• Do not provide an adequate model
• Disorganized	• Do not give constructive feedback
• Disengaged	• Are not an advocate for the profession
• Inflexible	• Display poor administrative skills
	• Display poor communication skills
	• Have a high need for control
	• Have a lack of trust

Adapted from Deluliis, E. (2017). Professionalism and fieldwork education. In E. Deluliis (Ed.), *Professionalism across occupational therapy practice* (pp. 201-221). SLACK Incorporated.

Evaluation

"... evaluates student performance to achieve entry-level practice in the fieldwork setting" (AOTA, 2009).

This competency is greater than just being knowledgeable about the AOTA Fieldwork Performance Evaluation (FWPE) or another comparable evaluation mechanisms used by an occupational therapy program. The evaluation process should be ongoing throughout the fieldwork experience and should promote self-reflection. Chapter 12 will provide various resources to guide the FWed to develop these competencies in evaluation.

Education

"... facilitates the student's development of professional clinical reasoning and its application to entry-level practice. The fieldwork educator assumes responsibility for ensuring her or his own competence as a fieldwork educator" (AOTA, 2009).

A critical perspective within this competency is that the FWed cannot adopt a one-size-fits-all mentality within their teaching style. Just like occupational therapy practitioners need to adapt their therapeutic approach based upon the needs of the client, FWeds need to adapt their teaching method based upon the students' knowledge, skill level, and learning style. Chapters 3 and 8 will provide various resources to guide the FWed to develop these competencies in education.

Supervision

"... facilitates student achievement of entry-level practice through a student-centered approach" (AOTA, 2009).

Understanding different types of supervision models and theories to support students' progress during Level II fieldwork is very important. In addition, creating site-specific learning assignments and objectives are beneficial to help the student achieve entry-level practice and promote student professional development. Chapter 2 will expose the FWed to various supervision models used in Level II fieldwork and provide various resources to guide the FWed to develop these competencies in supervision.

Professional Practice

"... demonstrates competencies in professional knowledge, skills, and judgment in occupational therapy practice that supports the clients in engagement in meaningful occupation" (AOTA, 2009).

This includes competencies including but not limited to the use of evidence to drive the occupational therapy process, the ability to engage in a therapeutic relationship with the client and coworkers, and having a solid understanding of the entry-level practice. Chapters 6 and 11 will provide various resources to guide the FWed to develop these competencies in professional practice.

BENEFITS AND PERCEIVED CHALLENGES OF LEVEL II FIELDWORK

Although serving as a FWed is an inherent professional responsibility as an occupational therapist, there are several intrinsic and extrinsic benefits. Intrinsic benefits have to do with nontangible benefits that help support the motivational success of the individual. Intrinsic benefits usually accompany a sense of personal achievement, satisfaction, and pride in the task performed. Extrinsic benefits are based upon tangible benefits given by superiors, such as a merit raise or promotion (Coccia, 2019). Various studies have been directed toward understanding factors that influence a practitioner's willingness to serve as a FWed (Tables 1-9 and 1-10).

Despite known benefits and incentives associated with serving as a FWed, there are also known challenges that hinder occupational therapy practitioners and/or practice settings from being open to fieldwork students. See Table 1-11.

TABLE 1-9

BENEFITS FOR FIELDWORK EDUCATORS

	BENEFIT	EXAMPLE
Intrinsic	Energizes career	Feelings of satisfaction and fulfillment in giving back to the profession.
	Personal satisfaction	
	Stay in tune with new/current practice	
	Develop professional relationships	
	Strengthen interpersonal skills	
	Deepen clinical reasoning abilities	
	Expand supervision and teaching skills	
	Increased motivation for practice	
Extrinsic	Earn professional development units	Level II: 1 unit per 1 week per student (up to 18 units per renewal cycle).
	Increased recognition	Potential to move up the clinical ladder due to engaging in advanced roles, such as FWed.
	Potential for adjunct instructor	During site visits, toot your horn when engaging with the AFWC. What specialty skills or practice do you have that would be of value in the classroom?
		Getting your toes wet with teaching as a guest lecturer or lab assistant may be a good first step.
	Engagement in research projects	The opportunity to collaborate with academic program faculty on research projects that may benefit the clients at your site.
	Incentives from academic institution	The academic institution may offer perks to the FWed, such as use of academic libraries and athletic facilities, reduced parking, or reduced tuition rate.

Data sources: Evenson et al., 2015; Hanson, 2011; NBCOT, 2020; Provident et al., 2009; Thomas et al., 2007.

TABLE 1-10

BENEFITS FOR FIELDWORK SITES

	BENEFIT	EXAMPLE
Intrinsic	Staff development	Develop staff skills in supervision, clinical reasoning, organization, and time management.
	Keeps clinician's skills current	Students bring knowledge about practice as well as a skillset about how to be an evidenced-based practitioner that can be a model to staff.
	Promotes workplace diversity	
Extrinsic	Increased productivity	
	Future employment potential (decrease recruitment costs)	
	Support quality/process improvement efforts	Assign a student project designed to accomplish an initiative of quality improvement (e.g., update to patient education materials).
	Students provide resources and inservices	Set a student requirement to deliver an evidenced-based presentation to expand the knowledge of your team.

Data sources: Evenson et al., 2015; Hanson, 2011; Provident et al., 2009; Thomas et al., 2007.

TABLE 1-11
POTENTIAL BARRIERS THAT MAY IMPACT A FIELDWORK EDUCATOR'S OPENNESS TO HAVING STUDENTS

	PERCEIVED CHALLENGE	STRATEGY TO REDUCE BARRIER
Fieldwork Educators	Feeling ill-prepared to be an educator	Self-educate. Network with academic programs. Seek out relevant continuing education on the FWed role such as the AOTA Fieldwork Certificate Program or attend the AOTA Education Summitt to further your service competency.
	Fear of difficult student interactions: • Learning styles clash • Student performance concerns • Fear of professionalism and social skills	Utilize learning style inventories to help match student to FWed. Implement placement interviews to ensure best fit (see examples in Chapter 5).
	Impact on productivity	Increase awareness about current evidence that debunks the myth that students negatively impact productivity. Here are two current studies completed within occupational therapy, and physical therapy: • Ozelie et al., 2015 *Supervision of Occupational Therapy Level II Fieldwork Students: Impact on and Predictors of Clinician Productivity* • Apke et al., 2020 *Effects of student physical therapists on clinical instructor productivity across settings in an academic medical center*
	Pressure from academic programs Workload pressures Time constraints Balance to review clinical concepts and complete job responsibilities	Although over the past decade, the number of occupational therapy programs across the United States has increased significantly, there are various strategies to help support the need for occupational therapy programs. One strategy is the use of nontraditional student supervision models that can successfully allow more than one student to be assigned to one FWed, such as the Collaborative Model. Continue to Chapter 2 to learn how to trial and implement these models.

(continued)

	PERCEIVED CHALLENGE	STRATEGY TO REDUCE BARRIER
	TABLE 1-11 (CONTINUED) POTENTIAL BARRIERS THAT MAY IMPACT A FIELDWORK EDUCATOR'S OPENNESS TO HAVING STUDENTS	
Sites	Facility constraints	Engage in a dialogue with your site administrators regarding studies that have demonstrated a positive impact on productivity as noted previously.
	Staffing issues	
	Lack of space/resources	
	Loss of reimbursement time	

Data sources: Apke et al., Hanson, 2011; Jensen & Daniel, 2010; Ozelie et al., 2015; Thomas et al., 2007; Varland et al., 2017.

SUMMARY

Preparing and developing the profession is a call to action within the strategic priorities of Vision 2025 set forth by the AOTA (2017). Fieldwork education, specifically, FWeds, play a central role in educating and activating students who will be future practitioners and eventually future FWeds. This chapter introduced the multidimensional role of the Level II FWed, emphasizing that it is grander than just clinical instruction. This concept will continue to be built upon in future chapters. As the landscape of education and health care settings remains dynamic, strengthening the skill set of the FWed is critical to the future success of the occupational therapy profession. Just like occupational therapy practitioners adapt their therapeutic use of self and intervention approaches to meet the needs of their clients, FWeds also need to adapt their teaching methods and align their teaching strategies to meet the students' developmental stage as well as their unique learning style. This book will provide unique resources for the Level II FWed, not just those developed by the occupational therapy profession. As experiential learning is a required curricular component within many professions, there are opportunities to learn from strategies that originated in other fields to enhance the FWed role in occupational therapy.

LEARNING ACTIVITIES

1. Reflect on your own Level II fieldwork education experiences. What were the skills and lessons learned?

2. Active recall: Brainstorm the members of the fieldwork education team and write down each of their key roles.

3. A Venn diagram is a visual that shows relationships between variables to highlight the similarities and differences. Create a Venn diagram to compare and contrast the differences between the Level I and Level II FWed roles.

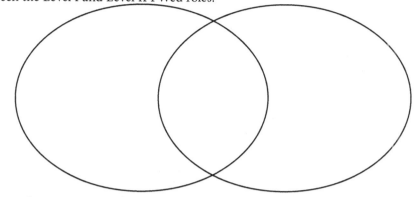

4. What academic programs does your facility have current affiliations with? Initiate a discussion with your administrator to learn more about the occupational therapy programs your site has affiliations with. Introduce yourself to the AFWC.

5. Create your personal pros and cons list for serving as a FWed annually.

REFERENCES

Accreditation Council for Occupational Therapy Education. (1998). Standards for an accredited educational program for the occupational therapist. *American Journal of Occupational Therapy, 53*(6), 575-582.

Accreditation Council for Occupational Therapy Education. (2006). *Standards and interpretative guide.* https://www.aota.org/~/media/Corporate/Files/EducationCareers/Accredit/StandardsReview/guide/2006ACOTEStandardsInterpretiveGuide8-2012.pdf

Accreditation Council for Occupational Therapy Education. (2011). *Standards and interpretative guide.* https://acoteonline.org/accreditation-explained/standards/

Accreditation Council for Occupational Therapy Education. (2018). *Standards and interpretative guide.* https://acoteonline.org/wp-content/uploads/2020/10/2018-ACOTE-Standards.pdf

American Medical Association. (1935). Essentials of an acceptable school of occupational therapy. *Journal of the American Medical Association, 107,* 683-684.

American Medical Association. (1943). Essentials of an acceptable school of occupational therapy. *Journal of the American Medical Association, 122,* 541-542.

American Medical Association. (1949). Essentials of an acceptable school of occupational therapy. *Journal of the American Medical Association, 141,* 1167-1169.

American Medical Association & American Occupational Therapy Association. (1965). Essentials of an accredited curriculum in occupational therapy. *American Journal of Occupational Therapy.*

American Medical Association & American Occupational Therapy Association. (1973). Essentials of an accredited educational program for the occupational therapist. *American Journal of Occupational Therapy, 29,* 485-496.

American Occupational Therapy Association. (1924). Minimum standards for courses of training in occupational therapy. *Archives of Occupational Therapy, 3*(4), 295-298.

American Occupational Therapy Association. (1983). Essentials of an accredited educational program for the occupational therapist. *American Journal of Occupational Therapy, 37,* 817-823.

American Occupational Therapy Association. (1991). Essentials and guidelines for an accredited educational program for the occupational therapist. *American Journal of Occupational Therapy, 45,* 1077-1084.

American Occupational Therapy Association. (1993). Occupational therapy roles. *American Journal of Occupational Therapy, 47*(12), 1087-1099. https://doi.org/10.5014/ajot.47.12.1087

American Occupational Therapy Association. (2009). Self-assessment tool for fieldwork educator competency. AOTA Press. https://www.aota.org/~/media/Corporate/Files/EducationCareers/Educators/Fieldwork/Supervisor/Forms/Self-Assessment%20Tool%20FW%20Ed%20Competency%20(2009).pdf

American Occupational Therapy Association. (2009). Guidelines for supervision, roles, and responsibilities during the delivery of occupational therapy services. *American Occupational Therapy Association, 63,* 797-803. https://doi.org/10.5014/ajot.63.6.797

American Occupational Therapy Association. (2017). Vision 2025. *American Journal of Occupational Therapy, 71*(3), 7103420010p7103420011-7103420010p7103420011. https://doi.org/10.5014/ajot.2017.713002

American Speech-Language-Hearing Association. (2018). 2020 Standards for the Certificate of Clinical Competence in Speech-Language Pathology. https://www.asha.org/certification/2020-SLP-Certification-Standards.

Amini, D., & Gupta, J. (2012). Fieldwork level II and occupational therapy students: A position paper. *American Journal of Occupational Therapy, 66*(Suppl. 6), S75-S77. https://doi.org/10.5014/ajot.2012.66S75

Apke, T. L., Whalen, M., & Buford, J. (2020). Effects of student physical therapists on clinical instructor productivity across settings in an academic medical center. *Physical Therapy, 100*(2), 209-216. https://doi.org/10.1093/ptj/pzz148

Coccia M. (2019). Intrinsic and extrinsic incentives to support motivation and performance of public organizations. *Journal of Economics Bibliography, 6*(1), 20-29. http://dx.doi.org/10.1453/jeb.v6i1.1795

Commission on Accreditation in Physical Therapy Education. (2017). Standards and required elements for accreditation of physical therapist education programs. http://www.capteonline.org/uploadedFiles/CAPTEorg/About_CAPTE/Resources/Accreditation_Handbook/CAPTE_PTStandardsEvidence.pdf

Commission of Collegiate Nursing Education. (2018). Standards for accreditation of baccalaureate and graduate nursing programs. https://www.aacnnursing.org/Portals/42/CCNE/PDF/Standards-Final-2018.pdf

Costa, D. (2008). The just-right challenge in fieldwork. *OT Practice, 13*(16), 10-24.

Council for the Accreditation of Educator Preparation. (2015.) CAEP accreditation standards. http://caepnet.org/~/media/Files/caep/standards/caep-2013-accreditation-standards.pdf

Crist, P. (2004). Ensuring FW outcomes: A call for reform. *Advance for Occupational Therapy Practitioners, 20*(20), 12.

DeIuliis, E. (2017). Professionalism and fieldwork education. In E. DeIuliis (Ed.), *Professionalism across occupational therapy practice* (pp. 201-221). SLACK Incorporated.

DeIuliis, E. D. (2023). Fostering the development of professionalism during level I fieldwork. In D. Hanson & E. D. DeIuliis (Eds.), *Fieldwork educator's guide to level I fieldwork* (pp. 109-142). SLACK Incorporated.

DeIuliis, E. D., Persons, K., Laverdure, P., & LeQuieu, E. D. (2021). A nationwide descriptive study: Understanding roles, expectations, and supports of academic fieldwork coordinators in occupational therapy programs. *Journal of Occupational Therapy Education, 5*(4). https://doi.org/10.26681/jote.2021.050415

Dickerson, A. E. (2006). Role competencies for a fieldwork educator. *American Journal of Occupational Therapy, 60*(6), 650-651. http://dx.doi.org/10.5014/ajot.60.6.650

Evenson, M. E., Roberts, M., Kaldenberg, J., Barnes, M. A., & Ozelie, R. (2015). National survey of fieldwork educators: Implications for occupational therapy education. *American Journal of Occupational Therapy, 69*(Suppl. 2), 1-5. https://doi.org/10.5014/ajot.2015.019265

Hanson, D. J. (2011). The perspectives of fieldwork educators regarding level II fieldwork students. *Occupational Therapy in Health Care, 25*(2-3), 164-177. https://doi.org.authenticate.library.duq.edu/10.3109/07380577.2011.561420

Hanson, D. J., & DeIuliis, E. D. (2015). The collaborative model of fieldwork education: A blueprint for group supervision of students. *Occupational Therapy in Health Care, 29*(2), 223-239. https://doi.org/10.3109/07380577.2015.1011297

Jensen, L. R., & Daniel, C. (2010). A descriptive study on level II fieldwork supervision in hospital settings. *Occupational Therapy in Health Care, 24*(4), 335-347. https://doi.org/10.3109/07380577.2010.502211

Jung, B., Salvatori, P., & Martin, A. (2008). Intraprofessional fieldwork education: Occupational therapy and occupational therapist assistant students learning together. *Canadian Journal of Occupational Therapy, 75*(1), 42–50. https://doi.org/10.2182/cjot.06.05x

Koski, K. J., Simon, R. L., & Dooley, N. R. (2013). Valuable occupational therapy fieldwork educator behaviors. *Work, 44*(3), 307-315. https://doi.org/10.3233/WOR-121507

Merriam-Webster. (n.d.a). Education. from https://www.merriam-webster.com/dictionary/education

Merriam-Webster. (n.d.b). Supervision. https://www.merriam-webster.com/dictionary/supervision

Musselman, L. (2007). Achieving AOTA's centennial vision: The role of educators. *Occupational Therapy in Health Care, 21*(1/2), 295-300. https://doi.org/10.1300/j003v21n01_29

National Board for Certification in Occupational Therapy. (2020). NBCOT Certification renewal activities chart. https://www.nbcot.org/-/media/NBCOT/PDFs/Renewal_Activity_Chart.ashx?la=en

Ozelie, R., Janow, J., Kreutz, C., Mulry, M. K., & Penkala, A. (2015). Supervision of occupational therapy level II fieldwork students: Impact on and predictors of clinician productivity. *American Journal of Occupational Therapy, 69*(1), 1-7. https://doi.org/10.5014/ajot.2015.013532

Provident, I., Leibold, M. L., Dolhi, C., & Jeffcoat, J. (2009). Becoming a fieldwork "educator": Enhancing your teaching skills. *OT Practice, 14*, 19.

Ryan, K., & Beck, M. (2018). Pennsylvania occupational therapy fieldwork educator practices and preferences in clinical education. *Open Journal of Occupational Therapy, 6*(1), 1-15. https://doiorg.prx-usa.lirn.net/10.15453/2168-6408.1362

Thomas, Y., Dickson, D., Broadbridge, J., Hopper, L., Hawkins, R., Edwards, A., & McBryde, C. (2007). Benefits and challenges of supervising occupational therapy fieldwork students: Supervisors' perspectives. *Australian Occupational Therapy Journal, 54*(Suppl. 1), S2-S12.

Varland, J., Cardell, E., Koski, J., & McFadden, M. (2017). Factors influencing occupational therapists' decision to supervise fieldwork students. *Occupational Therapy in Health Care, 31*(3), 238-254. https://doi.org/10.1080/07380577.2017.1328631

Wilding, C., & Whiteford, G. (2007). Occupation and occupational therapy: Knowledge paradigms and everyday practice. *Australian Occupational Therapy Journal, 54*(3), 185-193. https://doi.org/10.1111/j.1440-1630.2006.00621.x

Models for Level II Fieldwork Supervision

Michael Roberts, OTD, OT/L

Fieldwork, particularly Level II fieldwork, serves as a bridge between academic courses and professional practice. Just as bridges take a number of different forms, depending on the terrain, their function, and the features they span, Level II fieldwork models have taken a number of different forms around the world and throughout the years. With such a variety of models of fieldwork, it is unsurprising that there is not a perfect one-size-fits-all solution for every fieldwork experience or every student. The importance of finding the right fieldwork model fit can be a daunting task. Expectations of fieldwork students and their capacity for independent learning continue to increase steadily (Vogel et al., 2004). Greater expectations from fieldwork education coupled with multiple continuing trends toward a fieldwork supply bottleneck (Roberts & Simon, 2012) mean there has never been a greater emphasis on maximizing both supply and quality of fieldwork experiences.

Multiple models of fieldwork supervision have been developed and evaluated as a way to address the dilemma of maximizing quality and supply for fieldwork. Despite the development of these models, however, the one-to-one or apprenticeship model is still the most frequently used model in current practice in the United States (Evenson et al., 2015). In Canada, a one-to-one or apprenticeship model is used in 55% of fieldwork placements, while 32% of fieldwork experiences use two fieldwork educators (FWeds) to one student, 7% use more than two FWeds per student, and 6% of fieldwork experiences use other models, including multiple students per FWed (Mullholland & Hall, 2013). In Australia, Thomas et al. (2007) reported a more even distribution of supervision

DeIuliis, E. D., & Hanson, D. (Eds.).
Fieldwork Educator's Guide to Level II Fieldwork (pp. 29-83).

models, with 38% reporting use of a one-to-one model, 32% using multiple FWeds per student, and 30% using other models. This distribution may be due to universities offering multiple models of supervision for fieldwork as part of their programs. Gustafsson et al. (2017) surveyed Australian university programs and found all responding programs offered apprenticeship and multiple FWed models, and 95% offered collaborative model placements (multiple students per FWed).

Not only do most or all of the universities offer a variety of supervision models, 42% reported using role-emerging placements and a small number offered project placement fieldwork options (Gustafsson et al., 2017). In the United States, Evenson et al. (2015) found a greater reliance on traditional apprenticeship models for Level II fieldwork, with 68% of respondents reporting use of the one-to-one supervision model, 15% using a collaborative model (one FWed for two or more students), 2% using multiple FWeds per student, and 15% reporting use of other models. While the predominant fieldwork model may be a traditional apprenticeship model, a variety of models of supervision have been used since the early days of the profession, as evidenced by a description of multiple FWeds contributing to fieldwork evaluation in an article in the *American Journal of Occupational Therapy* in 1957 (Booth).

The variety of models leads to the question: which model is best? We answer this question much as we answer the question of which practice model is best for us to use with a client or practice. All models, including the popular apprenticeship model, have benefits and drawbacks. We identify the best model based on our practice, our setting, the population with which we are working, the skills and knowledge base of the practitioners, and the unique characteristics of the students with whom we are working.

An important consideration in the current setting for fieldwork is an understanding of the influence of the current shortages in fieldwork opportunities for students. A review of enrollment and licensure trends in the United States showed that the average number of available licensed practitioners per entry-level occupational therapy student is shrinking as enrollment increases outpace development of new eligible FWeds (Roberts & Simon, 2012). Site availability has been impacted negatively by reimbursement policy changes, higher enrollment trends, and, most recently, by once-in-a-century pandemics. Understanding the benefits and risks of different fieldwork models can provide the profession with flexibility and creativity that improve fieldwork site recruitment and retention.

In order to help with this process, it is important to define each model, and identify its unique qualities, benefits, challenges, and best uses. To that end, this chapter will define, describe, and compare each of the following models of fieldwork:

- Apprenticeship model, or traditional one-to-one student to FWed
- Project placement
- Role-emerging placement
- Multiple mentorship, or multiple FWeds with one or more students
- Collaborative model, or multiple students per FWed

LEARNING OBJECTIVES

By the end of reading this chapter and completing the learning activities, the reader should be able to:

1. Describe key characteristics of fieldwork supervision.
2. Recognize the primary features as well as similarities and differences between supervision models.
3. Describe the relative benefits and challenges of different models of fieldwork supervision.

4. Compare the evidence for the use of different models of fieldwork supervision in a variety of practice settings.

5. Identify resources available to FWeds to implement a variety of fieldwork supervision models.

KEY CHARACTERISTICS OF EFFECTIVE FIELDWORK SUPERVISION

Supervision is an innate feature across experiential learning in diverse professional degree programs. By definition, supervision refers to the action, process of supervising, watching, and direction of activities, which can also include oversight and/or surveillance (Merriam-Webster, n.d.a). In occupational therapy, supervision is clearly labeled as a key competency of the occupational therapy FWed (American Occupational Therapy Association [AOTA], 2009). As a construct, supervision can be described on a spectrum of direct to indirect supervision.

- *Direct supervision*: "Two-way communication that occurs in real-time and offers both audio and visual capabilities to ensure opportunities for timely feedback" (Accreditation Council for Occupational Therapy Education [ACOTE], 2018, p. 54). This can occur through observation, modeling, direct instruction, discussions, teleconferencing, etc.

- *Indirect supervision:* Supervision that occurs when the FWed gathers information from the supervisee **after performance** through a variety of methods, such as electronic, written, telephone communications, or interaction with other colleagues who have interacted with the student.

Within an experiential learning scenario, there are usually two key roles: a supervisor and a supervisee:

- *Supervisor*: "One who ensures that tasks assigned to others are performed correctly and efficiently" (ACOTE, 2018, p. 54).

- *Supervisee*: A person being supervised (Merriam-Webster, n.d.b).

While supervision is commonly described as a verb or action, it can also refer to a relationship or process that occurs between the supervisor and supervisee. A key aspect of effective supervision is that it is a **mutual** phenomenon, requiring ongoing participation from both the supervisor and the supervisee. In occupational therapy fieldwork, supervision is an intentional intervention used by the FWed aimed at helping students developing clinical and professional skills. At the core of the fieldwork education experience is the supervisory relationship between the FWed and the fieldwork student. While many practitioners can describe supervision in a practice sense, supervision in the context of fieldwork education is a unique construct.

In fieldwork, supervision serves many important purposes. Supervision promotes clinical reasoning, reflective practice, professional development, competence with career responsibilities, and ethical practice, which can match supervision provided to experienced practitioners. Fieldwork supervision builds on these efforts by adding components more directly tied to the developmental transition from student to professional, like sharing of the values and beliefs at the core of occupational therapy's professional identity, consumer protection, assessment of student progress toward the shared objectives of fieldwork experiences, effective use of resources, creativity, and innovation (ACOTE, 2018; AOTA, 2010, 2014). To effectively promote all these values, skills, and competencies, fieldwork supervision is necessarily a dynamic construct between educator and student. It requires the student and educator to share an understanding of each other's skills, knowledge, competencies, experience, and education (AOTA, 2014). It is a relationship built on communication and feedback that is meant to encourage and support the student to learn self-reflection and self-assessment about their strengths and opportunities, to grow as a professional toward their

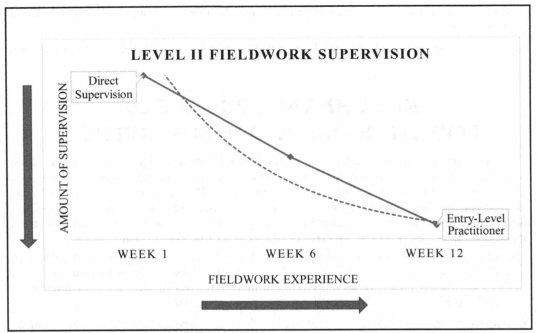

Figure 2-1. Structure of supervision.

shared objectives for the fieldwork experience, as well as empower the student to make the necessary changes to meet those objectives (AOTA, 2013).

Further adding to the dynamic nature of the relationship is its progressive format. Differing from language used in Level I fieldwork, Level II fieldwork specifies that supervision provided by the FWed starts out as direct, then becomes less direct as the fieldwork student demonstrates more competency with the skills necessary for professional practice (ACOTE, 2018). Figure 2-1 depicts how supervision becomes less direct as fieldwork progresses for the occupational therapy student.

However, this process is not linear. It changes and is modified, based on a number of different factors that the FWed must understand and assess continuously. These factors include the student's competence and confidence, the complexity of the needs of the client population, the number of clients, the diversity of the client population, the role of occupational therapy practitioner in that particular practice setting, and any unique requirements of that practice setting, including regulatory or reimbursement requirements (AOTA, 2012).

The FWed is primarily responsible for utilizing this dynamic relationship to achieve the goals of their practice as well as the shared objectives of the fieldwork experience. This means the FWed must retain the ultimate responsibility for all aspects of the occupational therapy service delivery for the client population, including the safety of the clients and the effectiveness of the occupational therapy interventions when services are provided by the fieldwork student (AOTA, 2010). While meeting these responsibilities, FWeds add on the additional requirements of ensuring their supervision of the student meets the student's current and advancing levels of competence as an occupational therapy student practitioner. This involves designing educational experiences to support student development, providing evaluation of the student's performance, adapting their own approach to align with the student's learning and communication style, as well as meeting the administrative requirements of the fieldwork program (AOTA, 2013).

The success of this dynamic and multifaceted supervision process is not the sole responsibility of the FWed. Successful supervision also requires that the student be an active participant in the supervision process. This includes developing and completing learning objectives, completing educational activities, seeking and incorporating feedback from the FWed, engaging in self-assessment and self-reflection, as well as participating in all evaluations by the FWed (AOTA, 2013).

While there are many facets and factors that influence success with the supervisory relationship, it is important to understand that these requirements and responsibilities are inclusive of all fieldwork supervision models. These general responsibilities described for the FWed and fieldwork student are expectations for all models of fieldwork supervision, and can be achieved in all models of fieldwork supervision. The foundation for that success is understanding the expectations and developing structures and experiences that meet the general requirements listed previously, and the unique requirements for each setting and supervision model used.

TYPES OF SUPERVISION MODELS

Outside of the mutual expectations and responsibilities of the supervisor and supervisee, there are different formats and models of how supervision can be utilized in Level II fieldwork. This next section will provide an overview of different types of supervision models used in occupational therapy. The structure of each supervision model will be described as well as inherent benefits and drawbacks; see Table 2-1 for a basic overview. Appendix A provides a deeper synthesis of the models presented in this chapter. Lastly, additional resources to support implementation of these models are provided for the reader in Appendix B.

One-to-One/Apprenticeship Model

The commonly used apprenticeship, or one-to-one (often referred to as the traditional model), model of fieldwork supervision resembles the structure of similar apprenticeship constructs in other trades, where an expert practitioner provides instruction and mentorship to the fledgling professional in a real-world context. This model provides an opportunity for the fieldwork student to learn skills, values, and behaviors through observing and modeling the practice of their FWed (Graves, 2019). The model is based on social learning and constructivist theories of professional development that underpin several aspects of occupational therapy education and practice (Hebert et al., 2013; Richard, 2008; Schwartz, 1984; Box 2-1).

For instance, the constructivist approach championed by Vygotsky (1978) features the concept of the Zone of Proximal Development, where an individual on the verge of achieving a developmental gain is recognized by a peer or collaborator, like a FWed, to be capable of progressing, and is guided or supported to make that developmental progress (Richard, 2008). Social learning, described by Wenger (2000), understands learning to be both a historical and social construct within a professional community, where learning takes place within the interplay between our experiences and competence defined by our professional community. Fieldwork students compare the established version of competency, from their FWed, with their lived experience as a practitioner and learn through resolving the similarities and differences observed (Wenger, 2000).

The apprenticeship model is easily the least complex model of fieldwork supervision, but that is not the sole reason for its ubiquity. It is hardly surprising that this model is used predominantly, as it allows the FWed to instruct the student directly about practice skills and knowledge, while also modeling professional behaviors and demonstrating norms of occupational therapy's professional culture. Richard (2008) describes an example of the process as described by a FWed:

I have [the student] go to a couple of orientation groups their first weeks so they can watch what I do and how I orient and assess. I'll model it for the student [modeling]. Then I

TABLE 2-1

OVERVIEW OF LEVEL II FIELDWORK SUPERVISION MODELS

SUPERVISION MODEL	NUMBER OF STUDENTS	NUMBER OF FIELDWORK EDUCATORS	ROLE OF THE FIELDWORK	STRUCTURE OF THE EXPERIENCE
One-to-one/ apprenticeship	1	1 (Generally employed within the fieldwork setting)	Provide direct supervision Model and facilitate student learning	Focus is on development of student skills for direct practice
Role emerging	1 (Could be more than 1 if also using a collaborative model at a role emerging site)	1 (May not be directly employed by the fieldwork setting)	Provide at least 8 hours of direct supervision per week; other indirect supervision and support provided as needed A staff member at the practice setting (who most likely is not an occupational therapist) provides day to day supervision	Focus is on development of student skills for direct practice and/or program development
Project placement	1	1 to 2 (Can be combination of on- and offsite staff)	Identification of potential projects Oversee completion of project	Focus is on development of project
Shared supervision/ multiple mentoring	1	2 (Generally employed within the fieldwork setting; could also be employed at different sites)	Provide direct supervision Model and facilitate student learning Collaborate with other FWeds	Focus is on skills for direct practice
Collaborative	2 or more (Could be from the same or different occupational therapy program)	1	Model and facilitate the coconstruction of knowledge (peer-learning) Guide clinical reasoning through different types of questioning approaches and foster student self-refection (see Chapter 8 for some example strategies in this area)	Focus is on skills for direct practice and interprofessional teamwork If used in a role-emerging setting, this might also include skills for program development

---

BOX 2-1

VIGNETTE USING ONE-TO-ONE/APPRENTICESHIP MODEL

"Becky? Hi, it's Sue. It was great running into you at the state conference last week. You were asking if I was ready to take on a Level II student, and after thinking about it, I decided I'm ready. I talked it over with my boss, and she said they would be able to adjust some staffing in the department to make sure I have the time to work with the student."

"That's great, Sue! You're going to do a wonderful job. I'll send over some paperwork by email after my meeting this afternoon. Would you be available this summer?"

"I was actually hoping for this fall. I have a vacation planned this summer and my caseload usually runs light during that time of year anyway. Is that okay?"

"Of course! I have a student who is going out on her first placement this summer, but just had her fall placement cancel. She's a strong student who did very well on her Level I placements. I know she's interested in working with a population like your clients, and I think her learning style and communication style will work well with you."

"That sounds perfect. By the way, I had heard at the conference about different models of fieldwork in use these days, and they sound interesting, but I think I'd rather keep it simple for my first time supervising a Level II. Is it okay if I just focus on a traditional one-on-one placement this time?"

"Of course! I think you would be able to do well with those models in the future, but I understand your wanting to start with the basics. I really appreciate your willingness to help us out. I'll get you connected with our student soon and make sure you have everything you need before she starts in September. As always, you know I'll be there to help out with anything you need. Thanks again for reaching out!"

"Thanks, I'm looking forward to it!"

---

usually have them assess me first, like, I'll present like a patient and have the student do a mock interview assessment with me [coach and scaffold]. Then we'll move to a patient, and I'll sit in, then give feedback and help them troubleshoot [coach and scaffold]. Then once they are comfortable and developed the skill, I let the student go [fading]. (p. 170)

This close relationship is a clear benefit to this model of supervision. Positive experiences with FWeds who are perceived as engaged and collaborative build positive, valued relationships with their students. Students appreciate their FWed's expertise and cooperative approach and strongly value their relationship with their FWed, even if they perceive their educator's practice as falling short of standards in occupation-based practice (Graves, 2019). More practically, the one-to-one model ensures that the student and their FWed observe each other regularly, work together, exchange feedback in a timely fashion, build a relationship, discuss practice, and reflect on experiences, all in a setting without competition or comparison with other students, and not contending with other students for time necessary for accurate assessment of their progress (Martin et al., 2004). Students in the one-to-one model see advantages in their individual attention from their FWeds, the clear and easy-to-understand expectations of their FWed, and the relatively easy logistic challenge of working with one FWed's schedule and caseload (Farrow et al., 2000).

Yet, while the model is commonly used across the occupational therapy practice world, its implementation is not without potential challenges. One identified challenge is fully allowing for independent practice by the students, when direct supervision is the expected model. Hengel and Romeo (1995) stated that:

The one-to-one approach tends to create an experience in which the student is more likely to imitate and rely on staff members than to develop his or her own clinical reasoning skills and individual style—both of which are necessary for competent practice. (p. 354)

This can be a particular concern when the nature of the caseload or the regulatory requirements of the community require more direct supervision. For example, up until recently, in 2020, the Commonwealth of Massachusetts in the United States required direct, on-site supervision of all occupational therapy students for any fieldwork activities. This represented a much more stringent standard for supervision than the contemporaneous standard of supervision, requiring a minimum of 8 hours of direct supervision per week for Level II fieldwork students (ACOTE, 2018). This was recently changed to reflect the national standard and thereby allow practitioners in Massachusetts to utilize nontraditional fieldwork supervision models (Massachusetts Board of Allied Health Professionals, 2020).

An additional challenge is the existence of FWeds who are limited in their collaborative approach and instead take a more hierarchical approach to fieldwork education. Given that the model is based on a dyad of a single student and single practitioner, the sole source of feedback, communication, modeling, and expertise for the student is their FWed. Thus, the quality of the experience rests exclusively on the quality of that relationship. Unfortunately, there are examples of suboptimal experiences in fieldwork. One example comes from an interview with a former fieldwork student:

Sylvia shared with me that her discomfort in the environment kept her from asking a lot of questions. She feared that her questions might sound stupid and her fieldwork educator would make fun of her and then talk about it in front of her co-workers when she thought Sylvia couldn't hear her. (Graves, 2019, p. 187)

When students experience disappointment in their fieldwork, their reactions can range from disappointment with the fieldwork experience, to emotional distress, to physical effects. In some cases, the student not only feels disappointed in the quality of their educational experience, but also doubts that their clients received the best possible care (Lew et al., 2007). Still, it is important to note that negative experiences like this are the exception rather than the rule with this model. Also, even students who have negative experiences with FWeds can derive positive results from their fieldwork experiences. These students report they become more self-reliant and stronger emotionally as a result of succeeding despite a negative relationship with their FWed (Lew et al., 2007).

See Table 2-2 for a snapshot of the benefits/challenges table for one-to-one/apprenticeship model.

See Box 2-2 for another vignette illustrating the one-to-one/apprenticeship supervision model.

TABLE 2-2
BENEFITS AND CHALLENGES FOR
ONE-TO ONE/APPRENTICESHIP MODEL

BENEFITS	CHALLENGES
• Direct one-to-one instruction about practice skills and knowledge.	• Fully independent practice by the student more difficult.
• Close, one-to-one relationship between student and FWed.	• Students tend to imitate and rely on other staff for development of clinical reasoning skills and individual therapeutic style.
• Ensures student and FWed observe each other, exchange feedback, discuss, and reflect on practice regularly.	
• No competition or contention with other students for time with FWeds.	• Only one source of feedback, communication, modeling, and expertise for student on fieldwork.
• Clear and easy to understand expectations communicated to student by FWed.	• Quality of fieldwork experience often depends on quality of relationship between student and FWed.
• Student only needs to attend to one FWed's schedule and caseload.	• Requires full-time commitment from an experienced FWed for each fieldwork student, most labor-intensive model, may limit supply of fieldwork experiences.

Multiple Mentorship/Shared Supervision Model

For decades, sites and practitioners have sought solutions for matching a variety of practice and staffing models to their goals of engaging in fieldwork education. Some sites have specialist practitioners who have a very specific caseload. These practitioners could provide a unique opportunity for fieldwork students to experience a rare and fascinating practice, but do not feel they have enough variety in their practice to provide a practical generalist experience for students as a foundation to their future work. Other excellent and qualified practitioners want to participate in fieldwork education, but work split or part-time schedules, so they cannot provide a full-time experience for students looking to complete their Level II full-time weeks in a timely fashion so they can begin their own professional careers. One solution to these challenges is to use an aggregate, shared supervision, or multiple mentorship model of fieldwork, where responsibility for the fieldwork student is split across specialty or part-time practitioners, resulting in a full-time experience but across multiple FWeds. See Boxes 2-3 and 2-4.

This is not a new idea in occupational therapy education. Mary Booth (1957) recommended using a combined rating from multiple FWeds for fieldwork students in her article about clinical training of occupational therapy students in just the 11th volume of the *American Journal of Occupational Therapy*. It has been utilized since then because of the perceived benefits from the sites and FWeds who use the model. The identified benefits are many, including allowing fieldwork sites to increase the number of students they accept for placements without increasing the stress on any particular FWed, spreading supervision across multiple practitioners or several practice areas, and offering support while putting more of the responsibility for learning on the

---

Box 2-2

Vignette From One-to-One/Apprenticeship Model

"Okay, let's pretend that I'm Mr. Lubomirski. Introduce yourself, and let's run through the upper extremity part of the eval one more time."

"All right. Hi, Mr. Lubomirski! I'm Katie. Today I want to test your arm strength. Are you ready?"

"Time out, quick thing: introduce yourself as 'Katie from occupational therapy' and explain why you need to test his arm strength. Relate it to occupation."

"Got it, sorry. Starting over … Hi Mr. Lubomirski! I'm Katie from occupational therapy. Today as part of your evaluation I'd like to test your arm strength. Knowing how strong your arms are will help me plan out how best to get you back to doing the cooking you love to do at home."

"Much better, continue …"

"Okay, Mr. Lubomirski. Would you please raise your arms straight up toward the ceiling? Good! And touch your shoulders. Good. Now can you do the movements I am doing? Great. Thanks. Now that I've seen how well you can move your arms, I'd like to see how strong you are. Go ahead and straighten out your arm away from your body like this. Good! Is it all right if I touch your arm? Thanks. I'm going to try and push your arm down toward the floor, but don't let me. Ready? Good! Nice and strong …"

"Okay, show me testing for elbow extension and shoulder external rotation …. Good, exactly right!"

"Thanks, better than last time, definitely …"

"You are doing much better; it just takes practice. You have a good interpersonal style with the clients, and you know all the procedures for the evaluation. Just remember to explain why you are doing each part, so the client understands the purpose of the evaluation, and relate it to his occupation-based goals for his return home. Are you feeling ready to go see Mr. Lubomirski?"

"Yes, I'm feeling a bit nervous, but I'm ready."

"Then let's go. I'll let you run the session, but I'll be there if you have any questions."

---

student (Nolinske, 1995). This model is also flexible enough to allow for combining both practice and research skills in less common practice areas, allowing for students to be prepared "not only as entry level therapists, but also as therapists who can add to the growing body of occupational therapy literature in this important time of best practice" (Precin, 2009, p. 75).

While the model has a great deal of flexibility built into the structure, there are still common defining characteristics of the model evident in practice. Essentially, it involves multiple FWeds providing supervision for one student or a group of multiple students (Graves & Hanson, 2014). Some examples involve the student working across practice settings with related populations, such as working with one FWed in an inpatient hospital setting and another FWed in community-based care (Engel et al., 2013). Other placements involved interdisciplinary groups of interns, including occupational therapy students, supervised by an interdisciplinary group of practitioners within a common practice setting (Precin, 2007). To ensure success, sites built in regular meeting time for FWeds to discuss supervision strategies and students' performance, while ensuring the students engage in self and peer evaluation and meet regularly to evaluate and support one another (Farrow et al., 2000). See Table 2-3 for recommendations from sites that successfully used the shared/multiple mentoring model. FWeds considered splitting a placement into consecutive blocks of time with different practices or practitioners, but recommend instead having students work with

---

BOX 2-3

VIGNETTE FROM MULTIPLE MENTORSHIP/
SHARED SUPERVISION MODEL

"Hi Camille! How are you enjoying the conference so far? Oh, and thanks for letting me know about that presentation your coworker, Deb, was doing on inpatient pediatric splinting. That is such a fascinating niche practice, and she is such an engaging speaker."

"No problem! I knew you would find her presentation to be excellent and so informative. Those splints are so tiny! It blows my mind how she does that work. She's amazing."

"I agree. I know at least a few of my students were there as well, and I'll likely have them asking me about Level II fieldwork with her or someone like her. Do you know if she takes fieldwork students?"

"I wish she would, it would be such a great experience and she's so good at teaching her practice. Only thing is, that practice only takes up about 10 to 15 hours per week, and she's not there full time. So, it doesn't work."

"Actually, that's not necessarily true. Would you be willing to consider a shared supervision model Level II placement with her? We could combine your practice with her practice and you'd share the supervision of the student."

"How would that work?"

"Just like the name implies, you would share supervision of the student. You work full time and have a more consistent caseload at the same facility, but she has the unique practice. You would work out in advance how to split the student caseload, what the learning objectives for the student would be, who would complete the fieldwork performance evaluation (FWPE), and how you would collaborate on supervision. The student works most of her case load with you, but has a set percentage of her caseload with your colleague. The student gets the benefit of learning the unique practice, your colleague gets the benefits of working as a FWed, and your collaboration with her ensures you cover all the bases for Level II fieldwork responsibilities. It takes some initial planning and ongoing communication between the two of you, but I doubt that would be a problem."

"That's really interesting. I didn't know we could split a student like that. Sounds like the perfect arrangement for her and for me. What are our next steps?"

"I send you some resources and examples of materials other shared supervision placements have used, as well as some evidence for the model. You can review that with your coworker and decide if it's the right decision for you both. Once you've agreed to move forward, I can send along additional resources with our student when they come by for an interview. We'll make sure you've got a student that you think will be a good match to both practices and the shared supervision model. Then, we finally get to see your coworker as a FWed!"

"That would be such a great opportunity for a student. I am very excited about this idea and I have a funny feeling Deb will be excited about it, too. I'll talk about it with her when she's back at work on Monday and I'll let you know what she says. Thanks for this great idea!"

"Thanks for considering the opportunity. I'm looking forward to hearing from you soon."

---

multiple FWeds concurrently to achieve greater repetition with skills necessary for effective practice (Gaiptman & Forma, 1991). See Figures 2-2 and 2-3 for two illustrations of how to split a Level II fieldwork experience across FWeds and/or fieldwork sites.

Box 2-4

Vignette From Multiple Mentorship/ Shared Supervision Model

"Hey, Linda! Another busy day today, and another two evals coming in. I think Erika can take them both to get her up to five by midterm next week. One is pretty straight-forward, a client status post–hip replacement with a history of chronic obstructive pulmonary disease and congestive heart failure, the second one is for your caseload, stage 3 glioblastoma, getting radiation for another 2 weeks. What do you think? Can she handle adding those two to her caseload?"

"Oh, sure. She did great with the eval and treatment plan on last week's new eval, the client with the non–small cell lung cancer. They were pretty complex, with pain issues, radiation, a course of chemo wrapping up. She had lots of questions, but they were good questions, so I felt confident she wasn't missing anything. She had a great interpersonal style with the client, they think Erika's the best. If they come in tomorrow, Thursday, that's great because I'm on-site Thursday, Friday, Monday for the next month or so. This way I can help supervise the eval and the write-up, then we can meet at our regular time after department meeting on Monday to plan for the rest of the week."

"Sounds good, Dan. It will be helpful for us to meet so I know what the two of you have planned for that new client with the brain tumor and I can be available through Wednesday while you're at the other site. Oh, and remember, we need to schedule a meeting the following week so we can collaborate on her midterm evaluation. I'll meet with her to discuss all of our feedback, but I have some specific questions to ask you about her performance so far. That will help me make sure she's getting all the necessary information for her assessment."

"Yes, that works. Do me a favor and send me an email with the specific questions you have and I'll work on them and have them ready for next week. Does that work for you?"

"Yes, that's perfect. Anything else you need me to keep an eye on while you're off-site next week with the new client?"

"Just make sure she checks physician orders and labs or blood work every day. Oh, and make sure she knows the radiation schedule, especially if it's b.i.d. That will do it."

"Thanks! We make a great team."

"It helps that we got a great student … See you tomorrow!"

Having built the fieldwork program around the recommendations in Table 2-3, what benefits can be expected with its utilization? Returning to intentions in developing the model, multiple mentorship was designed to allow access to multiple practice areas, FWeds with a narrow but valuable practice area, FWeds who work less than full time, and multiple practice settings. In multiple placement settings across the globe, practitioners find exactly these benefits (Avi-Itzhak & Kellner, 1996; Copley & Nelson, 2012; Engel et al., 2013; Farrow et al., 2000; Gaiptman & Forma, 1991; Precin, 2009). The model is also shown to increase opportunities for contact with clients, developing professional skills, and working collaboratively, while demanding less of the FWed's time if organized effectively (Farrow et al., 2000). Other sites that utilized the model cited additional benefits, such as FWeds perceiving the shared supervision as less "draining," additional students expanded the services they could provide to their clients, and the students finished fieldwork with greater competency than in use with individual supervision (Copley & Nelson, 2012). Significantly, sites also reported that students' greater autonomy and responsibility led to the students experiencing a less dependent relationship with their FWed (Gaiptman & Forma, 1991). Students' teamwork skills developed quickly as the students relied on each other and supported each other's learning

TABLE 2-3
RECOMMENDATIONS FOR MULTIPLE MENTORSHIP/SHARED SUPERVISION FIELDWORK SITES

SOURCE	RECOMMENDATIONS
Copley & Nelson, 2012	Set up structures in advance to manage logistics, track students' learning and performance, and monitor student caseloads.
	Require students to prepare written materials for supervision meetings in advance.
	Share a clearly defined list of expected competencies for the students, so that current performance can be compared with the list to generate timely feedback.
	Use a structured system for recording feedback for each student.
	Encourage students to work with peers to support each other's knowledge and learning, as they would not expect to always have a FWed by their side.
	Monitor team dynamics among the multiple students in practice.
Precin, 2009	Provide manual, binders, workbooks, or other evidence-based resources for the students to use independently in their preparations for practice.
	Collaborate with the university in advance to ensure consistency in understanding of the unique characteristics of the model.
Graves & Hanson, 2014	Identify clinical reasoning differences before supervision begins.
	Learning contracts clarify expectations and encourage students to take ownership of their fieldwork assignments. (Refer to Chapter 10 for a detailed view of learning contracts.)
Farrow et al., 2000	Occupational therapy programs should address the differences of the roles and responsibilities of the students and FWeds in this model in advance.
	Methods of evaluation and strategies to facilitate group learning clearly articulated.

processes (Copley & Nelson, 2012). FWeds reported the students in the multiple mentorship model learned and processed more information at a faster rate and at a deeper level, as well as collaborating more with staff (Precin, 2009), while being exposed to a statistically significantly greater number of practice areas (Farrow et al., 2000).

Challenges or risks were also identified in the use of this model, including managing expectations from multiple FWeds or any potential contradictions or inconsistencies from different FWeds (Copley & Nelson, 2012; Graves & Hanson, 2014), a larger initial investment of time related to the need for advanced organization to ensure a smooth process, as well as a concern about having less control of their caseload (Copley & Nelson, 2012). Lengthy orientation processes, possible preference for a particular FWed over others, the pressure of learning more than one practice area (Engel et al., 2013; Gaiptman & Forma, 1991), as well as the logistical challenges of different schedules are factors that can impact implementation of this model (Farrow et al., 2000). See Table 2-4 for the advantages and challenges of the shared supervision model.

Figure 2-2. Splitting the fieldwork experience between sites and FWeds.

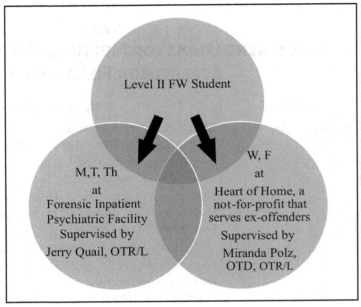

Figure 2-3. Splitting the fieldwork experience between FWeds (same site).

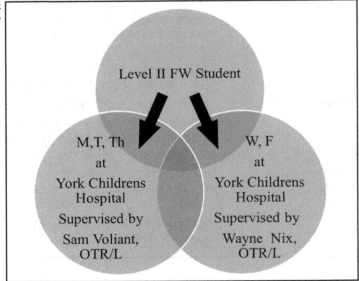

Collaborative Student Supervision Model

The collaborative model is also garnering particular attention in the world of occupational therapy fieldwork, with one source referring to it as "... likely to be a model of choice in the future" (Price & Whiteside, 2016, p. 123). A collaborative model placement involves two or more students working under the supervision of a one primary FWed (Box 2-6). While gaining in popularity currently, it is not a new idea, as the Mayo Clinic was using the model for physical therapy clinical education as far back as the 1930s (Rindflesch et al., 2009). The most notable difference between the collaborative model and traditional apprenticeship fieldwork is the expectation that students will take an autonomous and independent approach to learning in cooperation with their student peers (Bartholomai & Fitzgerald, 2007). This collaborative approach is informed primarily by the

TABLE 2-4
ADVANTAGES AND CHALLENGES OF MULTIPLE MENTORSHIP/ SHARED SUPERVISION MODEL

PERSPECTIVES	ADVANTAGES	CHALLENGES
Student	Quick development of teamwork skills. Inclusion as team member (rather than intern). Fast clinical reasoning and decision-making skills. Allows access to multiple practice areas, FWeds with narrow but valuable practice areas, and FWeds who work part time. Students' greater autonomy and responsibility leads to experiencing a less dependent relationship with their FWed. Increased opportunities for contact with clients and working collaboratively.	Managing expectations from multiple FWeds (inconsistencies or contradictions). Pressure of learning more than one practice area. Preference of one FWed over others. Less control of caseload. Logistical challenges of different FWeds' schedules.
FWed	Students process and learn at a faster and deeper level. Students collaborate with more staff members. Students are exposed to more practice areas. Less demand on the FWed's time. More access for students means expanded services available for clients in a practice setting.	Longer orientation process. Coordination of different FWeds' schedules. Larger initial investment of time for advanced organization and lengthy orientation process to ensure a smooth placement. At times, preference for one FWed over another.

Data sources: Copley & Nelson, 2012; Engel et al., 2013; Farrow et al., 2000; Gaiptman & Forma, 1991; Graves & Hanson, 2014; Precin, 2009.

social constructivist theories on learning espoused by Lev Vygostsky at the end of the 20th century. Vygotsky posited several important theories about learning, including that all expressions of cognitive functions are products of social interactions, that all learning is a movement toward integration into a knowledge community, and that cognitive development takes place in a social context (1978). Vygotsky described cognitive development as movement from a state of actual development, where an individual can solve problems independently, into a zone of proximal development, where the individual can achieve a higher level of cognitive skill development or maturation within a social context through collaboration with peers (1978). This theoretical foundation is expressed in the collaborative model as the structure of collaborative peers helping each other achieve development they could not achieve on their own, through modeling, guidance, and cooperation within a shared social context.

Box 2-5
VIGNETTE USING ROLE-EMERGING SUPERVISION MODEL

"This is Suzanne."

"Hi, it's Judy! Calling to talk about the evaluation?"

"Great, thought it might be you. Okay, so your email said we have a new client intake coming in tomorrow morning. What time do you plan to meet with him for the evaluation? Do you have all of his intake paperwork yet?"

"Yes, I have the paperwork, at least all the stuff that the new client filled out. Kyle gave it to me. I might not have caught the new client name on the board, but I had asked Kyle to let me know if any new clients are going to be coming in. He was going to do the social work side of the intake, then let me go in after he's done. I'll probably go in just before lunch after the B-period groups. He offered to chat with me about the client before I go in. Do you think that's okay?"

"Sure! I picked him as your primary contact when I'm not there because he has a very client-focused and functional approach to his social work practice. I always joke with him that he's secretly another occupational therapist … Anyway, definitely chat with him about the client. When I'm there tomorrow morning, we can talk about what questions would be most helpful for you to ask in that meeting. Speaking of tomorrow, what is your plan for your evaluation of the client tomorrow? I'll be there as a resource if you need me, but I'm expecting you'll run this one on your own."

"I've been going over records from other clients and thinking about what the best approach would be. I've decided I will use the Canadian Occupational Performance Model (COPM) and develop an occupational profile using the AOTA template from their website."

"Good plan. What areas are going to be your primary focus in discussing occupational performance with the client?"

"I'm going to make sure I cover instrumental activities of daily living, leisure interests, coping strategies, and ask about any compensatory techniques he is using in the community. I'll obviously also cover the content from the COPM."

"Good! I like the plan. Give yourself a little time to build in anything you feel you need to address after talking to Kyle as well. Great, so I will be in at 8 as usual. Let's meet to review how today's groups went, then talk plans for the meeting with Kyle, and we can go over how best to assess the content you will evaluate with the intake of the new client. Again, I'll be there but I'm sure you can handle this one with me just shadowing in the background."

"Great! I like the plan, too. I'll have the coffee ready for us when you get here. Thank you!"

Implementation of the model, like any fieldwork model, requires conscientious preparation. A clear and concise model for implementation of a collaborative model fieldwork experience was developed by Hanson and colleagues (2019) based on a factor analysis of a national survey of stakeholders in occupational therapy fieldwork education. This model neatly ties together the perceived value, site/client considerations, FWed considerations, and pragmatic considerations necessary for utilization of the Collaborative Model (Hanson et al., 2019). Successful implementation of the model depends on the use of specific recommendations and resources described in current literature. Sites must collaborate with the academic fieldwork coordinator (AFWC) from the university, educate the practice site and staff on the philosophy of the model, update or revise student internship materials, and engage the students in efforts to self-evaluate and take ownership of their

---

Box 2-6

Vignette Using
Collaborative Student Supervision Model

"Well, Mary, thanks for submitting Jaynee's final FWPE. You included some really helpful feedback, and Jaynee said she thought the experience was wonderful. Of course, you're used to the positive experiences and high praise at this point. It's such an asset to the program to know we can count on you consistently to take Level II students. And thanks for agreeing to take Caryn starting next week! Honestly, we really do appreciate all you do for our students and the program."

"You know I love working with the students, Scott. And I love showing students that they don't need to be afraid of working in practice with mental health clients. I think that's so important."

"Oh, I absolutely agree. We both know how critical it is to the future of the profession to ensure students have access to mental health practice. And your program is so interesting and high quality, no wonder the students love it every time."

"Thank you, and yes, we need to make sure our model of practice is celebrated and students are aware of what it's like to work as an occupational therapist in this way. I just wish I could do more. Sometimes I worry that taking three or four students a year is just a drop in the bucket, that it's not making a real difference."

"You are doing so much already between all the Level I and Level II students over the last couple of years. And you are making a big difference in the professional lives of the students you work with. They all talk about how they love working with you and many of them choose to consider mental health practice after graduation, likely because of their experience at your practice."

"That's so good to hear. Thank you. I hope some of those students do go into mental health practice and work with students of their own someday. That way we can keep paying it forward and expand the practice even more. Just seems like it will take forever to make that impact."

(continued)

---

learning (Hanson & DeIuliis, 2015). Preparations in advance of the placement can include training inservices that describe the model, discuss feedback strategies, and the importance of cooperative peer learning (Kinsella & Piersol, 2018). Sharing the evidence for the model in advance to staff, FWeds, and students can help with buy-in from stakeholders (Cohn et al., 2009; Price & Whiteside, 2016). Sites can also identify cooperative learning activities to incorporate into the placement, or other activities to encourage student autonomy, and develop learning contracts in collaboration with the students before beginning the placement (Price & Whiteside, 2016). Caseload challenges can be managed by cooperative work with other occupational therapy practitioners in the department, if available (Kinsella & Piersol, 2018). Staff can be educated about the administrative expectations and best ways to support students within the model. Timetables can also be helpful to develop in advance so students have a realistic picture of their FWed's work and administrative duties, and to allocate particular times to structured supervision meetings. This and other information, like outlines for supervision sessions or lists of available educational resources on site, can be combined in a student manual as a resource for students, and sites can even dedicate a workspace for the students if available (Bartholomai & Fitzgerald, 2007).

Box 2-6 (continued)
Vignette Using
Collaborative Student Supervision Model

"Actually, that's why I was calling today. Again, thanks for all the work you've done with our students. You know I share your goal of providing students with a well-rounded fieldwork experience and honoring mental health practice in the profession. And, I also would love to have you work with even more students in the future. That's why I'd like to propose we try a collaborative model placement in the spring. It would involve sending a pair of students to do their placements simultaneously, working together as a team with you."

"I've heard of that, but wouldn't that mean double the work for me? With the new programming we're rolling out next year, I don't know if I'll have a lot of extra time for double the supervision …"

"That's a common question about the model, but it doesn't translate into double the work, because the students utilize each other as resources instead of coming to you with all of their needs. The students can practice skills and assessments on each other, give each other feedback, review each other's work, and help each other with questions they might feel awkward bringing to their FWed. You still supervise their work and development, but they become more independent, show more initiative, and feel more responsibility for their own professional development by being less directly reliant on you for every part of the experience."

"That actually sounds like a really interesting idea. Could they co-lead groups, or would I have to find separate programming for each student?"

"Having them co-lead groups is actually a great idea. They can give each other feedback and collaborate directly every day because they're observing each other in real time with every intervention."

"I'd still meet with each one individually as needed, right?"

"Yes, but you would also meet with them as a pair to address both their individual performance and their performance as a team. It's a great way to get students ready for working in interdisciplinary teams."

"So, I could essentially double the number of students I work with, in the same amount of time, but do it in a way that requires less time for me on the little things, and more time where the students are learning to be independent, self-directed occupational therapists who can work well in teams? That sounds like a great idea!"

"I was so hoping you'd think so! Let's meet next week and I can show you some resources that are specific to the model, including sample timelines, new content for your student manual, and evidence for both you and your students about the model. Does that work for you?"

"I'm looking forward to it. And tell Caryn I'm looking forward to working with her next week, too."

"Will do. Talk soon!"

Clear communication about the model does not end with the preparations in advance of the students' arrival. The expectation of collaboration between students must be emphasized clearly and concretely. Students should be provided with time in their schedules specifically for collaboration, and make it clear this cooperation is expected, not "cheating." Students should have cooperative supervision meetings, cooperative work-related activities with specified roles, co-lead

TABLE 2-5
PREPARING FOR FIELDWORK SUCCESS

EDUCATORS/FIELDWORK SITE	STUDENTS
• Collaboration between site and school.	• Engage in self-evaluation and take ownership of their learning.
• Educate practice staff on the philosophy of the model, feedback strategies, and the importance of cooperative peer learning.	• View themselves as equally responsible with their FWeds for their learning successes.
• Update or revise student internship materials.	• Be familiar with the Collaborative Model and its evidence.
• Engage students in self-evaluation.	• Demonstrate mutual respect for other students in their cohort.
• Share evidence for the model in advance with stakeholders.	• Utilize peers as resources instead of exclusively relying on their direct FWed.
• Incorporate cooperative learning activities into the placement to encourage student autonomy.	• Take initiative with their own problem solving and clinical reasoning with questions related to their caseload.
• Develop learning contracts in collaboration with the students before the placement.	• Be prepared to provide peer evaluation on interpersonal skills and be comfortable giving and receiving feedback on collaborative skills.
• Develop and share timetables and/or schedules in advance.	
• Emphasize the expectation of collaboration clearly and concretely.	• Participate in cooperative work-related activities with specified roles.
• Clarify that students will be evaluated and supervised on their own needs and merit.	• Review each other's documentation.
• Provide high-quality orientation experience, manage delegation of caseload to students, and role-model collaboration in practice settings.	
• Explicitly establish collaboration as a learning outcome for the fieldwork students.	
• Identify necessary resources from the occupational therapy school to maximize success.	

individual and/or group treatment sessions, and review each other's documentation (Collier & O'Connor, 1998). Students should be informed that, while they are working concurrently, there is no rivalry or competition. Each student will be evaluated and supervised on their own needs and merit (Wilske, 2016). See Table 2-5 for summary for fieldwork preparation.

Students have their own expectations to ensure success with a collaborative model placement. The student should view themselves as equally responsible with their FWeds for their learning successes. They should be familiar with the model and have mutual respect for the other students in their cohort. They must manage their individual and shared clients, utilize their peers as resources instead of exclusively relying on their direct FWed, and take initiative with their own problem solving and clinical reasoning with questions related to their caseload. They should be prepared to provide peer evaluation on interpersonal skills and be comfortable giving and receiving feedback on collaborative skills (Hanson & DeIuliis, 2015).

The FWed responsible for the collaborating fieldwork students should focus on particular strategies to ensure success. They should provide a high-quality orientation experience, delegate the caseload to the students, ensure learning activities and feedback to maximize student development, serve as a resource for legislative and third-party payer requirements, role model collaboration in practice settings, and provide evaluation of the students. This will involve conducting both individual and group supervision sessions, monitoring student performance, and collaborating with the university's AFWC as necessary (Bartholomai & Fitzgerald, 2007; Hanson & DeIuliis, 2015). The idea of collaboration as a learning outcome needs to be made explicit with the students and evaluation of collaboration should be incorporated into supervision of the students (Boshoff et al., 2019). FWeds also need to focus on being positive but pragmatic, and ensure they set boundaries as needed (Price & Whiteside, 2016), as a FWed may have difficulty "letting go" of the familiar traditional fieldwork models in order to trust in the collaborative model (Flood et al., 2010).

The AFWC should serve as a resource for examples of materials for student manuals, collaborative learning activities, evidence to support the collaborative model, and resources for training FWeds (Hanson & DeIuliis, 2015). They should also ensure that appropriate students are recommended for a collaborative model placement, including students with the requisite collaborative and communication skills, as well as knowledge preparation for practice within the model (Hanson & DeIuliis, 2015; Price & Whiteside, 2016).

All of these preparations and expectations may seem like a daunting workload for students and FWeds. Why then go through all these efforts? What are the expected benefits of the use of the collaborative model for fieldwork? Are there challenges that must be answered in order to maximize the value of the experience for the student, university, and fieldwork site?

Practitioners and students identify a wide variety of benefits associated with this model. The experience leads to development of teamwork skills, independent learning, and self-confidence (Kinsella & Piersol, 2018; Rindflesch et al., 2009; Wilske, 2016). Students report feeling less intimidated talking out issues with peers than with the FWed, allowing for initial processing to lead to more substantive and advanced conversations in supervision (Wilske, 2016). Students report increased self-reliance and FWeds saw greater creative thinking by students (Collier & O'Connor, 1998), with some students appreciating the opportunity to develop their own practice style without the close supervision in traditional fieldwork (Flood et al., 2010). Work with peers can also provide unique opportunities for motivation and encouragement that would not be possible during traditional fieldwork (Price & Whiteside, 2016), including opportunities to practice techniques together, ask questions without judgment, and give feedback after observing each other with clients (Martin et al., 2004). Skills in communication, collaboration, conflict resolution, and compromise around intervention planning are identified as positive outcomes in this model, all necessary skills for work in interprofessional settings (Boshoff et al., 2019). One FWed described the collaborative model as "... as close an experience as possible to the real world" (Flood et al., 2010, p. 26). From the site's and profession's perspective, use of the model increases the student experience for each FWed, translates into additional contact for patients, creates additional fieldwork opportunities, and may be financially positive in certain settings (Floor et al., 2010; Rindflesch et al., 2009; Box 2-7). See Box 2-8 for a list of benefits of the Collaborative Student Supervision Model.

Of course, challenges and barriers must be overcome to fully realize these benefits in a collaborative model placement. Some are unavoidable but necessary, such as additional planning work and additional paperwork (Rindflesch et al., 2009), while some identified issues, like adequate workspace (Kinsella & Piersol, 2018), require greater creativity. Without prior experience with the model, FWeds may have concerns about increased workload, student competition, or needing to attend to all of a student's needs, but these are generally based on a misperception of a collaborative model as concurrent traditional fieldwork experiences, instead of a unique collaborative model of supervision (Bartholomai & Fitzgerald, 2007; Hanson, 2011a; Martin et al., 2004; Wilske, 2016).

BOX 2-7

VIGNETTE USING
COLLABORATIVE STUDENT SUPERVISION MODEL

"Okay, second evaluation. We got this!"

"Absolutely. Look out, Mrs. Bozyck, here we come! Okay, Ash, did you review the medications and the past medical history from the referral?"

"Yes, the medication we didn't know was a blood thinner, so we have to be careful with mobility and any bumps or bruises during the ADL eval. The past medical history was significant for a triple bypass 5 years ago, a diagnosis of bronchitis 2 years ago, and a history of angina. We'll want to keep an eye on heart rate, blood pressure, and O_2 sats."

"Yes. And didn't Mary Jean mention a blood test we would have to check?"

"Right! Pro-time I think and … one other one. Hang on, I'll check the manual for the protocol. Yes, here it is … okay, we'll check that before we go in. Okay … so last time, I did the morning ADL and you did sensation, cognition, and perception in the afternoon. This time we switch, right? Did Mary Jean have feedback for you from last time?"

"Yes, she recommended I make sure I have all the supplies for the sensory eval before I started, and the supplies for the vision test. I ended up having to hunt around for the stuff last time and I felt so self-conscious because the client was just sitting there watching me poke around in the closet."

"Okay, I'll do that. Will you show me where the materials are in the closet so I can get them before I do the afternoon part of the eval?"

"I'll trade you the location of the supplies for 10 minutes of helping me practice manual blood pressures."

"It's a deal! Is Mary Jean going to be with us for both parts of the eval?"

"She's going to check in on each of us, but won't be staying with us for the whole thing."

"Okay … so will you need an extra pair of hands for the ADL eval?"

"Sure, why not? I won't keep you there the whole time, just for some of the mobility assessment and maybe while I get posturals."

"Sounds good … regroup at 8 tomorrow morning?"

"Yes, 8 a.m. And I'll check the blood values in the morning before we go in."

"I'll remind you, since it's pretty important. We don't want to miss it."

"We won't, we're quite a team!"

Students expressed concerns that FWeds would not be able to assess them effectively, especially when three or more students were supervised by one FWed, which becomes a legitimate issue to be addressed as early as possible by the FWed (Martin et al., 2004). Challenges associated with varying levels of preparation or styles of learning in students can be met with flexibility and accommodation by the FWeds (Wilske, 2016). Concerns about reduced clinical exposure, specifically repetition with practice skills, were identified in some settings, especially those that do not have a great deal of consistency and repetition in the available caseload, which would require greater caseload management by both the FWed and the rest of the occupational therapist staff on site (Martin et al., 2004; Price & Whiteside, 2016). Table 2-6 outlines the benefits and challenges for the collaborative supervision model.

> **BOX 2-8**
>
> Collaborative Model fieldwork placements have many benefits:
>
> - Students develop teamwork skills, learn more independently, gain self-confidence, and exhibit greater creative thinking.
> - Students develop a unique practice style more independent of their FWed's practice style.
> - Peer collaboration around questions and issues leads to better, more efficient meetings with FWeds, as well as opportunities for students to motivate and encourage each other.
> - Students can practice skills and assessments on one another, ask questions free of fear of judgment, and practice giving and receiving feedback in practice sessions or after observations with clients.
> - Encourages and reinforces communication, collaboration, conflict resolution, and compromise around intervention planning with students, necessary for any interprofessional practice.
> - Provides more students and, therefore, more experience for FWeds in a shorter time.
> - Increases service contact with clients, which may be financially positive in some settings.
> - Increases fieldwork opportunities per FWed, reducing a supply bottleneck in some areas.

Role-Emerging Model

Another fieldwork model used around the world is the role-emerging fieldwork placement. While traditional fieldwork placements involve a student working under direct supervision of an experienced practitioner in an established practice setting, role-emerging placements are fieldwork experiences in sites or settings where there is no currently established occupational therapy service. Frequently, this involves supervision from an off-site occupational therapist and an on-site mentor, usually from another profession (Thomson & Thompson, 2013; Box 2-9).

In the United States, ACOTE (2018) specifies that supervision of fieldwork students in settings where occupational therapy services do not exist must include plans for provision of services and supervision of the students before the placement begins. Supervision must be provided by a licensed occupational therapist with the equivalent of 3 full-time years of experience. That supervision must be a combination of at least 8 hours per week of direct supervision, availability of the FWed through a variety of contact methods during all working hours, and on-site supervision by an assigned practitioner from another profession when the occupational therapist FWed is off site (ACOTE, 2018).

The structure of traditional fieldwork experiences is well-established over decades of occupational therapy education history. Role-emerging placements do not benefit from having a well-established template for organization and structure, especially given that there generally is not even an existing occupational therapy practice at the site before the fieldwork experience begins. Over the last decade, however, multiple universities and their practice partners have developed functional models for these placements with quantifiable benefits. Their experience has provided a variety of important recommendations and features for utilization of role-emerging fieldwork. Successful versions of this model have included content that requires initiative and engagement, like the use of goal attainment scaling to set learning goals, individual and group reflection sessions, and self-reflective journaling (Phelps, 2017). The structure of successful role-emerging placements also included on-site observations and structured off-site weekly group meetings at

TABLE 2-6
BENEFITS AND CHALLENGES IN COLLABORATIVE MODEL

BENEFITS	CHALLENGES
• Development of teamwork skills, independent learning, and self-confidence.	• Additional planning and paperwork for FWed.
• Students report feeling less intimidated talking out issues with peers than with the FWed, leading to more substantive and advanced conversations in supervision meetings.	• Student concerns over adequate assessment of their performance with more students per FWed.
• Greater self-reliance and creative thinking by students.	• Levels of preparation or styles of learning within collaborating groups of students may vary.
• Students have more freedom to develop their own practice style without the close supervision in traditional fieldwork.	• Reduced repetition with practice skills.
• Students have opportunities to practice techniques together, ask questions without judgment, and give feedback after observing each other with clients	
• Improved skills with communication, collaboration, conflict resolution, and compromise around intervention planning.	
• Increased student experience for each FWed.	
• Additional contact for clients.	
• Additional fieldwork opportunities.	

the occupational therapy school to allow for detailed case reviews and discussion related to common themes in reflective journal content (Thomson & Thompson, 2013). This clearly requires increased communication among the school, students, and site, which is possible only where time and scheduling will allow for this (Mulholland & Derdall, 2005). One comprehensive resource for helpful tools to facilitate the use of a role-emerging fieldwork model was developed by Hanson and Nielson (2015) for the second edition of *The Essential Guide to Occupational Therapy: Fieldwork Education Resources for Educators and Practitioners* from AOTA Press (Costa, 2015). Their chapter, "Introduction to Role-Emerging Fieldwork," includes many valuable resources that help educators understand, implement, and evaluate role-emerging fieldwork. These resources include comparisons between traditional and role-emerging fieldwork, assessment of interpersonal abilities, eligibility requirements and application processes, and summative reflective questions for students and FWeds (Hanson & Nielson, 2015).

Resources like these are valuable for FWeds looking to utilize this model of fieldwork and are available from a variety of sources. Clear communication and continuous review of expectations are very important in this model, in alignment with adult learning theories, so online student manuals and orientation information include the variety of student responsibilities associated with the fieldwork experience (Phelps, 2017; Thomson & Thompson, 2013). These responsibilities include skills and application of clinical reasoning, including expectations to collaborate with other practitioners, facilitate inservices for other students and staff, recruit client participation in

---

BOX 2-9
VIGNETTE ON ROLE-EMERGING MODEL

"Thanks again for coming in to speak to our students about your practice, Shirish. It sounds so fascinating, and the students were really interested in hearing about what you are doing in assisted living. They don't hear a lot about a practice like yours. I mean, they may occasionally hear about community-based programs in that setting that also do reminiscence groups and cooking groups, arts and crafts, but not programs that use exergaming and yoga like you do. So interesting!"

"Thanks for having me come in, Patty. I love talking about what we're doing in our practice, but it's not just me. Having an experienced nurse and really creative therapeutic recreation specialist makes it much easier and keeps me challenging myself to do new things with our clients. Plus, it's ideal for me working just 30 hours per week so I can do my volunteer work and all my other things I love outside of work."

"Well, I'm sure I will have a dozen students emailing me or at my office door this week asking about Level II fieldwork with you and your practice. Would that be a possibility for you later this year?"

"I've thought about that recently. I remember having students at my previous job at the skilled nursing facility, and how it really made me think about my own practice. It made me a better occupational therapist, honestly. Then, with my current job, I think about how bringing in students would help us expand the variety and number of programs we can run, bring in new evidence and ideas, and bring in new energy. Our residents would love having some fresh new faces around. Only problem is, I don't work full-time, so it wouldn't work."

"Actually, that's not true. You don't need to be working full-time to take on a Level II student. In fact, since you have some clinical experience and you've had students before, you could use a role-emerging model for fieldwork at your facility."

"Role-emerging? What does that mean?"

"Well, for settings where there isn't a full-time occupational therapist available for practice, but there is a clear role for occupational therapy, you use a combination of an occupational therapist FWed and on-site experienced professionals to provide supervision for the student. You still meet regularly with the students, review their performance, provide feedback, and guide their development in the practice. On days you are not there, they have an experienced contact person, like your therapeutic recreation specialist or the nurse you work with, and the student can contact them for questions or guidance. That way, you get the benefits of having the student on site, the student learns an interesting new way to be an occupational therapist, and they get prepared for whatever the future brings in occupational therapy, because they've worked more independently in a setting where they define their own practice more directly."

"I can actually see that working for us. With the right student and help from you if I have any questions, that could be a great opportunity for us and the student … and the residents! I like this idea. What are our next steps?"

(continued)

services, conduct assessments, design new programs, compile needs assessments, complete typical documentation, including occupational profiles, and implement individual and group interventions (Phelps, 2017).

This model also functions best when students exhibit certain characteristics, such as a comfort level with the greater degree of autonomy featured in this model (Thomson & Thompson, 2013). To address this, fieldwork sites have used a variety of methods, including student preplacement

> **BOX 2-9 (CONTINUED)**
> ## VIGNETTE ON ROLE-EMERGING MODEL
>
> "I would get you some more evidence and resources for the use of the model and send that to you for your review. You and I could then collaborate on how to structure and plan for the experience before the first student arrives. Then, I pick a student who would do well at your practice and send them over with paperwork for an interview. If you're happy with the student and the support, we get started. I think this could be a win-win-win, for you, the student, and your facility. Do you have time next week to talk more and start planning?"
>
> "When I'm back at work, I'll check my calendar and we'll set it up. I might do some reading on my own in the meantime. Thanks for bringing this up, I thought fieldwork wasn't a possibility for us. This is exciting!"
>
> "I know our students will be excited to work with you, too. Glad we had this chat. I'll check in with you soon about setting up that meeting. Thanks again!"

interviews and student learning contracts with details of the model (Martin et al., 2004; McGill University, 2020; Phelps, 2017). Because of the challenges of working more independently and without the benefit of established practice structures on site, students who succeed in role-emerging settings are those who exhibit initiative and autonomy but also have adequate insight to know their own limitations (Rodger et al., 2009). Students must also be able to work effectively in a context of deferred feedback, as compared with the nearly immediate feedback associated with the traditional apprenticeship model (Thomson & Thompson, 2013).

In many ways, traditional direct delivery skills are learned in role-emerging placements. In a program described by Tyminski (2018), students developed an evidence-based curriculum of activity-based groups that addressed areas of interest to the community at the shelter, including independent living skills, community reintegration skills, and health and wellness concerns. Students used needs assessment to determine topics of groups the shelter clients felt would be most valuable. Evaluation and intervention followed traditional outlines, with the students using the COPM as an evaluation tool and developed an intervention plan for each client consisting of recommended activity groups and individual interventions built around client objectives. Short- and long-term objectives were developed with each client to ensure focus on progress with areas of concern identified by the client. The students who completed the final evaluation tool at the end of the experience reported a significant increase in their ability to implement occupation-based interventions and improvement in communication skills with the population at the shelter.

There are also unique benefits in direct delivery skill development in this model. Bossers et al. (1997) found that working in a nontraditional setting also encourages more flexibility in a student's approach. Not starting from a diagnosis or disability, one student described they focused more on "their strengths and their areas of need. You don't see them as psychiatric patients, you see them as people who just need some skill building" (Bossers et al., 1997, p. 74). Students also identified greater comfort working with clients, greater compassion, and greater personal maturity. Stereotypes and fears students associated with the population were reduced with greater contact with the clients.

An important consideration for this model is that its benefits can be seen as two sides of the same coin. On one side, students grow in their direct service delivery competencies in unique ways, given the unique structure of the supervision and placement. On the other side is the growth that occurs in program development, a natural outcome of use of this fieldwork model. That growth in program development involves the professional skills for program development, as well as expanding the reach and scope of service delivery in the communities potentially served by occupational therapy. Students perceive a number of benefits to their skills in direct delivery when participating in role-emerging placements. Mattila (2019) found students identified multiple areas of growth, including seeking information, development of creativity in using their own ideas in practice, organizing time effectively when faced with unexpected changes, and adjusting to new settings and the challenges that come with them.

Lau and Ravanek's (2019) review of literature pertaining to student perspectives on role-emerging placements found that students experienced some challenges, such as a perceived lack of structure and support, and high levels of personal responsibility. They also found students perceived numerous benefits and opportunities, including development of professional and personal skills, independence and autonomy, a client-centered focus reducing the impact of diagnosis or disability on student's approach, and changed perspectives on their future in the profession, including a greater likelihood of working in a similar setting in the future. Similarly, Mattila et al. (2018) found student confidence improved significantly after a Level I role-emerging experience, including in communication, adaptation, innovation, risk-taking, supervision, clinical practice, and professional competency subscores.

All of these improvements in direct delivery skills, as well as the benefits unique to the model, are important and valuable to future practitioners. The model's context also challenges students to develop skills related to program development, as well as demonstrates the value of occupational therapy to the community at large. These unique characteristics of the model are particularly valuable in facilitating growth in the profession moving forward. For example, Fleming et al. (2014) described the resources and skills students developed in a role-emerging placement collaborating with a community sport organization. Students designed a gross motor skills assessment for the program, proposed a research project for future students to evaluate program outcomes. They developed charts that correlated developmental milestones with specific skills taught in sports activities in the program. They developed inclusion resources for coaches to use with children in the program. Students also developed promotional/marketing materials for the program. Students learned how to develop outcome measures to allow for evidence-based program evaluation, necessary for growth of community-based practice. Students were successful not just because they passed the placement but also because they developed and implemented new resources to enhance the work of the coaches, developed marketing and other business skills not typically utilized in traditional fieldwork settings, and demonstrated the impact of occupational therapy on community-based programming (Fleming et al., 2014). These skills are necessary for program development, but importantly, the process of developing these programs through fieldwork increases the availability and scope of occupational therapy practice in the communities. New practices are developed, new clients served, and more communities become aware of the unique value of occupational therapy.

An additional important consideration for this model is the skills and competencies of the FWeds utilizing this model. First, the FWed must have a clear understanding and acceptance of the accountability and risk issues that are more prevalent in this model than in traditional fieldwork (Thomson & Thompson, 2013). The FWed is seen more as a facilitator than as a resident expert or oracle. They should be committed to student learning and a collaborative approach, utilizing an open, trusting, approachable, and nonjudgmental style. They should be able to recognize different learning styles, encourage independent problem solving and reflection, and provide balanced feedback in a timely fashion (Gat & Ratzon, 2014; Phelps, 2017; Rodger et al., 2009). One Canadian program went so far as to hire a Fieldwork Educator for Independent Community Placements to ensure a high quality of communication and competency in a liaison between the practice setting and the occupational therapy program (Mulholland & Derdall, 2005, p. 32). This educator facilitated student learning at the site, provided direct support to the student and site, and ensured a clear communication of the occupational therapy perspective through the students' practice. This significantly increased communication with the site and ensured clearer expectations for students from the outset of the fieldwork experience (Mulholland & Derdall, 2005).

The role-emerging model has been utilized to achieve specific benefits for the students and site. The unique approach and challenges, addressed in a model that requires more autonomy from students, lead to improvements and some intangible fieldwork benefits, like competencies with social responsibility, initiative, self-directed learning, and self-awareness, all of which are seen as critical skills for developing successful relationships with clients in the future (Mattila & Dolhi, 2016). Students themselves report an appreciation for the opportunity to grow the practice of occupational therapy in a setting where it had not yet taken root, which required challenging themselves to confidently and clearly articulate the role and value of occupational therapy in a practice environment (Thomson & Thompson, 2013). These experiences also had a positive impact on the capacity of the students to succeed in a role on a collaborative interdisciplinary team. Students also learned more practical skills, such as developing skills related to initiative, time management, organization, and effective use of supervision, all leading to an opportunity to work with greater autonomy and independence than would be available in traditional apprenticeship fieldwork (Rodger et al., 2009). All of this experience with a more independent placement led to greater confidence in their practice skills going forward. The need for flexibility and creativity led to measurable growth in adaptability, dealing with challenges, adjusting to new settings, and using their own ideas in practice (Mattila et al., 2018). In fact, when directly compared to students in traditional fieldwork experiences, there were no significant differences between role-emerging and traditional placement students in perceptions of personal and professional skills, but those students in a true role-emerging site with no active occupational therapist present on site scored significantly higher on their perception of personal responsibility, cultural competence, and overall personal skills than those with an active occupational therapist on site (Gat & Ratzon, 2014).

All of these benefits do come with specific challenges that must be addressed to access the unique benefits of this model. Students and FWeds in these fieldwork experiences recognize that the absence of an established occupational therapy presence on site creates a disadvantage for the students. The students themselves identified specific challenges, including managing the expectations of multiple FWeds, educating on-site staff about the role of occupational therapy, and limited opportunities to develop clinical knowledge or specific occupational therapist skills (Rodger et al., 2009). While the limited opportunities for technical or clinical skill development were a common concern by students at the onset of a role-emerging placement, some students addressed their concerns by using evidence-based resources or role-play with peers, turning a challenge into a rewarding aspect of the placement (Thomson & Thompson, 2013). See Table 2-7 for the benefits and challenges associated with the role-emerging placement model.

Project Placements

Some iterations of role-emerging fieldwork use the completion of a specific project by the students as an integral part of the placement. When used as the exclusive component of the fieldwork experience in countries where 12-week placements are not the norm, these are called *project placements*. Much like the name implies, this model of fieldwork features the completion of a project that is needed by a fieldwork site, rather than a student taking over a FWed's caseload or practice. These projects are developed and completed under the supervision of an occupational therapist and can be completed as either a full- or part-time placement. Many occupational therapy schools and practice sites offer the practice placement as an option for students, but Prigg and Mackenzie (2002) in New South Wales, Australia, and Thew et al. (2008) from Leeds, United Kingdom, gave the clearest examples of how to structure these placements and ensure a good result for all stakeholders. Project placements are not utilized in the United States as they are usually much shorter in duration (4 to 6 weeks) compared to the ACOTE requirement for Level II fieldwork.

In Australia, they utilized a clear and intentional structure. They sought confirmation from local fieldwork sites that they preferred project placements as a nontraditional placement model. They gathered the stakeholders together, including fieldwork coordinators and academics from

Box 2-10
VIGNETTE USING PROJECT PLACEMENT MODEL

"I think you're still on mute …"

"Sorry, can you hear me now?"

"Yes! Thank you! So, Friday of week 8 … I know you're busy but it must feel good to be approaching the finish line."

"I am really busy, yes, but I'm really enjoying it. The time is flying by! I am so going to miss these clients. I really grew attached to them. I've learned so much …"

"Actually, that is the big theme I wanted to discuss today. You've put in all this work developing the programming, the groups, the activities, and they're really appreciative of all the resources you've brought to Shiretown Village. Assisted living facilities often have activities, but they've never had an occupational therapist there before and I think they are starting to see the unique value we bring to their residents. Louise, the Wellness Director, even called me to ask how they can keep your programs going after you leave."

"They could just hire me, that would be the easiest solution …"

"True, not sure if that is in their budget, but maybe we can work together on a proposal before your final week. Meanwhile, how did your new Reminiscing Group go? You ran it for the first time yesterday, right?"

"Yes, it went great! A little clumsy at the start but everyone connected with the activity and they seemed to be having fun with the old music. I had no idea what a good voice Mel had!"

"How did you know to try a group like that?"

"Same as the previous groups. After week 6, I knew I had room and resources to add two more groups. I cleared the use of the space with Louise, then did a needs assessment survey. I asked what types of content they wanted, as well as areas they would like to improve in their daily routine, and what activities they enjoyed generally. Then, I just looked at the results for common threads. Socializing, improving memory, and music were the most common themes, so I built a group around that. We had eight residents at the first group, I expect more at the next one."

"You said it went well. How do you know?"

"I asked everyone for feedback at the end and asked how likely they were to try this group again in the future. Everyone said they liked it and wanted to know when it would meet again so they won't miss it. I'm going to make a feedback form like I did for the other groups, so I can collect outcomes and make sure I'm matching the content to what the residents want."

"How does this fit with your overall program model for your work at the Village?"

"My original goals included reducing isolation among residents and developing client-centered group programming, so I thought this group was a perfect fit."

"I agree. So, send me a copy of the outcome measure before you distribute it at the next group. That way I can make sure it fits your logic model and it is structured to give you data that's clearly useful for you. Let's also start thinking about how to present all the valuable outcomes you planned to collect in your program evaluation model. That will help with demonstrating the value of the programming to the residents and to the Village. Outcome data from the residents themselves will be particularly compelling, so let's make sure we've got that in a clear format. You'll need to put together the program evaluation over the next 2 weeks, so let's get started on that. Contact me or send me drafts if you have any questions."

(continued)

Box 2-10 (continued)
Vignette Using Project Placement Model

"Wow, yes, I can't believe I'm talking about the end already ... unless they want to hire me, of course ..."

"One step at a time, let's show the outcomes and the value to the community. If they're interested, I'm sure they'll approach you in the next couple of weeks. If not, at least they'll have group protocols to use going forward, and you'll have a template for developing high-quality resources for another community that would like to add occupational therapy to the team. Okay! Good to talk to you again, let's talk again at our regular time on Tuesday and I'll swing by the Village in person on Wednesday. Let me know if anything else comes up in the meantime, call or email."

"Will do, thanks!"

"Goodbye!"

Table 2-7
Benefits and Challenges for Role-Emerging Model

BENEFITS	CHALLENGES
• Encourages more flexibility in student's approach.	• Perceived lack of structure and support is possible.
• Develops comfort working with clients, compassion, and personal maturity.	• Higher levels of personal responsibility for students.
• Client-focused, rather than diagnosis-/disability-focused.	• Managing expectations of multiple FWeds and on-site staff.
• Students develop creativity in using their own ideas in practice.	• Educating on-site staff about the role of occupational therapy.
• Greater independence and autonomy for students.	
• Significant improvements in student confidence.	• Limited opportunities to develop particular clinical skills.
• Changed perspective on student's future in the profession.	
• Students learn program development skills, including program evaluation, promoting the profession, development of outcome measures, and interprofessional collaboration.	
• Improvements in social responsibility, initiative, self-directed learning, and self-awareness.	
• Potential to expand scope and reach of practice in the community.	

Box 2-11

As referred to in Figure 2-1, related to Level II fieldwork, supervision is a continuum. In occupational therapy practice, specifically referring to the supervisor relationship between an occupational therapist and occupational therapy assistant practitioner or the competency development from a novice to experienced practitioner, there are a variety of levels of supervision. The type of supervision utilized may be dependent on a variety of factors, such as the level of experience or competency level of the supervisee, the expectations and complexity of the practice setting, and parameters from state licensure boards or reimbursement bodies. Some other terms used along with supervision are:

- *Close* or *direct*: Daily, direct, contact at the practice setting (refers to face-to-face on-site supervision). Direct supervision can be further described as *direct personal supervision*, which pertains to being in line of sight.

- *Routine*: Direct contact that occurs at least every 2 weeks.

- *General*: Direct contact that occurs monthly.

- *Minimal*: Direct contact only on an as needed basis.

- *Distant* or *indirect*: Involves communication over phone, email, written notes, video conferencing, etc.

Disclaimer: FWeds should also be aware and compliant with any supervision guidelines inherent within their state practice act or dictated by their licensure board for fieldwork. Supervision requirements set by third-party payers, such as the Centers for Medicare & Medicaid Services, should also be attended to.

the occupational therapy schools, senior clinicians in the community, and students. That group developed strategies for placement recruitment, criteria for preapproval of projects, matching students to projects/sites, designing a student assessment, and criteria for evaluating placements. Information was also distributed to FWeds about the benefits and process of project placements. Seminars for local clinicians increased awareness, and information sessions for eligible students were produced at the end of the previous year. Once potential projects were identified by fieldwork sites and approved by the fieldwork coordinator at the occupational therapy program, information about each project was made available to students, and students then assigned themselves to each placement in small groups. Finally, 1 week before the placement was scheduled to begin, students and FWeds for each project met to clarify the nature of the project, make expectations clear, review documentation to be used in the experience, including for student assessment, and to collect information on assessment and interpretation of attitudes toward the placement (Prigg & Mackenzie, 2002).

In the United Kingdom, they identified possible sites through charity group partners or contacts through networking with local occupational therapy practitioners. Once identified, a representative from the university would arrange a visit, where an information packet was shared and used to facilitate cooperation in the program. Sites were also checked to ensure they were capable of providing health, safety, and supervision requirements of the program. Distant supervision (Box 2-11) was then provided by occupational therapists, with on-site staff responsibilities discussed in advance (Thew et al., 2008).

On-site staff were expected to prepare the site for the student placement, oversee onboarding, serve as the practice setting expert, communicate with the university about student performance and progress, review relevant policies and procedures, and provide regular student supervision. Meanwhile, the off-site occupational therapy FWed is expected to support the student to ensure they incorporate an occupational practice in their work, help the student define the occupational therapy role on site, provide practice guidance, support student reflection, offer evaluation and

TABLE 2-8
PROJECT PLACEMENT EXAMPLES

PRACTICE AREA	PROJECTS
Pediatric	Review standardized assessments and recommendations for purchase.
	Develop a sensory floor mat for children with severe sensory disabilities.
	Develop a manual of methods to adapt the Department of Education Physical Education curriculum for children with developmental disability.
	Make suggestions to encourage participation in meaningful occupations for boys to promote social participation.
Occupation-based	Review hospital staff procedures for use of health hoists and other manual handling equipment, and develop educational material.
	Task analysis and recommendations for safe practice for school kitchen duties.
	Task analysis and recommendations for safe practice for cleaners at a nursing home.
	Make a video of service users describing the benefits from participation in organic gardening.
Physical dysfunction	Develop an educational package and audio-visual resources about multiple sclerosis and vision.
	Adapt horticultural activities for adults with physical disabilities in a community setting.
Mental health	Make session plans for an anxiety management group.
	Make an activity analysis of tasks in a service user craft group.

feedback, discuss outcomes with the student and the university staff, provide guidance on incorporating theory into practice, and act as a role model for the profession (Thew et al., 2008).

Whether used as a stand-alone experience in educational systems that allow this, or as components of a role-emerging fieldwork placement, project placements can address a variety of needs identified by the fieldwork site. In the examples from Australia (Prigg & Mackenzie, 2002) and the United Kingdom (Thew et al., 2008), there were a wide range of activities, resources, and services provided to the sites (Table 2-8).

These examples represent many different valuable resources for the fieldwork sites, their staff, and their clients. Work on these projects can be expected to offer valuable training, skills, client contact, application of occupational therapy theory, and utilization of professional reasoning. But what were the perceived benefits and challenges of the use of the projects in these examples?

There were several identified benefits reported by students and site FWeds in the use of the previously identified project. Participants appreciated the opportunity to work independently, gain knowledge, improve time management, and demonstrate creativity. They appreciated working collaboratively toward a finished product that gave them satisfaction and a sense of pride, including students working collaboratively with their FWeds, rather than feeling subordinate, and feeling that their eventual product was valued by the department or program they were working with. They appreciated the freedom to try new things, the challenge of learning how to develop and satisfy an unmet needs assessment, and the opportunity to teach the value of engagement in meaningful occupation. Students felt they had more responsibility, flexibility, and an opportunity to develop presentation skills and self-confidence. Students also felt like they learned to be more resourceful, learned more in-depth information about a particular area of practice, felt respected, and felt people believed in what they were doing (Prigg & Mackenzie, 2002; Thew et al., 2008).

These positive results and perceptions were tempered by some of the aspects of these projects that were identified as challenging by the participants. Students were concerned in some instances with their initial lack of direction and lack of feedback from FWeds in the context of a short time frame for completion of the projects. Some students were disappointed if they did not know how their proposal/project had been utilized after they left, and some students were disappointed to see a great deal of need but few available resources at some sites (Prigg & Mackenzie, 2002; Thew et al., 2008).

Perceptions of the students in these examples are an important outcome, but equally important are the perceptions of the sites and their FWeds. FWeds generally appreciated having fewer supervisory demands on them, while still resulting in a useful outcome for their practice. They hoped to gain resources and useful information, and all reported they had benefitted from the students' contributions (Prigg & Mackenzie, 2002; Thew et al., 2008).

The third entity focused on effective use of this model are the occupational therapy schools themselves. These project placements can represent a way to help bridge the perceived gap between the academic world and the practice community in a tangible, practical way (Bonsaksen et al., 2013). Important lessons were learned from the experiment in New South Wales to help ensure the maximum value derived from the use of the projects, and these recommended strategies can be facilitated through the occupational therapy schools. The recommendations mirror those for role-emerging fieldwork in general, and include (Prigg & Mackenzie, 2002):

- Providing additional training on the unique supervision and evaluation strategies with the projects.
- More student preparation, including regular academic support and clear expectations for a more self-directed fieldwork placement.
- Encouraging FWeds to plan sufficient time for supervision, identify the general practice skills students can acquire through the projects, and clearly recognizing the students' contributions.
- Approving only projects that provide relevant learning and professional development experiences that are of interest to students, and include direct or hands-on client contact.

As currently utilized, there are additional steps to be taken, extra work and communication among all stakeholders, and assurances for the sites, FWeds, schools, and students to maximize the value of the use of projects in fieldwork. Given these additional challenges, there are also unique benefits to be harvested from this additional work for all stakeholders in fieldwork education. See Table 2-9 for the benefits and challenges for the project placement model.

CHOOSING THE BEST MODEL FOR YOUR PRACTICE SETTING

More than 25 years ago, U.S. practitioners publicized that there are limitations to the traditional one-to-one/apprenticeship model. Hengel and Romeo (1995) pointed out that the model assumes the FWed has the "knowledge, experience, and attitudes that make for a competent fieldwork educator and role model" and that is not always the case (p. 354). They also claimed the one-to-one model led students to imitate and rely on practitioners on site rather than develop their own skills and style. The "unnecessary demands on staff members" were also identified

TABLE 2-9

BENEFITS AND CHALLENGES FOR PROJECT PLACEMENT MODEL

BENEFITS	CHALLENGES
• Opportunity to work independently, gain knowledge, improve time management, and demonstrate creativity. • Students work collaboratively with FWeds on a shared product valued by the department or program. • More responsibility and flexibility. • Opportunity to develop presentation skills and self-confidence. • Students learn to be more resourceful and learn more in-depth information about a particular area of practice. • Fewer supervisory demands on FWeds.	• At times, an initial lack of direction and lack of feedback in the context of a short time frame for completion of a project. • Students may not learn if the resources they developed were utilized after the placement ended. • At times, students encountered a great deal of need but few available resources. • More student preparation required in advance, as well as more input from stakeholders on potential projects.

as problematic for use of the model (Hengel & Romeo, 1995, p. 354). Their interpretation of the limitations of traditional models led them to develop a group approach to supervision, based on several assumptions, including that the students "need supported freedom to discover and verify their abilities" and "will function competently if the environment is open and supportive" (Hengel & Romeo, 1995, p. 355).

Meanwhile, Canadian practitioners envisioned a similar model featuring shared supervision (Jung et al., 1994). They recognized the value of the traditional one-to-one model, especially the focused learning within a particular practice setting and caseload, a FWed providing knowledge, therapeutic skills, learning opportunities, feedback, and clinical reasoning training on a full-time basis, specifically for that student. Direct one-to-one interaction with the FWed is the well-controlled conduit for learning. Yet, they also appreciated the value of a group approach to fieldwork supervision, including facilitating collaboration within the fieldwork experience, exposing the student to a variety of approaches in a variety of practice areas, more control of the learning process and learning plan by students, and teaching students how to integrate knowledge from FWeds, clinical experts, and peers.

Fast forward 10 years and practitioners in Australia were describing how occupational therapy practice was changing from a more medical model to a community-based practice model (Thomas et al., 2005) and that students needed to be prepared through fieldwork to practice in that new reality. This led them to explore and utilize nontraditional supervision models, including collaborative models and role-emerging models. They agreed that traditional one-to-one models help students directly learn skills necessary for succeeding in a setting with a well-established role, while the FWed can directly adjust caseloads and supervision to match the students' learning styles or different needs. At the same time, envisioning the challenges facing students and the profession in the 21st century, the practitioners felt that students needed to be exposed to "… a fuller spectrum of occupational learning opportunities" (Thomas et al., 2005, p. 80).

Fast forward again, and AOTA's *OT Practice* features a description of how practitioners are using collaborative model fieldwork and project placement models successfully in the United Kingdom, describing the positive impacts of self-directed learning, self-knowledge of students, especially in therapeutic use of self and comfort with defining occupational therapy's role in interdisciplinary settings (Hanson, 2011b). Researchers are also seeing these nontraditional models as a possible solution to an increasing shortage of fieldwork placements in the United States, as one of the top five factors that positively influenced the decision to supervise fieldwork students was "if there was an opportunity to share student supervision with another occupational therapist" (Varland et al., 2017, p. 247). Outside of prevailing fieldwork site shortages due to the number of occupational therapy programs growing across the United States, the global pandemic has been exceptionally traumatic to the world of fieldwork. Site capacity restrictions, site closures, personnel shortages, and practitioner burnout further exacerbate existing challenges. The use of alternative supervision models can be a win-win scenario.

Here is a logic model to help guide a selection of the ideal supervision model for you and your setting.

First, use the following questions to engage in a self-reflection:

- What can the FWeds at your organization contribute to fieldwork education?
- What benefits and unique characteristics are available to fieldwork students through your practice?
- What do you want your fieldwork students to learn, and what professional competencies should they develop through fieldwork education with you and your colleagues?
- Which model do you believe is most appropriate for your practice, setting, and fieldwork education resources?
- What does your ideal "fieldwork culture" look like for students working with you?
- How will your practice, site, or facility be different, or better, having provided a quality fieldwork education experience?

Next, review a summary of factors you might consider in choosing a model in Figure 2-4. When reviewing Figure 2-4, look through each of the benefits listed. For each benefit you feel is important, note the models that provide that benefit by tracking to the top of the chart, and ideally, record the models that provide the fieldwork results you want. After you have run through the list of benefits and recorded the models that match your desired outcomes, review the results to learn which models appear most frequently in your list. Consider utilizing or further investigating the model that provides most of your desired fieldwork outcomes.

SUMMARY

Within this chapter, several supervision models have been described, including its recommended structure, the benefits, and challenges faced with implementing the model in practice. Experiences with the use of the various models from around the world have been shared to help inform the professional reasoning of those involved in fieldwork education. Yet, despite all of these descriptions and details, one may still be left with uncertainty about which type of bridge should be built to connect students to professional practice. There is general guidance available from the AOTA in its *COE Guidelines for an Occupational Therapy Fieldwork Experience–Level II* (AOTA, 2013). In that document, the AOTA identifies that a variety of fieldwork models exists and that they should be implemented "… depending on the preferences of the fieldwork educator, the nature of the fieldwork site, and the learning needs of the students …" and that "the more collaborative the fieldwork model, the more active student learning occurs" (AOTA, 2013, p. 4). This leaves the practitioners and educators to evaluate their site, their practice, their team of FWeds,

APPRENTICESHIP TRADITIONAL ONE-TO-ONE	SHARED SUPERVISION MULTIPLE MENTOR	ROLE-EMERGING	COLLABORATIVE MODEL
Individual attention for student			
No comparisons with other students			
Simpler to identify one FWed's expectations			
Easier organization with one practitioner's schedule			
Well-established single role for occuptional therapy for students to learn			
Student questions help with FWed's reflective practice			
Compatible model for novice practitioners			
	Broader practice experience and more access to specialty practice areas		
	More autonomy and responsibility for students with less one-to-one dependence on a particular FWed		
	More FWed can be involved, including those with limited schedules or specialty practices		
	Multiple perspectives with evaluation and feedback		
	Promotes initiative and problem-solving in students		
	Opportunity for students to develop their own therapeutic style, rather than copying style from single FWed		
	Less supervision time commitment per FWed		
	Collaboration facilitates development of clinical reasoning among FWeds		
	Can allow for less experienced FWeds to develop confidence within reduced supervision role		
		Collaboration with peers on practice reflections and skills reviews allows for more focused and direct use of FWeds time	
		More students on site means more added benefit and resources for fieldwork site	
		Students are more autonomous and independent, with greater professional growth	

Figure 2-4. Considerations when choosing a supervision model. (*continued*)

APPRENTICESHIP TRADITIONAL ONE-TO-ONE	SHARED SUPERVISION MULTIPLE MENTOR	ROLE-EMERGING	COLLABORATIVE MODEL
		Greater opportunities for creativity and developing time management skills	
	Prepares students for greater variety of practice options in the future		
		Higher student perception of personal responsibility, cultural competence, and personal skills when compared with one-to-one model	
	Prepares students for professional challenges that classroom or traditional fieldwork cannot provide		
		Students are more active learners, with increased independence, improved problem-solving skills, and more effective teamwork skills	
			More work with peers leads students to feel more comfortable, confident, relaxed, less intimidated

Figure 2-4 (continued). Considerations when choosing a supervision model. (*continued*)

their resources, and the students and schools with whom they work to find the right model for them based on the best evidence available at the time. Just as there is no right approach or bridge for every situation, every situation has a best approach or best type of bridge to connect students to their destination.

LEARNING ACTIVITIES

1. What are the unique skills, knowledge, or competencies that students develop during a role-emerging or collaborative model fieldwork that they likely will not develop during a traditional one-to-one model fieldwork experience?

2. Imagine you are working full time as an experienced occupational therapy practitioner in a multidisciplinary community-based adult traumatic brain injury program, operating on a clubhouse model. Which supervision model would be the best fit for your practice? Who would be your ideal students? What would you need from your AFWC?

APPRENTICESHIP TRADITIONAL ONE-TO-ONE	SHARED SUPERVISION MULTIPLE MENTOR	ROLE-EMERGING	COLLABORATIVE MODEL
			Students can practice techniques together, discuss plans and clients, bounce ideas off each other, and ask questions they are reluctant to ask their FWed
			Students provide each other with motivation, encouragement, feedback, and shared observations of one another's practice
	Reduced practice load for FWed, can increase departmental productivity		
			Additional available student work for departmental projects
Provides skills needed for students to work within multidisciplinary teams			

Figure 2-4 (continued). Considerations when choosing a supervision model.

3. Traditional fieldwork evaluation methods, like the FWPE, assess the professional competencies common to all Level II fieldwork experiences. Role-emerging placements require unique skills from students and FWeds. These unique skills are required because of the dual characteristics of developing practice where limited or no services are currently available, as well as expanding or justifying future practice in a setting. How would you assess a student's competency with critical skills for a role-emerging practice? For example, how would you assess a student's skills in the following competencies?

   a. Accurately identifying opportunities for expanding occupational therapy services in a setting?

   b. Justifying occupational therapy services to internal stakeholders in an organization?

   c. Developing programming that is consistent with the mission and vision of an organization?

   d. Developing outcome measures for established and new occupational therapy services?

   e. Addressing long-term sustainability of new occupational therapy programming or services?

   f. Articulating the evidence-based, client-centered, and occupation-based nature of proposed new occupational therapy services or programming?

4. Utilizing the multiple-mentorship model requires clear communication practices and procedures for both students and FWeds. What are the structures, procedures, or methods you can use to ensure clear, effective communication around expectations, feedback, and evaluation when using this model?

5. Telesupervision can provide a level of access and flexibility for students and FWeds in a number of different practice models. See Appendix C for a brief overview on telesupervision. After reviewing Appendix C, consider these questions about the use of telesupervision technologies in Level II fieldwork:

   a. What unique challenges and skills are necessary for a FWed in using these technologies?

   b. How would you ensure communication is timely, accessible, and effective using these technologies?

   c. What is the back-up plan in case of technology glitches?

   d. How will you determine the right mix of in-person communication, email, phone contact, and video calls for your student in your practice setting?

   e. How will you set limits on accessibility through these technologies? Will you set limits on times or days when specific technologies are not used? For instance, will you allow students to send emails at any time, with an agreement about how quickly you will respond? Will certain days or times be off-limits for phone calls or video calls? How can you make these limits and expectations as clear as possible?

   f. What issues may arise in the use of these technologies that are unique to your practice setting or population? For instance, are there limits on video calls involving observation of pediatric clients or forensic clients? How will you identify these issues and develop solutions that ensure safety and confidentiality?

REFERENCES

Accreditation Council for Occupational Therapy Education. (2018). Standards and interpretive guide (effective July 31, 2020), December 2020 interpretive guide version. https://honline.org/download/3332/

American Occupational Therapy Association. (2009). Self-assessment tool for fieldwork educator competency. AOTA Press. https://www.aota.org/~/media/Corporate/Files/EducationCareers/Educators/Fieldwork/Supervisor/Forms/Self-Assessment%20Tool%20FW%20Ed%20Competency%20(2009).pdf

American Occupational Therapy Association. (2010). Practice advisory: Services provided by students in fieldwork level II settings. https://www.aota.org//media/Corporate/Files/EducationCareers/Educators/Fieldwork/StuSuprvsn/Practice%20Advisory%20Services%20provided%20by%20students%20in%20FW%20Level%20II%20final.pdf

American Occupational Therapy Association. (2012). Fieldwork level II and occupational therapy students: A position paper. *American Journal of Occupational Therapy, 66*(Suppl.,S75-S77). https://doi.org/10.5014/ajot.2012.66S75

American Occupational Therapy Association. (2013). COE guidelines for an occupational therapy fieldwork experience–level II. https://www.aota.org/Education-Careers/Fieldwork/LevelII.aspx

American Occupational Therapy Association. (2014). Guidelines for supervision, roles, and responsibilities during the delivery of occupational therapy services. *American Journal of Occupational Therapy, 68*, 516-522. https://doi.org/10.5014/ajot.2014.686S03

Avi-Itzhak, T. E., & Kellner, H. (1996). Fieldwork centers approach: Supervisors' perceptions of a fieldwork education alternative. *Israeli Journal of Occupational Therapy, 5*(4), E205-E221.

Bartholomai, S., & Fitzgerald, C. (2007). The collaborative model of fieldwork education: Implementation of the model in a regional hospital rehabilitation setting. *Australian Occupational Therapy Journal, 54*. https://doi.org/10.1111/j.1440-1630.2007.00702.x

Bonsaksen, T., Celo, C., Myraunet, I., Granå, K. E., & Ellingham, B. (2013). Promoting academic-practice partnerships through students' practice placement. *International Journal of Therapy and Rehabilitation, 20*(1), 33-39. https://doi.org/10.12968/ijtr.2013.20.1.33

Booth M. D. (1957). A study of the relationship between certain personality factors and success in clinical training of occupational therapy students. *American Journal of Occupational Therapy, 11*(2 Part 2), 93-96.

Boshoff, K., Murray, C., Worley, A., & Berndt, A. (2019). Interprofessional education placements in allied health: A scoping review. *Scandinavian Journal of Occupational Therapy, 27*(2), 80-97. https://doi.org/10.1080/11038128.2019.164 2955

Bossers, A., Cook, J., Polatajko, H., & Laine, C. (1997). Understanding the role-emerging fieldwork placement. *Canadian Journal of Occupational Therapy, 64*(1), 70-81. https://doi.org/10.1177/000841749706400107

Cameron, D., Cockburn, L., Nixon, S., Parnes, P., Garcia, L., Leotaud, J., MacPherson, K., Mashaka, P. M., Mlay, R., Wango, J., & Williams, T. (2013). Global partnerships for international fieldwork in occupational therapy: Reflection and innovation. *Occupational Therapy International, 20*(2), 88-96. https://doi.org/10.1002/oti.1352

Chipchase, L., Hill, A., Dunwoodie, R., Allen, S., Kane, Y., Piper, K., & Russell, T. (2016). Evaluating telesupervision as a support for clinical learning: An action research project. *International Journal of Practice-Based Learning in Health and Social Care, 2*(2), 40-53.

Collier, G. F., & O'Connor, L. (1998, April). Collaborative supervision, real-life skills. *OT Practice, 3*(4), 46-48.

Copley, J., & Nelson, A. (2012). Practice educator perspectives of multiple mentoring in diverse clinical settings. *British Journal of Occupational Therapy, 75*(10), 456-462. https://doi.org/10.4276/030802212x13496921049662

Costa, D. (Ed.). (2015). *The essential guide to fieldwork education* (2nd ed.). AOTA.

Costa, D., Molinsky, R., & Sauerwald, C. (2012). Collaborative intraprofessional education with occupational therapy and occupational therapy assistant students. *OT Practice, 17*(21), CE-1-CE-8.

Diler, R., Regev, S, Kastner, L, & Stoler, M. (2012). Supervision for occupational therapy students in the 21st century: Correspondence via electronic mail as a supplementary means for fieldwork education. *Israeli Journal of Occupational Therapy, 21*(3), E72. https//doi.org/132.174.255.153.

Dudding, C. (2012). Focusing in on tele-supervision. America Speech-Language-Hearing Association: Information to Academic Programs and Faculty. https://academy.pubs.asha.org/2012/12/focusing-in-on-tele-supervision/.

Engel, L., Gillespie, H., & Lundberg, J. (2013). Integrated-split placement: Optimizing opportunities and enhancing learning. *Occupational Therapy Now, 15*(1), 24-26.

Evenson, M. E., Roberts, M., Kaldenberg, J., Barnes, M. A., & Ozelie, R. (2015). National survey of fieldwork educators: Implications for occupational therapy education. *American Journal of Occupational Therapy, 69*(Suppl. 2), 1-5. https://doi.org/10.5014/ajot.2015.019265

Farrow, S., Gaiptman, B., & Rudman, D. (2000). Exploration of a group model in fieldwork education. *Canadian Journal of Occupational Therapy, 67*(4), 239-249. https://doi.org/10.1177/000841740006700406

Fleming, S., Kasner, M., D'Rocha, J., & Noble, S. (2014). Occupational therapy in a community sport organization: Supporting a vision of social inclusion. *Occupational Therapy Now, 16*(2), 8-9.

Flood, B., Haslam, L., & Hocking, C. (2010). Implementing a collaborative model of student supervision in New Zealand: Enhancing therapist and student experiences. *New Zealand Journal of Occupational Therapy, 57*(1), 22-26. https://doi.org/10.12691/education-7-11-13

Gaiptman, B., & Forma, L. (1991). The split placement model for fieldwork placements. *Canadian Journal of Occupational Therapy, 58*(2), 85-88. https://doi.org/10.1177/000841749105800206

Gat, S., & Ratzon, N. Z. (2014). Comparison of occupational therapy students' perceived skills after traditional and nontraditional fieldwork. *American Journal of Occupational Therapy, 68*(2), e47-e54. https://doi.org/10.5014/ajot.2014.007732

Graves, C. (2019). Integrating best practice into fieldwork: A narrative inquiry into the level II experiences of occupational therapy students (Publication No. 2556) [Doctoral dissertation, University of North Dakota]. https://commons.und.edu/theses/2556

Graves, C., & Hanson, D. (2014). The multiple mentoring model of student supervision: A fit for contemporary practice. *OT Practice, 19*(8), 20-32.

Gustafsson, L., Brown, T., McKinstry, C., & Caine, A. (2016). Practice education: A snapshot from Australian university programmes. *Australian Occupational Therapy Journal, 64*(2), 159-169. https://doi.org/10.1111/1440-1630.12337

Hanson, D. (2011a). Collaborative supervision models: Are two (or more) students better than one? *OT Practice, 16*(1), 25-26.

Hanson, D. (2011b). Expanding practice borders: The value of nontraditional fieldwork models. *OT Practice, 16*(20), 6-8.

Hanson, D. (2012). Collaborative fieldwork education: Intraprofessional and interprofessional learning. *OT Practice, 16*(9), 16-23.

Hanson, D. J., & DeIuliis, E. D. (2015). The collaborative model of fieldwork education: A blueprint for group supervision of students. *Occupational Therapy in Health Care, 29*(2), 223-239. https://doi.org/10.3109/07380577.2015.1011297

Hanson, D., & Nielsen, S. K, (2015). Introduction to role-emerging fieldwork. In D. Costa (Ed.), *The essential guide to fieldwork education* (2nd ed.). AOTA.

Hanson, D., Stutz-Tanenbaum, P., Rogers, O., Turner, T., Graves, C., & Klug, M. (2019) Collaborative fieldwork supervision: A process model for program effectiveness. *American Journal of Educational Research, 7*(11), 837-844. https://doi.org/10.12691/education-7-11-13

Hebert, M., Beaudoin, J., Grandisson, M., Al-Azourri, G., Thibeault, R., Tremblay, M., Savard, J., & Guitard, P. (2013). Preparing occupational therapy students for professional practice. *Occupational Therapy Now, 15*(3), 22-24.

Hengel, J. L., & Romeo, J. L. (1995). A group approach to mental health fieldwork. *American Journal of Occupational Therapy, 49*(4), 354-358. https://doi.org/10.5014/ajot.49.4.354

Jung, B., Martin, A., Graden, L., & Awrey, J. (1994). Fieldwork education: A shared supervision model. *Canadian Journal of Occupational Therapy, 61*(1), 12-19. https://doi.org/10.1177/000841749406100105

Kinsella, A. T., & Piersol, C. V. (2018). Development and evaluation of a collaborative model level II fieldwork program. *The Open Journal of Occupational Therapy, 6*(3). https://doi.org/10.15453/2168-6408.1448

Lau, M., & Ravenek, M. (2019). The student perspective on role-emerging fieldwork placements in occupational therapy: A review of the literature. *The Open Journal of Occupational Therapy, 7*(3), 1-21. https://doi.org/10.15453/2168-6408.1544

Lew, N., Cara, E., & Richardson, P. (2007). When fieldwork takes a detour. *Occupational Therapy in Health Care, 21*(1), 105-122. https://doi.org/10.1300/j003v21n01_08

Martin, M., Morris, J., Moore, A., Sadlo, G., & Crouch, V. (2004). Evaluating practice education models in occupational therapy: Comparing 1:1, 2:1 and 3:1 placements. *British Journal of Occupational Therapy, 67*(5), 192-200. https://doi.org/10.1177/030802260406700502

Martin, P., Kumar, S., Lizarondo, L., & VanErp, A. (2015). Enablers of and barriers to high quality clinical supervision among occupational therapists across Queensland in Australia: Findings from a qualitative study. *BMC Health Sciences Research, 15*(413), 1-8. https://doi.org/10.1186/s12913-015-1085-8

Massachusetts Board of Allied Health Professionals. (2020). 259 CMR 3: Occupational therapists. Commonwealth of Massachusetts Board of Allied Health Professionals. https://www.mass.gov/doc/259-cmr-3-occupational-therapists/download

Mattila, A. (2019). Perceptions and outcomes of occupational therapy students participating in community engaged learning: A mixed-methods approach. *The Open Journal of Occupational Therapy, 7*(4), 1-17. https://doi.org/10.15453/2168-6408.1612

Mattila, A., Deiuliis, E. D., & Cook, A. B. (2018). Increasing self-efficacy through role emerging placements: Implications for occupational therapy experiential learning. *Journal of Occupational Therapy Education, 2*(3). https://doi.org/10.26681/jote.2018.020303

Mattila, A. M., & Dolhi, C. (2016). Transformative experience of master of occupational therapy students in a non-traditional fieldwork setting. *Occupational Therapy in Mental Health, 32*(1), 16-31. https://doi.org/10.1080/0164212x.2015.1088424

McGill University. (2020). Role emerging community fieldwork handbook. School of Physical & Occupational Therapy, McGill University. https://www.mcgill.ca/spot/files/spot/role-emerging_community_fieldwork_handbook.pdf

Merriam-Webster. (n.d.a). Supervision. https://www.merriam-webster.com/dictionary/supervision

Merriam-Webster. (n.d.b). Supervisee. https://www.merriam-webster.com/dictionary/supervisee

Mulholland, S., & Derdall, M. (2005). A strategy for supervising occupational therapy students at community sites. *Occupational Therapy International, 12*(1), 28-43. https://doi.org/10.1002/oti.13

Nagarajan, S., McAllister, L., McFarlane, L., Hall, M., Schmitz, C., Roots, R., Drynan, D., Avery, L., Murphy, S., & Lam, M. (2016). Telesupervision benefits for placements: Allied health students' and supervisors' perceptions. *International Journal of Practice-Based Learning in Health and Social Care, 4*(1), 16–27. https://doi.org/10.18552/ijpblhsc.v4i1.326

Nolinske, T. (1995). Multiple mentoring relationships facilitate learning during fieldwork. *American Journal of Occupational Therapy, 49*(1), 39-43. https://doi.org/10.5014/ajot.49.1.39

Peel, N. M., Russel, T. G., & Gray, L. C. (2011). Feasibility of using an in-home video conferencing system in geriatric rehabilitation. *Journal of Rehabilitation Medicine, 43*, 364-366. https://doi.10.2340/16501977-0675.

Phelps, G. K. (2017). Best practice model for a community-based level II fieldwork program (Publication No. 6723). [Doctoral dissertation, Boston University]. Boston University Libraries.

Precin, P. (2007). An aggregate fieldwork model: Interdisciplinary training/intervention component. *Occupational Therapy In Health Care, 21*(1), 123-131. https://doi.org/10.1300/j003v21n01_09

Precin, P. (2009). An aggregate fieldwork model: Cooperative learning, research, and clinical project publication components. *Occupational Therapy in Mental Health, 25*(1), 62-82. https://doi.org/10.1080/01642120802647691

Price, D., & Whiteside, M. (2016). Implementing the 2:1 student placement model in occupational therapy: Strategies for practice. *Australian Occupational Therapy Journal, 63*(2), 123-129. https://doi.org/10.1111/1440-1630.12257

Prigg, A., & Mackenzie, L. (2002). Project placements for undergraduate occupational therapy students: Design, implementation and evaluation. *Occupational Therapy International, 9*(3), 210-236. https://doi.org/10.1002/oti.166

Richard, L. F. (2008). Exploring connections between theory and practice: Stories from fieldwork supervisors. *Occupational Therapy in Mental Health, 24*(2), 154-175. https://doi.org/10.1080/01642120802055259

Rindflesch, A. B., Dunfee, H. J., Cieslak, K. R., Eischen, S. L., Trenary, T., Calley, D. Q., & Heinle, D. K. (2009). Collaborative model of clinical education in physical and occupational therapy at the Mayo Clinic. *Journal of Allied Health, 38*(3), 132-142.

Roberts, M., & Simon, R. (2012). Fieldwork challenge 2012. *OT Practice, 17*(6), 20.

Rodger, S., Thomas, Y., Holley, S., Springfield, E., Edwards, A., Broadbridge, J., Greber, C., McBryde, C., Banks, R., & Hawkins, R. (2009). Increasing the occupational therapy mental health workforce through innovative practice education: A pilot project. *Australian Occupational Therapy Journal, 56*(6), 409-417. https://doi.org/10.1111/j.1440-1630.2009.00806.x

Schwartz, K. B. (1984). An approach to supervision of students on fieldwork. *American Journal of Occupational Therapy, 38*(6), 393-397. https://doi.org/10.5014/ajot.38.6.393

Thew, M., Hargreaves, A., & Cronin-Davis, J. (2008). An evaluation of a role-emerging practice placement model for a full cohort of occupational therapy students. *British Journal of Occupational Therapy, 71*(8), 348-353.https://doi.org/10.1177/030802260807100809

Thomas, Y., Dickson, D., Broadbridge, J., Hopper, L., Hawkins, R., Edwards, A., & Mcbryde, C. (2007). Benefits and challenges of supervising occupational therapy fieldwork students: Supervisors' perspectives. *Australian Occupational Therapy Journal, 54*, S2-S-12. https://doi.org/10.1111/j.1440-1630.2007.00694.x

Thomas, Y., Penman, M., & Williamson, P. (2005). Australian and New Zealand fieldwork: Charting the territory for future practice. *Australian Occupational Therapy Journal, 52*(1), 78-81. https://doi.org/10.1111/j.1440-1630.2004.00452.x

Thomson, N. A., & Thompson, L. (2013). Reflections on a role-emerging fieldwork placement using a collaborative model of supervision. *Occupational Therapy Now, 15*(3), 17-20.

Thomure, R., Cendejas, R., & Roe, D. (2021). Supporting level II occupational therapy fieldwork students over telehealth in community mental health. *Communique, 1*, 17-18.

Tyminski, Q. (2018). The development of a role-emerging fieldwork placement in a homeless shelter. *Journal of Occupational Therapy Education, 2*(2), 1-13. https://doi.org/10.26681/jote.2018.020207

Varland, J., Cardell, E., Koski, J., & McFadden, M. (2017). Factors influencing occupational therapists' decision to supervise fieldwork students. *Occupational Therapy in Health Care, 31*(3), 238-254. https://doi.org/10.1080/07380577.2017.1328631

Vogel, K., Grice, K. O., Hill, S., & Moody, J. (2004). Supervisor and student expectations of level II fieldwork. *Occupational Therapy in Health Care, 18*(1), 5-19. https://doi.org/10.1300/j003v18n0102

Vygotsky, L. S. (1978). *Mind in society: The development of higher psychological processes.* In M. Cole, V. John-Steiner, S. Scribner, & E. Souberman (Eds.). Harvard University Press.

Wenger, E. (2000). Communities of practice and social learning systems. *Organization, 7*(2), 225-246. http://org.sagepub.com/content/7/2/225

Wilske, G. (2016). A personal viewpoint on the collaborative model. *OT Practice, 21*(3), 19-20.

APPENDIX A

Synthesis of Level II Fieldwork Supervision Models

MODEL	ROLE OF FIELDWORK EDUCATOR	ROLE OF STUDENT	BENEFITS	DRAWBACKS	PREPARATIONS
Apprenticeship	Provides feedback in one-to-one contact with student. Develops learning opportunities for each student. Develops learning plan and objectives. Communicates with occupational therapy program about student performance. FWed serves as expert; in control of time, content, and structure.	Active participation in placement to develop knowledge and skills. Implement individual and group interventions and complete documentation. Address learning needs through one-to-one contact with FWed.	Individual attention for student. No comparisons with other students. Simpler to identify one FWed's expectations. Easier organization with one practitioner's schedule. Well-established single role for occupational therapist for students to learn. Student questions help with FWed's reflective practice. Compatible model for novice practitioners.	Quality of placement may depend on quality of relationship with one FWed. Little opportunity for peer feedback or collaboration. Limited to one practitioner's practice area. Learning opportunities limited by FWed's caseload and practice setting. Risk of developing or reinforcing dependency. Student opportunities to practice skills, share ideas, ask questions, or reflect on practice are limited by FWed's availability.	Ensure FWed has necessary skills, knowledge, qualifications, and resources for supervision of Level II students. Develop a student manual to be used as a resource for the FWed and student, describing policies, procedures, schedules, and expectations.

(continued)

MODEL	ROLE OF FIELDWORK EDUCATOR	ROLE OF STUDENT	BENEFITS	DRAWBACKS	PREPARATIONS
Shared supervision/ multiple mentorship	Provides learning opportunities to pair or group students. Provides performance feedback to students. Facilitates effective collaboration. Develops learning plan and objectives. Communicates with occupational therapy program about student performance. Collaborate with other FWeds within specific shared supervision plan.	Meets learning objectives through interactions with a variety of practitioners. Utilize peers as resources and learning partners. Integrate knowledge with peers, FWeds, and in group supervision. Develop learning plan and share with FWed and peers. Demonstrate maturity, flexibility, and self-direction in learning.	Broader practice experience and more access to specialty practice areas. More autonomy and responsibility for students with less one-to-one dependence on a particular FWed. More FWeds can be involved, including those with limited schedules or specialty practices. Multiple perspectives with evaluation and feedback. Promotes initiative and problem-solving in students.	Additional orientation and on-boarding time if more than one unit or practice area. Potential for better relationship with one FWed than the other. Potential for more difficulty developing rapport with multiple FWeds. Possible perceived comparison or competition between students. Perception of increased workload of shared supervision vs. apprenticeship.	Shared supervision plan for FWeds, including determination of educator primarily responsible for formal performance evaluation. Works best with set schedule, especially with multiple practices. Students should exhibit motivation, self-confidence, independence, and problem-solving skills. Fieldwork sites should offer orientation to available resources, FWed teaching styles, schedules, and preferred communication methods.

(continued)

MODEL	ROLE OF FIELDWORK EDUCATOR	ROLE OF STUDENT	BENEFITS	DRAWBACKS	PREPARATIONS
Shared supervision/ multiple mentorship	Shared supervision, not full-time supervision of students. Communicate with peers about assigned tasks, feedback, and performance to improve efficiency and decrease duplication of feedback.	Be more proactive in identifying needs. Implement individual and group interventions and complete documentation.	Opportunity for students to develop their own therapeutic style, rather than copying style from single FWed. Less supervision time commitment per FWed. Collaboration between FWeds facilitates development of clinical reasoning among FWeds. Can allow for less experienced FWeds to develop confidence within reduced supervision role. Collaboration with peers on practice reflections and skills reviews allows for more focused and direct use of FWed's time. More students on site means more added benefit and resources for fieldwork site.	Depends in part on quality of organization of experience in advance of student arrival. Inconsistency among educators can be stressful for students.	Collaborate with students and other FWeds to develop learning objectives and performance expectations, including use of learning contracts. Establish structures like weekly group supervision meetings with all FWeds and students, tracking for student caseload and progress, and consistent scheduled meetings for regular communication.
Role-emerging/ project placement	Supervise and manage students. Establish and monitor occupational therapy programming at practice site.	Need to identify the role of occupational therapist in the setting and articulate the role effectively.	More autonomous and independent, with greater professional growth. Greater opportunities for creativity and developing time management skills. Prepares students for greater variety of practice options in the future.	Set-up and monitoring can be more demanding. Can be challenging for students with limited knowledge of occupational therapist's role in a setting.	Complete a needs assessment for the practice if applicable Clearly establish process for supervision, feedback, and evaluation of students.

(continued)

MODEL	ROLE OF FIELDWORK EDUCATOR	ROLE OF STUDENT	BENEFITS	DRAWBACKS	PREPARATIONS
Role-emerging/ project placement	Supervise and manage students. Establish and monitor occupational therapy programming at practice site. Serve as liaison between fieldwork site and educational institution. Provide 8 hours per week of direct supervision and additional consults as needed in compliance with ACOTE standards. Must have 3 years' full-time work experience at a minimum. Serve as facilitator of development, encouraging autonomy and independence while providing support as needed, not serving exclusively as an expert. Promote learning opportunities, learning, reflection, and independent problem solving. Provide clear instructions and continue reviews of expectations. Collaborate with on-site interprofessional mentor. Facilitate productive student relationships with site staff and clients. Communicates with occupational therapy program about student performance.	Collaborate with other service providers. Implement individual and group interventions. Design new programs for clients as needed. Complete needs assessments, documentation, and learning goals for themselves as needed. Demonstrate initiative, self-directed learning, and self-awareness.	Higher student perception of personal responsibility, cultural competence, and personal skills when compared with traditional model fieldwork. Prepares students for professional challenges that classroom or traditional fieldwork cannot provide.	Time with FWed is more limited. Greater emphasis on clarity with expectations. Concerns regarding liability may exist. Students may be concerned about performance evaluation when on-site occupational therapy supervision is limited.	Develop resources in advance, such as a student binder that includes policies and procedures, site-specific objectives, usernames and passwords, required readings, and other relevant information for the setting.

(continued)

MODEL	ROLE OF FIELDWORK EDUCATOR	ROLE OF STUDENT	BENEFITS	DRAWBACKS	PREPARATIONS
Collaborative model	Develop learning activities and joint practice tasks that students can complete together. Ensure organizational support, especially from FWed's peers. Keep positive, pragmatic approach to experience as a FWed. Provides performance feedback to students. Facilitates effective peer collaboration. Develops learning plan and objectives. Communicates with occupational therapy program about student performance. Adapt to differences in rates of development of students and different student learning or communication styles. Provide group and individual supervision.	Utilize peers as resources and learning partners Integrate knowledge with peers, FWeds, and in group supervision. Develop learning plan and share with FWed and peers. Demonstrate maturity, flexibility, and self-direction in learning. Be more proactive in identifying needs. Meet formally with FWed one-to-one weekly. Share experiences with peers and learn from mistakes.	Students are more active learners, with increased independence, improved problem-solving skills, and more effective teamwork skills. More work with peers leads students to feel more comfortable, confident, and relaxed, and less intimidated. Students can practice techniques together, discuss plans and clients, bounce ideas off each other, and ask questions they are reluctant to ask their FWed. Students provide each other with motivation, encouragement, feedback, and shared observations of one another's practice.	May be difficult managing multiple different learning styles, communication styles, and needs of students. Maintaining student privacy can be challenging. Monitoring multiple students' strengths, weaknesses, and progress is more challenging. Can take longer for students and FWeds to build a relationship. Space for students can be restricted.	Ensure adequate caseload for multiple students. Develop learning activities and joint practice tasks that students can complete together. Ensure organizational support, especially from FWed's peers. Keep positive, pragmatic approach to experience as a FWed. Review evidence for the model in advance. Collaborate with occupational therapy school to ensure student compatibility with peers, model, and practice.

(continued)

MODEL	ROLE OF FIELDWORK EDUCATOR	ROLE OF STUDENT	BENEFITS	DRAWBACKS	PREPARATIONS
Collaborative model	Delegate workload and client assignments. Include assessment of collaboration as an outcome measure.	Serve as role model for peers, give and incorporate peer feedback. Implement individual and group interventions and complete documentation.	Reduced practice load for FWed, can increase departmental productivity. Additional available student work for departmental projects. Provides skills needed for students to work within multidisciplinary teams.	Some clients may be reluctant to work with more students. Possible student incompatibility. May be more challenging for novice practitioners.	Develop a clear timetable and schedule for the fieldwork experience. Identify space for students to use for room and privacy while working. Develop how-to references for common tasks in the practice setting.

ADAPTED FROM

Bartholomai, S., & Fitzgerald, C. (2007). The collaborative model of fieldwork education: Implementation of the model in a regional hospital rehabilitation setting. *Australian Occupational Therapy Journal, 54*, S23-S30. https://doi.org/10.1111/j.1440-1630.2007.00702.x

Boshoff, K., Murray, C., Worley, A., & Berndt, A. (2019). Interprofessional education placements in allied health: A scoping review. *Scandinavian Journal of Occupational Therapy, 27*(2), 80-97. https://doi.org/10.1080/11038128.2019.1642955

Copley, J., & Nelson, A. (2012). Practice educator perspectives of multiple mentoring in diverse clinical settings. *British Journal of Occupational Therapy, 75*(10), 456-462. https://doi.org/10.4276/030802212x13496921049662

Costa, D., Molinsky, R., & Sauerwald, C. (2012). Collaborative intraprofessional education with occupational therapy and occupational therapy assistant students. *OT Practice, 17*(21), CE-1-CE-8.

Farrow, S., Gaiptman, B., & Rudman, D. (2000). Exploration of a group model in fieldwork education. *Canadian Journal of Occupational Therapy, 67*(4), 239-249. https://doi.org/10.1177/000841740006700406

Flood, B., Haslam, L., & Hocking, C. (2010). Implementing a collaborative model of student supervision in New Zealand: Enhancing therapist and student experiences. *New Zealand Journal of Occupational Therapy, 57*(1), 22-26. https://doi.org/10.12691/education-7-11-13

Gaiptman, B., & Forma, L. (1991). The split placement model for fieldwork placements. *Canadian Journal of Occupational Therapy, 58*(2), 85-88. https://doi.org/10.1177/000841749105800206

Gat, S., & Ratzon, N. Z. (2014). Comparison of occupational therapy students' perceived skills after traditional and nontraditional fieldwork. *American Journal of Occupational Therapy, 68*(2), e47-e54. https://doi.org/10.5014/ajot.2014.007732

Graves, C., & Hanson, D. (2014). The multiple mentoring model of student supervision: A fit for contemporary practice. *OT Practice, 19*(8), 20-32.

Hengel, J. L., & Romeo, J. L. (1995). A group approach to mental health fieldwork. *American Journal of Occupational Therapy, 49*(4), 354-358. https://doi.org/10.5014/ajot.49.4.354

Jung, B., Martin, A., Graden, L., & Awrey, J. (1994). Fieldwork education: A shared supervision model. *Canadian Journal of Occupational Therapy, 61*(1), 12-19. https://doi.org/10.1177/000841749406100105

Martin, M., Morris, J., Moore, A., Sadlo, G., & Crouch, V. (2004). Evaluating practice education models in occupational therapy: Comparing 1:1, 2:1 and 3:1 placements. *British Journal of Occupational Therapy, 67*(5), 192-200. https://doi.org/10.1177/030802260406700502

Mattila, A. M., & Dolhi, C. (2016). Transformative experience of master of occupational therapy ttudents in a nontraditional fieldwork setting. *Occupational Therapy in Mental Health, 32*(1), 16-31. https://doi.org/10.1080/0164212x.2015.1088424

Mulholland, S., & Derdall, M. (2005). A strategy for supervising occupational therapy students at community sites. *Occupational Therapy International, 12*(1), 28-43. https://doi.org/10.1002/oti.13

Phelps, G. K. (2017). Best practice model for a community-based level II fieldwork program (Publication No. 6723). [Doctoral dissertation, Boston University]. Boston University Libraries.

Price, D., & Whiteside, M. (2016). Implementing the 2:1 student placement model in occupational therapy: Strategies for practice. *Australian Occupational Therapy Journal, 63*(2), 123-129. https://doi.org/10.1111/1440-1630.12257

Prigg, A., & Mackenzie, L. (2002). Project placements for undergraduate occupational therapy students: Design, implementation and evaluation. *Occupational Therapy International, 9*(3), 210-236. https://doi.org/10.1002/oti.166

Thomas, Y., Penman, M., & Williamson, P. (2005). Australian and New Zealand fieldwork: Charting the territory for future practice. *Australian Occupational Therapy Journal, 52*(1), 78-81. https://doi.org/10.1111/j.1440-1630.2004.00452.x

Thomson, N. A., & Thompson, L. (2013). Reflections on a role-emerging fieldwork placement using a collaborative model of supervision. *Occupational Therapy Now, 15*(3), 17-20.

Wilske, G. (2016). A personal viewpoint on the collaborative model. *OT Practice, 21*(3), 19-20.

APPENDIX B
Additional Resources on Models of Supervision

The University of Queensland Clinical Educator's Resource Kit

Available from: https://otpecq.group.uq.edu.au/resources-publications/clinical-educators-resource-kit

Use: Researching a wide variety of resources for occupational therapy fieldwork. This resource was originally developed by the Queensland Occupational Therapy Fieldwork Collaborative to engage practitioners more directly and consistently into fieldwork education. The information is organized into five components: preplacement considerations, setting up and sustaining a positive student clinical placement, approaches to clinical education, the feedback process and evaluation, and working with students who are experiencing difficulty. There are also three particularly useful sections with easy-to-use resources: useful fact sheets, templates and worksheets, and publications and presentations. The useful fact sheets include short documents, including "Benefits of Collaborative Placements," "Benefits of Role Emerging Placements," "Benefits of Multiple Mentoring Placements," and documents on setting up and managing placements with all nontraditional supervision models. The templates and worksheets include orientation checklists and action plans for setting up student placements. The publications and presentations section is a comprehensive bibliography of resources relating to fieldwork education.

Supervision model: All, with particular resources dedicated to Collaborative Model, Role-Emerging Fieldwork, and Shared Supervision Model.

AOTA Fieldwork Experience Assessment Tool

Available from: https://www.aota.org/-/media/Corporate/Files/EducationCareers/Accredit/FEATCHARTMidterm.pdf

Use: Helping to ensure both the student and the FWed share the same perception of the expectations and objectives of the fieldwork experience. Can be completed at midterm or at any time a discussion around fieldwork expectations is helpful.

Supervision model: All

Midterm Level II Feedback form

Available from: https://www.aota.org/-/media/Corporate/Files/EducationCareers/Educators/Fieldwork/LevelII/level2midfd.pdf

Use: Providing a platform to ensure communication about necessary information and resources for the Level II fieldwork student, as well as a check on the adequacy of the preparations and resources provided by the site. Includes sections on orientation, assignments, client caseload, supervision, communication, professionalism, and professional development.

Supervision model: All

Weekly Review Form

Available from: https://www.aota.org/-/media/Corporate/Files/EducationCareers/Educators/Fieldwork/LevelII/level2weekrev.pdf

Use: A format for structuring regular weekly supervision meetings. This form includes sections on strengths, growth areas, goals, and meetings/assignments. This format can be completed by the student in advance, then reviewed by the FWed. Feedback may be provided on the same form, and these weekly forms can be collected and reviewed by the student and FWed at regular intervals during the fieldwork experience.

Supervision model: All

Personal Data Sheet

Available from: https://www.aota.org/-/media/Corporate/Files/EducationCareers/Educators/Fieldwork/Supervisor/Forms/persdata.doc

Use: A general snapshot for a student to complete and submit in advance of their placement. Covers basic demographic and contact information, previous work/volunteer experience, strengths, areas of growth, special skills, preferred learning style, preferred supervision style, and other fieldwork experience. Can help with matching students with FWeds or to match students with particular programs, practice settings, or peers for collaborative model placements.

Supervision model: All

Self-Assessment Tool for Fieldwork Educator Competency

Available from: https://www.aota.org/-/media/Corporate/Files/EducationCareers/Educators/Fieldwork/Supervisor/Forms/Self-Assessment%20Tool%20FW%20Ed%20Competency%20(2009).pdf

Use: Self-assessment (that can be shared with peers or supervisors) of five areas of competency, including professional practice, education, supervision, evaluation, and administration. The tool concludes with a format for a professional development plan to help facilitate growth in competency areas before accepting a student. The tool can also be used on a regular basis by FWeds to ensure continual improvement between student placements. It can also be used to help match FWeds as collaborators in shared supervision model fieldwork.

Supervision model: All

Student Evaluation of Fieldwork Experience

Available from: https://www.aota.org/-/media/Corporate/Files/EducationCareers/Educators/Fieldwork/StuSuprvsn/Student-Evaluation-Fieldwork-Experience-2016.docx

Use: Gathering subjective information from students after completion of the fieldwork experience. This form collects information from the student about the site's orientation process, evaluations, interventions, population served, outcomes, training opportunities, documentation, contextual issues, expectations, and collaboration with the FWeds. Information about the lived experience of the fieldwork student is collected and can be compared with the structure and objectives of the experience. This can also be used to provide feedback on supervision for the FWed's professional development.

Supervision model: All

Steps for Implementing the Collaborative Model

Available from: Hanson, D. J., & Deluliis, E. D. (2015). The collaborative model of fieldwork education: A blueprint for group supervision of students. *Occupational Therapy in Health Care, 29*(2), 223-239. https://doi.org/10.3109/07380577.2015.1011297 (Table 1 on page 226 and Table 5 on page 234)

Use: Understanding the preparation and implementation steps, as well as the outcomes to evaluate, in developing a collaborative model fieldwork experience. Includes important areas to consider in developing the experience, including collaboration with the AFWC, preparing staff for the experience, and sources of feedback for evaluating the experience. Also includes how to operationalize the valuable elements of collaborative model fieldwork, like positive interdependence, accountability, and teamwork skills.

Supervision model: Collaborative Model

Preparation and Implementation of Collaborative Model Level II Fieldwork

Available from: Kinsella, A. T., & Piersol, C. V. (2018). Development and evaluation of a collaborative model level II fieldwork program. *The Open Journal of Occupational Therapy, 6*(3). https://doi.org/10.15453/2168-6408.1448 (Pages 2 and 3)

Use: Reviewing effective strategies for preparing staff and students for maximizing the value of their experience in collaborative model fieldwork. Includes specific content to be used for education before commencement of the experience and formats for monitoring the effectiveness of the supervision model during fieldwork.

Supervision model: Collaborative Model

Strategies for Maximizing Opportunities Available in Collaborative Model Fieldwork

Available from: Price, D., & Whiteside, M. (2016). Implementing the 2:1 student placement model in occupational therapy: Strategies for practice. *Australian Occupational Therapy Journal, 63*(2), 123-129. https://doi.org/10.1111/1440-1630.12257 (Pages 6 and 7)

Use: Specific strategies to use to maximize the benefits and possibilities of collaborative model fieldwork. Includes features to include in student learning plans, strategies for FWeds, and recommendations for organizational support.

Supervision model: Collaborative Model

Recommendations for Collaborative Model Fieldwork

Available from: Wilske, G. (2016). A personal viewpoint on the collaborative model. *OT Practice, 21*(3), 19-20. (Practical tips on page 2)

Use: Practical everyday tips to enhance the benefits of the collaborative model fieldwork experience, including recommendations for supervision meetings, recommended information to share with students, and ways to foster collaboration among students.

Supervision model: Collaborative Model

Considerations for Implementation of the Collaborative Model of Fieldwork Education

Available from: Bartholomai, S., & Fitzgerald, C. (2007). The collaborative model of fieldwork education: Implementation of the model in a regional hospital rehabilitation setting. *Australian Occupational Therapy Journal, 54*, S23-S30. https://doi.org/10.1111/j.1440-1630.2007.00702.x (Graphical representation of model on page S25, roles and responsibilities pages S25-S29)

Use: Articulating the model for collaborative supervision, as well as specific information on the roles and responsibilities for stakeholders, including students, FWeds, AFWCs, the university, and other occupational therapy staff. Also includes important considerations in developing and implementing the program, such as students' previous clinical experience, appropriate caseload, support, and resources.

Supervision model: Collaborative Model

Typical Timeline for Clinical Experience with Collaborative Model Fieldwork

Available from: Rindflesch, A. B., Dunfee, H. J., Cieslak, K. R., Eischen, S. L., Trenary, T., Calley, D. Q., & Heinle, D. K. (2009). Collaborative model of clinical education in physical and occupational therapy at the Mayo Clinic. *Journal of Allied Health, 38*(3), 132-142. (Timeline available in Table 1 on page 135)

Use: Examples of scheduling important activities throughout a collaborative model fieldwork experience, and their associated educational focus. Provides a week-by-week guide for assignments and progression of responsibilities in fieldwork, albeit with a 9-week model, rather than a typical 12-week model. This schedule also articulates the expectations and opportunities associated with the progression through the experience.

Supervision model: Collaborative Model

Ways for Fieldwork Educators to Facilitate Collaboration

Available from: Collier, G. F., & O'Connor, L. (1998). Collaborative supervision, real-life skills. *OT Practice, 3*(4), 46-48. (Figure 2 on page 47)

Use: Simple and practical ways to encourage collaboration between students and to be successful in a collaborative model fieldwork experience, including contents for orientation and the importance of role modeling collaboration with other health care professionals.

Supervision model: Collaborative Model

Interview Resource for Nontraditional Fieldwork Models

Available from: Martin, M., Morris, J., Moore, A., Sadlo, G., & Crouch, V. (2004). Evaluating practice education models in occupational therapy: Comparing 1:1, 2:1 and 3:1 placements. *British Journal of Occupational Therapy, 67*(5), 192-200. https://doi.org/10.1177/030802260406700502 (Interviews section on page 194)

Use: Informational interviewing of students and FWeds before beginning a nontraditional model fieldwork experience. The recommended topics for the semi-structured interview cover a range of topics including feedback to students, advantages and disadvantages of current supervision model, and student learning.

Supervision model: Collaborative Model, Role-Emerging Fieldwork, Shared Supervision Model

Best Practice Model for Community-Based Level II Fieldwork

Available from: Phelps, G.K. (2017). *Best practice model for a community-based level II fieldwork program* (Publication No. 6723). [Doctoral dissertation, Boston University]. Boston University Libraries. (Orientation checklist page 101, content of student manual page 113)

Use: Examples of orientation material and the contents of a student manual for a role-emerging community-based Level II fieldwork experience. Sample slides from orientation materials include content on adult learning theory and recommendations on reflective practice. The sample student manual content provides examples of many important resources for a student to have on-hand or available throughout the experience, including both general information about fieldwork from AOTA and categories of site-specific information.

Supervision model: Role-Emerging Fieldwork

Resource for Program Development Role-Emerging Level II Fieldwork

Available from: Hanson, D., & Nielsen, S.K, (2016). Introduction to role-emerging fieldwork. In D. Costa (Ed.), *The essential guide to fieldwork education* (2nd ed.). AOTA.

Use: A concise introduction to structure and value of role-emerging fieldwork with a focus on many valuable resources that help educators understand, implement, and evaluate role-emerging fieldwork. These resources include comparisons between traditional and role-emerging fieldwork, assessment of interpersonal abilities, eligibility requirements and application processes, sample schedules and assignments, a case study showing progression from role-emerging fieldwork to program development, and summative reflective questions for students and FWeds.

Supervision model: Role-Emerging Fieldwork, including program development

Role-Emerging Community Fieldwork Handbook From McGill University in Canada

Available from: https://www.mcgill.ca/spot/files/spot/role-emerging_community_fieldwork_handbook.pdf

Use: A handy resource with sample schedules, readings, evaluation forms, checklists for FWeds and students, sample fieldwork experience student contracts, and information on adult learning principles. The document was published originally in 1997 and is updated regularly. The document is 45 pages of essential resources, examples, and templates for use with the role-emerging model.

Supervision model: Role-Emerging Fieldwork

Intern Resource Manual Table of Contents

Available from: Precin, P. (2009). An aggregate fieldwork model: Cooperative learning, research, and clinical project publication components. *Occupational Therapy in Mental Health, 25*(1), 62-82. https://doi.org/10.1080/01642120802647691

Use: Ensuring communication of the important considerations for both multiple FWeds and students in a Shared Supervision Model fieldwork experience. The sample resource manual outline includes a very comprehensive list of resources and information used during the fieldwork experience. The list recommends including information related to the facility and surrounding community, steps for on-boarding students, relevant policies and procedures, information about the specific unit where the student will be working, expectations for fieldwork, documentation, supervision, instructional videos, assessments to be used, and lists of appropriate interventions.

Supervision model: Shared Supervision Model

APPENDIX C
Overview of Telesupervision

Advances in telecommunications have made connections in fieldwork education easier and more convenient. Email, videoconferencing, tablets, smartphones, and the proliferation of broadband internet access have enabled students, FWeds, and AFWCs to get connected and stay connected. For more than a decade, these technologies have been incorporated into supervision and fieldwork education. Telesupervision, as it is described in the literature, generally involves directly observing students via video conferencing technology, students and educators consulting over distance technologies about the fieldwork experience, or a FWed reviewing video, audio, or other materials, then discussing feedback with students through email, phone, or video conference (Diler et al., 2012; Dudding, 2012).

Importantly, these technologies were always used as a component of supervision, to enhance the quality and availability of the collaboration between educator and student, without serving as the sole method of communication. Martin et al. (2015) found there was a definite benefit to supplementing phone supervision with video conferencing because there was value in a face-to-face communication, even if it was in a virtual space. The quality of the supervision was perceived as improved through the video conferencing, likely because the nonverbal communication was retained as part of the supervision process (Martin et al., 2015). The technique has proven valuable across multiple practice settings, as it was used effectively in a metropolitan setting, a regional city, and a rural town (Chipchase et al., 2014). In that study, the combination of telesupervision and face-to-face supervision did not compromise student learning and students were satisfied with the process, provided the ratios were kept to four educators or fewer per student (Chipchase et al., 2014).

An interesting component of the work by Chipchase and colleagues was the use of a portable video conferencing device, called the E-HAB. This device "includes a laptop with software, camera and echo-cancelling microphone in a lockable case …. The system uses a wireless mobile phone connection (3G) and can be battery powered for two-three hours" (Chiphase et al., 2014, p. 43). The portable system was innovative at the time because it allowed for remote camera control, video- or audiotaping of student interactions for future feedback, instant real-time feedback, and the sharing of educational resources or video clips. These functions all enhanced the educational capacity of the educators, including allowing for FWeds to work with students in underserved, understaffed, or role-emerging settings, provided FWeds and fieldwork coordinators completed targeted training in advance (Chipchase et al., 2014; Peel et al., 2011).

Today, students don't need to be provided with a suitcase-sized portable videoconferencing device, because the smartphone in their pocket may be able to record crystal-clear sound and 8K video, sharing the content on 5G broadband networks. One study examined the experience of a multidisciplinary group of students using their own personal devices for telesupervision. Nagarajan et al. (2015) worked with a group of physical therapy, speech-language pathology, and occupational therapy students from Australian and Canadian universities to analyze their experience using smartphones and computers for telesupervision in role-emerging or community-based practice settings. While technology challenges and limited confidence in using technologies caused some barriers to participation, prior training and a willingness by FWeds to use the technology helped reduce the impact of these barriers (Nagarajan et al., 2015). Students reported the primary benefits as readily available support and expertise, while FWeds reported enhanced student learning outcomes, supplemental support for students having difficulties, and greater opportunity to provide feedback for professional development for the students as most beneficial (Nagarajan et al., 2015).

The dramatic advances in technology over the last 10 years have made the full range of benefits of telesupervision accessible to a wide variety of students, FWeds, fieldwork coordinators, and fieldwork sites. Ideally, this technology will continue to enhance the quality of collaboration between FWeds and students, open a greater variety of sites in underserved areas and practices for fieldwork, and ultimately, lead to more practice opportunities for students in a greater variety of settings, increasing the impact and growth of the profession in the near future.

In 2020, the COVID pandemic caused many FWeds and students to utilize this technology as a matter of necessity. Instead of abandoning their fieldwork experiences, some practitioners and students adapted and thrived. One example is the intraprofessional pair of FWeds, Ryan Thomure, OTD, LCSW, OTR/L and Ray Cendejas, COTA/L, who collaborated on a community-based telehealth Level II experience for student Danielle Roe at AMITA Health Housing and Health Alliance in Illinois in the summer of 2020. Thomure et al. (2021) say:

> If you had told me in the Spring of 2019 that I would have the ability to support a Level II fieldwork student who spent all 12 weeks of her internship 2000 miles away, I'd have laughed you out of the room. As we all know by now though, there are a lot of things that we never would have imagined wanting to or being able to do even 1 year ago that have now become part of our everyday routine. (p. 17)

Ryan, Ray, and Danielle collaborated throughout the 12-week experience using a telesupervision approach. The FWeds had advice for succeeding in the virtual context for fieldwork:

> One of the primary suggestions that I would share with others who are preparing to supervise a student virtually is to be as available and present as possible. I've always felt that moments outside of groups or individual sessions have helped me to better understand a student, build rapport, and learn how I can be of the most support. Without being able to have those moments, I wanted to make sure that ample time was available to not only discuss and plan for interventions, but to "just talk" sometimes. Fieldwork experiences lay the foundation for who we become as practitioners, so being ready to help our student through the ups and downs of this process was important to me. (Thomure et al., 2021, p. 17)

Danielle, the fieldwork student, also had advice on success with the new, unfamiliar format:

> Organization is always important, but when you are not physically on-site with clinical supervisors by your side to remind you of schedules, meetings, etc., it becomes even more crucial to stay organized! A planner, watch, and daily checklists quickly became my best friend. Also, ensuring that you and your supervisors have frequent, daily communication can reduce stress and enhance cohesion. (Thomure et al., 2021, p. 18)

Ryan, Ray, and Danielle found themselves in a challenging situation, but, like all good occupational therapy practitioners, adaptation was a key to their success. They embraced the new technology and by doing so, not only ensured successful completion of a fieldwork placement, but also ensured their clients received the high-quality services they deserved and demonstrated the unique value and contributions of our profession.

The expansion of telesupervision in Level II fieldwork might not only address the historical fieldwork shortage dilemma or limitations to certain practice settings due to geographics, but also enhance student learning and satisfaction and the essential collaboration between the FWed and fieldwork student. Are you up to trialing serving as a FWed in a telesupervision model?

Learning to Think Like an Educator

Julie A. Bednarski, OTD, MHS, OTR

"When you learn, teach. When you get, give."
—Maya Angelou

This Maya Angelou quote emulates the professional responsibility of occupational therapy practitioners to essentially pay it forward and share their knowledge and skills with others. As clinicians, occupational therapy practitioners use their knowledge and skill among persons, groups, and populations to influence engagement in occupation, health, and well-being. Likewise, this information-sharing process is enacted while assuming the role of fieldwork educator (FWed) and done so to intentionally influence the future of the profession. Supervision of others and education are within the scope of an occupational therapy practitioner's toolkit and should be part of their philosophy and professional responsibility. According to the American Occupational Therapy Association (AOTA), "supervision is based on mutual understanding between the supervisor and the supervisee about each other's education, experience, credentials, and competence" (2020a, p. 1). This process, or relationship, if executed properly in a practice setting, should consist of "education and support, foster[ing] growth and development, promot[ing] effective utilization of resources, and encourag[ing] creativity and innovation" (AOTA, 2020a, p. 1).

REFLECTION QUESTION

What do the educational theoretical underpinnings that guide this collaborative process and relationship between a FWed (teacher) and the fieldwork student (learner) look like?

DeIuliis, E. D., & Hanson, D. (Eds.).
Fieldwork Educator's Guide to Level II Fieldwork (pp. 85-109).
© 2023 Taylor & Francis Group.

As part of the Accreditation Council for Occupational Therapy Education (ACOTE) *Standards and Interpretive Guidelines* (2018), Standard B.6.6. requires that occupational therapy and occupational therapy assistant programs prepare students with the skills to work in an academic setting. The content of this standard should include education on instructional design as well as the essential skills to best facilitate the teaching/learning process. This standard specifically emphasizes preparation for an academic setting, yet how is the FWed role introduced and developed in the classroom? Previously, ACOTE (2011) required occupational therapy programs to teach ongoing professional responsibility for providing fieldwork education and supervision; however, this requirement in occupational therapy education is no longer indicated. Some FWeds might only have their own unique fieldwork experience as a student to draw from in regard to how to perform in the role of FWed. As part of their academic preparation, many occupational therapy practitioners are fully equipped to serve as a novice FWed and to provide general supervision to students on fieldwork. However, just like clinical practice skills are strengthened with continuing education and professional development, being an effective FWed requires a commitment from the practitioner to also develop their teaching and learning skills further.

The purpose of this book and reading of this chapter indicates that you, the FWed, are seeking ways to improve your effectiveness as a FWed and have a commitment to developing your skills in this role. This chapter will allow you to begin to answer the following questions:

- How do I begin the process of becoming an effective FWed?
- How do I optimize my student's learning and performance and how do I make adjustments to fit the student?
- How do I gather information about the learning preferences of my fieldwork student?
- What is my philosophy of teaching that informs how I provide supervision and education to my fieldwork students?

Just as we go into our clinical practice toolbox to grade and modify our intervention approaches based upon the needs of our clients and with an aim of creating a just-right challenge, these same beliefs also hold true for fieldwork education. But, how do we expand this concept of the FWed as an educator or instructional designer? More so, what steps should be taken to develop knowledge and use best practice teaching and learning approaches to foster a healthy, transparent, and transformative relationship with the fieldwork student?

While this process is intuitive to some, new and seasoned FWeds may benefit from gaining a deeper understanding of the intricacies associated with the teaching/learning process, as well as the theoretical underpinnings that can serve to guide the unique relationship between a FWed and the Level II fieldwork student. The purpose of this chapter is to help you, as a FWed, to think like an educator and dive deeper into this realm of understanding theory behind adult learning and specific teaching and learning styles. Strengthening your understanding of teaching and learning principles and components of adult learning theory will in turn strengthen your effectiveness as a FWed.

LEARNING OBJECTIVES

By the end of reading this chapter and completing the learning activities, the reader should be able to:

1. Appreciate the occupational therapy practitioner's role as a FWed.
2. Recognize how the philosophy of occupational therapy aligns with best practices in the field of education and teaching and learning.

3. Compare and contrast diverse learning theories that can be used to support and optimize a Level II fieldwork student's performance and growth.

4. Identify actions steps and resources that will enhance an occupational therapy practitioner's ability to use best practice teaching and learning principles as a Level II FWed.

UNDERSTANDING THE OCCUPATIONAL THERAPIST AS AN EDUCATOR

REFLECTION QUESTION
How should I begin the process of becoming an effective FWed?

Although not every occupational therapy practitioner becomes attracted to the occupational therapy profession with the desire of becoming a teacher, as practitioners we use elements of teaching and learning theory in clinical practice on a routine basis across the lifespan and across practice settings. We may teach our clients how to perform their activities of daily living in an adaptive way to conserve energy or maintain ergonomic principles. We may educate family members or caregivers on how to support safe swallowing during bottle feeding with a premature infant. We train occupational therapy aides or volunteers how to perform rote tasks in various practice settings to support the flow of service delivery. Despite this, practitioners may not consider themselves fully as educators, nor have been exposed to best practices in adult learning theory and teaching and learning principles.

Much of what is done in the role of the FWed aligns with what you do as a clinician with a client. Think of your fieldwork student as a client. With a client, you provide client-centered interventions that you can grade up/down based on a just-right challenge to ensure the client's occupational engagement goals are attained. As a FWed, working with an occupational therapy fieldwork student, you will be doing the same. Oftentimes you grade your support and supervision up or down based on your student's level of competency, and you work with the student with the end goal that they will achieve entry-level competency in your practice setting. In both relationships, the therapeutic use of self, a cornerstone of occupational therapy practice (AOTA, 2020b), becomes important to build the trust within the relationship while engaging in occupations or learning. Table 3-1 further illustrates a comparison between the skills of the occupational therapy practitioner and the FWed, which may assist you in your thinking as we move forward in this chapter.

As shown in Table 3-1, occupational therapy practitioners utilize theories or models of practice to guide their practice. The *Occupational Therapy Practice Framework: Domain and Process, Fourth Edition (OTPF-4)* is a fundamental paradigm that guides occupational therapy practice (AOTA, 2020b; Cole & Tufano, 2008). Occupation-based models that explain the interaction between the person, environment, and occupational performance are overarching theories. Some examples include Person-Environment-Occupational Performance Model, Model of Human Occupation, and the Ecology of Human Performance. Frames of references assist practitioners in applying theory to clients, explaining how theory works in practice (Cole & Tufano, 2008), such as the Biomechanical Frame of Reference or Neurodevelopmental Treatment Approach. Each individual occupational therapy practitioner determines the optimal theory and frame of reference to serve as the lens in guiding evaluation sessions, planning and implementing interventions, and determining outcomes for clients in their practice setting. These choices are based on the theory's assumptions, generalizations, and hypotheses and how the practitioner determines best application to the client. You can probably remember your occupational therapy studies and think about

TABLE 3-1
OCCUPATIONAL THERAPY CLINICAL PRACTICE SKILLS COMPARED TO FIELDWORK EDUCATOR SKILLS

OCCUPATIONAL THERAPY CLINICAL PRACTICE SKILLS	EXAMPLES AS A FIELDWORK EDUCATOR
Ability to grade tasks or activities to influence client performance and provide the just-right challenge.	Grade up or down student activities to challenge and/or support student learning at the level of student need.
Consideration of the impact from environment and context on the client and their performance.	Setting matters! Pace and engagement will depend on student skill set, client needs, and general expectations of the setting.
Client-centered approach.	Student-centered approach.
Occupation is "doing."	Learning occurs through "doing/experiencing."
Therapeutic use of self is a cornerstone (AOTA, 2020b) of occupational therapy practice.	Therapeutic use of self can facilitate a stronger bond between FWed and fieldwork student.
Goal setting to reflect the client's attainment of treatment goals that reflect engagement in occupation.	Goal setting to reflect the student's ability to achieve entry-level competency.
Clinicians are guided by occupational therapy theories, models of practices, and frames of reference.	Educators are guided by learning theories.

Data sources: AOTA, 2020b; Deluliis, 2017.

a foundational theory course where you were required to intentionally apply theories, occupation-based models, and frames of reference to clinical scenarios or case studies. As you delved further into your occupational therapy education, application of theory became a thread throughout your curriculum. At this point in your career, you may be integrating theories at an expert level and no longer consciously think about specifics that are guiding you, or you may still feel you are at a novice level and are consciously making determinations for theory application when choosing assessments and initiating interventions. Take a moment to reflect:

- Think about a client (define your client). Is your client a person diagnosed with a spinal cord injury (SCI), a community organization, or maybe a population?
- How will you evaluate your client? Will you utilize an occupational profile for an individual, a group, or population? What assessment tool will you utilize? What outcome measure did you utilize? Think about why you made that choice.
- What will guide your intervention sessions?
- How will you determine discharge and how will you assess outcomes?
- As you were thinking about these prompts, can you determine a theory that guided you throughout or were multiple theories guiding you?

It is interesting to move through a reflective exercise such as this to bring to the forefront what is guiding your practice as a clinician. It is the same process you might use when thinking about yourself as a FWed. Educators provide instruction to students and occupational therapy practitioners inherently incorporate instruction to clients via the occupational therapy process (AOTA, 2020b); FWeds provide this same instruction to students to facilitate the development and achievement of entry-level practice skills. Occupational therapy practitioners are inherently teachers and learners, making fieldwork education a natural role for an occupational therapy practitioner. To facilitate the process of serving as a FWed, the application of teaching/learning and higher education theories can support the process. Let us delve into some of the educational learning theories so that you can begin applying these theories to enhance your role as a FWed.

TEACHING AND LEARNING THEORIES

> **REFLECTION QUESTION**
>
> What frameworks do I consciously use to optimize my fieldwork student's learning and how do I, as the educator, make adjustments to fit the needs of my student?

In trying to answer this reflection question, you need to take a closer look at educational learning theories and relate them to yourself as an educator of a fieldwork student. You have a theory that guides you in your occupational therapy practice and you have a solid base for understanding for that theory. You may adjust your models and theories based on client needs and this requires an understanding of each. This is the same for educational learning theories. As you begin to think about yourself as an educator, first it may be helpful to understand learning theories and then determine what theory will best guide you as you further develop your FWed skills. Educational learning theories were first developed to understand children and how children learn, and have evolved into theories about how adults learn. It will be most helpful to discuss first the meaning of **pedagogy** vs. **andragogy** and then move on to discuss the evolution of educational learning theories and application to fieldwork education.

Pedagogy

Pedagogy can be defined as the art and science of teaching children (Knowles et al., 2020). Pedagogy evolved between the 7th and 12th centuries in the education of young boys. In the 19th century, the pedagogical model was utilized in U.S. K-12 school setting. Until fairly recently, this was the only model of education (Knowles et al., 2020). In the pedagogical model of education, the teacher takes full responsibility for all that will be learned by students. The assumptions of this model include (Knowles et al., 2020):

- Teachers have full responsibility.
- Learners need to know what the teacher teaches.
- Learners' self-concept is dependent.
- Learners' experience is not relevant.
- Learners are ready to learn what the teacher knows.
- Learners learn by subject.
- Learners' motivation is extrinsic.

If you align with these pedagogical assumptions, as a FWed:

- You are the expert and take responsibility to make sure your student is competent in each area.
- Your student learns from you and needs to know what your site needs them to know.
- You believe your student is dependent on you at the start of the fieldwork and slowly the student will become self-directed.
- Discussions of the student's prior experience are of little value—it is important that they learn the site-specific methods.
- You determine when the student is ready to move to the next skill.
- You have your student learn based on a logical sequence of skills and content.
- You believe your student will be motivated to learn because they need to pass the fieldwork experience.

Some of these assumptions may be appropriate to apply to a fieldwork student; however, because an occupational therapy fieldwork student is considered an adult learner and not a child learner, it is important to investigate how adults best learn, which is known as *andragogy*. This, in turn, presents different assumptions for the role of the Level II FWed.

Andragogy

Andragogy is a science that studies the teaching and learning of adults. After the end of World War I, scholars in the United States and Europe began investigating adult learners and their unique learning needs (Knowles et al., 2020). The overall basic assumptions of andragogy include (Knowles et al., 2020):

- Adults need to know why they need to learn what they learn and the educator needs to help the adult become aware of what they need to know.
- Adults' self-concept—taking responsibility for learning, decisions—they need to be seen as someone who is capable of self-direction.
- Adults bring in their own experiences—experiential techniques and greater emphasis of peer-helping activities.
- Adults become ready to learn when they need to know—timing to coincide with developmental tasks.
- Adults' orientation to learning is that they are motivated to learn when learning helps them with a task—connect to real-life situations.
- Adult learners are more motivated by internal factors.

As a FWed for occupational therapy students, you will be working with adult learners. Understanding how to utilize principles of adult learning when engaging with your fieldwork student can have a positive effect on student learning. Here are some ways to engage your fieldwork student using adult learning principles:

- **Take on a facilitator role.** You will let the student discover gaps between what they know and what they still need to know. For example, have the student do a self-assessment of their skills after a completion of an evaluation session in a patient room. This allows the student to think about strengths as well as areas of weakness without you as the FWed giving the feedback. You will discuss this assessment with the student to facilitate a discussion of what the student will continue to need to work on, but the student is taking the lead. This is a great way for students to take in feedback, and it reduces those defensive statements that students may make when they are given direct feedback from the FWed prior to be given the option and time to self-reflect.

- **Provide experiences that enable the student to move from dependency to self-direction.** For example, after the student has proven competency on a skill, such as the ability to complete a self-care session focused on incorporation of hip precaution techniques, focus your supervision on questions promoting self-reflection after the completion of the session and provide less guidance during the session.

- **Value their past experiences and who they are as a person.** You are not trying to make them into a "mini you," and you know that they bring in their prior life experiences and these are important to their learning. Ask the student about their prior experiences when they begin their experience with you and take time to understand your student as a person just as you get to know your client as a person.

- **Understand the developmental cycle of the 8- (occupational therapy assistant) or 12- (occupational therapist) week Level II fieldwork experience and provide them with learning experiences appropriate to their developmental level.** For instance, you do not assume that by the end of week 1 they can independently complete an evaluation for a client who sustained a high-level SCI.

- **Believe the student is motivated to learn.** Taking time to discuss and collaborate on goals the student has for learning during their time in fieldwork will facilitate the motivation to learn. The student has come to the fieldwork experience wanting to apply what they learned in the classroom to real-life contexts. For example, a student learned in the classroom how to identify and fabricate an orthosis for a client with a specific diagnosis so now the student is motivated to apply this learning to a client in an outpatient fieldwork setting.

- **Believe the student is motivated by intrinsic factors.** Understand the student's internal motivators through discussions. Asking the student why they chose this site for one of their fieldwork experiences, goals for the experience, and what opportunities and experiences they hope to have during their time with you will assist in your understanding the student's intrinsic motivators.

As a FWed, reflect on these foundational principles of pedagogy and andragogy. Because you are working with students who are adult learners, hopefully you feel better aligned with the andragogy principles. Take a moment to reflect on how you can begin to integrate principles of adult learning into your role as a FWed by answering and reflecting on the questions in Table 3-2.

You should now understand the foundational adult learning principles to apply to your students in order to promote a better fieldwork learning environment. Now let us delve into educational learning theories and the application to the practice of fieldwork education. In the following sections, we will examine some well-known educational learning theories and how you can apply them to your role as a FWed.

Behavioral Learning Theory

In the 1920s, John B. Watson developed the behaviorism approach to learning. "Behaviorists believe that human behavior is the result of the arrangement of particular stimuli in the environment" (Merriam & Bierema, 2014, p. 26). The basic assumption is if a behavior is reinforced it will continue and if it is not reinforced it will likely disappear. Behaviorists believe that learning occurs when a response happens based on an environmental stimulus. The key elements are the stimulus and response (Ertmer & Newby, 2013). An example of the use of a behavioral learning theory may be the use of behavioral learning objectives, mastery of steps—learn a skill, move on to the next skill, use a competency check off. The focus of learning within this model is on the individual learner's experience. The use of a letter grade system is an example in which the summative points are attached to student performance and are used as a positive or negative reinforcement (Mukhalalati & Taylor, 2019). As a FWed, you will be utilizing a summative assessment of

TABLE 3-2
FACILITATING ADULT LEARNING PRINCIPLES

QUESTIONS TO ASK YOURSELF	FOLLOW PRINCIPLES OF ANDRAGOGY BY ...
How do I describe my role as a FWed?	Being a facilitator. Allow students to take the lead in their own learning.
How do I facilitate self-direction in my student?	Allowing your students to develop goals for their learning. Be open to the student when they ask for resources and experiences to gain knowledge in specific areas and/or have opportunities within other departments or with other practitioners.
How can I better understand my students' past experiences?	As part of orientation phase, asking questions about experiences and try to understand their reasoning for choosing the fieldwork site, population, or practice setting.
How am I providing experiences that meet the developmental level of my student?	Making sure you are not providing too much or not enough oversight. Be responsive to the student's level of understanding and try to match to the supervision you are providing.
How am I facilitating the transition of learning from the classroom to the clinic?	Asking what the student learned in the classroom and what they are excited about now applying to clients.
What are the internal learning motivations for my student?	Asking the student what motivates them and how they are become and stay motivated.

student learning that allows you to give a score to indicate how the student was able to achieve certain behavioral objectives and pass the overall experience. Utilization of the AOTA Fieldwork Performance Evaluation (FWPE) to evaluate the fieldwork student is a behavioral approach to grading the student on their fieldwork experience. It is a summative performance evaluation and has a rating scale of 1 (unsatisfactory) through 4 (exemplary) and requires a score of 111 to pass the fieldwork experience (AOTA, 2020c). Use of a summative assessment of the student is an example of being guided by behavioral learning theory.

As a FWed using the behavioral learning theory, you will want to find out what motivates your student and how you may be able to provide reinforcement to achieve learning. A learning contract that is oftentimes developed between a FWed, the academic fieldwork coordinator (AFWC), and the student when there is a problem behavior that arises is an example of using a behavioral learning strategy to help guide student performance. Further guidance on how to create a learning contract will be discussed in Chapter 10. More on best practice approaches to evaluate student learning and performance on Level II fieldwork will be covered in Chapter 12 of this book. See Vignette 1 for an illustration of this teaching and learning theory in action.

VIGNETTE 1: BEHAVIORAL APPROACH

Prior to the start of fieldwork, the student was given information on where to park and to arrive at 7:00 a.m. each day. On the first day, the student arrived 15 minutes late. The student apologized and stated there was more traffic than expected and locating a place to park took time. The FWed, knowing it was only the first day, said "It's ok, it is just the first day and things are still new to you, just make sure tomorrow you are here by 7:00, now let's get started …". During the first 2 weeks, the student was late four more times, sometimes just by 5 minutes. This was a behavior not acceptable at the site and is deemed unprofessional. A meeting was set with the student at the end of week 2 to discuss these behaviors. The student apologized again and said that she just had a difficult time getting up so early and she had a 45-minute drive, but she promised to do better. The FWed decided to take a behavioral approach in trying to find a solution for this problem, so a learning contract was established. Together, the student and FWed worked on developing goals and identifying action steps to achieve the desired performance level with time and attendance. The student agreed that being late was an unprofessional behavior and understood it was not acceptable and did want to change her behavior. They agreed upon the following goal:

I will demonstrate professional behavior by arriving on site by 6:50 a.m. in order to be ready to start the day by 7:00 a.m. I understand that this behavior needs to occur each day without exception unless there is an emergency at which time I will call my FWed prior to 6:50 a.m.

The FWed asked the student how she could support the student with goal achievement. The student said it was just a matter of organizing the evening to better prepare for the next day. Through continued discussion, the student stated she would take 1 hour each evening to review materials/resources needed for the next day and pack her lunch in order to leave her apartment at 6 a.m. They discussed and documented that if this goal was not met the FWed would call the AFWC at the school to arrange a meeting to develop a new plan. The student understood the behavior of being late is not acceptable and continuing the behavior of being late to fieldwork could result in a failure of the fieldwork. The student signed the contract.

Two weeks later, the student was doing well and had not been late since the contract was established. In this instance, the student required feedback that being late, even 5 minutes, was not acceptable and she was demonstrating unprofessional behaviors. Taking the time to create even a simple contract can assist a student in understanding the expectations and promote positive outcomes.

Humanistic Learning Theory

Humanism was developed through the works of humanistic psychologists, Rogers and Maslow. "Underpinning this perspective is the assumption that human beings have the potential for growth and development and that people are free to make choices and determine their behavior" (Merriam & Bierema, 2014, p. 29). Learning focuses on the whole person, including the mind, body, and spirit. You can see how this correlates to our occupational therapy beliefs in that we place importance on understanding the whole person when providing services to our clients. Occupational therapists gather "information about the client's wants, needs, strengths, contexts, limitations, and occupational risks" (AOTA, 2020b, p. 2). Valuing your student as a whole being and allowing your student to be more self-directed to guide their learning experiences is taking a humanistic approach as a FWed. Utilization of this approach requires communication and conversation to develop plans for the fieldwork experience. Other critical elements of this theory

---

VIGNETTE 2: HUMANISTIC APPROACH

A FWed working in an acute care teaching hospital on the cardiopulmonary unit is meeting with a new student. The FWed takes a humanistic approach and feels it is important to let the student guide their learning during the fieldwork rotation. The FWed asks the student, "What do you want to learn and experience during this Level II fieldwork experience and how can I best assist you in your learning?" The student responds that he wants to take full advantage of all that is offered at this hospital and learn as much as possible. The FWed delves further into what the student means when stating "learning as much as possible." The student states, "the opportunity to observe a surgery would be amazing and also being able to spend time with other occupational therapists on other units." The FWed knows that she will be on vacation for 1 week during the student's experience so they discuss that would be a good week to set a time to observe surgery and plan to work alongside other occupational therapists in different units. The student is excited and says he will assist with the learning plan.

The FWed goes on to ask what skills the student wants to address during the first weeks of the experience. The student reflects on what he learned while in the classroom as related to evaluation and intervention with patients diagnosed with cardiopulmonary disorders and states the need to study metabolic equivalent (MET) levels and application to interventions. The FWed then asks the student to write a learning plan that outlines the goals he has for his learning while at the site. The student thinks this is a good idea and says he will have that developed by the next day.

The FWed would like to know how to best support the student and asks the student directly, "How can I best support your learning while you are with me on your Level II fieldwork"? The student says by just having this conversation there is a feeling of support. The student goes on to state that anxiety has been an issue but is receiving the help needed. The FWed thanks the student for this disclosure and asks the student to voice any problems that may arise. They decide to meet each morning during the first 2 weeks to plan the day together and discuss any issues or questions the student may have.

---

include the importance of an opportunity to work and learn from peers. The collaborative model of supervision and providing a safe environment for learning aligns with the humanistic approach to learning. Oftentimes peer interactions facilitate the learning process and in fieldwork, a collaborative model of supervision, in which one FWed is the supervisor for two to four students, can facilitate a positive student learning environment. The model facilitates students utilizing each other for a resource and often leads to more risk taking and exploration with learning (DeIuliis, 2017). In a collaborative supervision model, the FWed is the facilitator and the students are the self-directed learners. In this environment, the students are increasing their own responsibility for learning and professional development (DeIuliis, 2017). Concepts of self-directed learning, andragogy, and transformational learning are all built from humanistic concepts (Merriam & Bierema, 2014). See Vignette 2 for a situational example using the Humanistic Approach.

Cognitive Learning Theory

Cognitive learning theory places the educational emphasis on promoting mental processing. Vygotsky and Piaget influenced the development of the cognitive learning theory. Vygotsky was influenced by developmental psychology, while Piaget focused on the cognitive development of children (Stevens-Fulbrook, 2021). The **Zone of Proximal Development** and **scaffolding** are Vygotsky's key concepts related to how children learn. The term *Zone of Proximal Development* is considered a zone surrounding a child's current level of understanding (Stevens-Fulbrook, 2021).

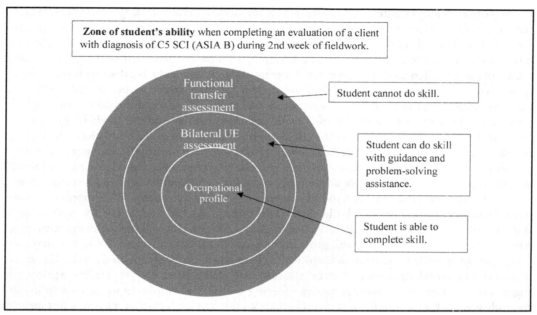

Figure 3-1. Zones of proximal development. (ASIA=American Spinal Cord Injury Association; SCI=spinal cord injury; UE=upper extremity.)

The lower limit surrounding the learner is what the learner can learn through their own efforts; the upper zone is what can be learned when someone, such as a teacher, steps in and without this person stepping in the learner would not learn the information (Stevens-Fulbrook, 2021). This process of learning fosters the cognitive development of a child. Applying this concept to your role as an educator, it is important that you are there to provide education to your student in order for them to grasp the highest levels of content. For example, a student may be able to understand concepts of Neurodevelopmental Treatment techniques, but may not fully grasp implementation with clients and handling techniques unless you guide the student in applying techniques to clients to facilitate engagement in occupation. As you work with the student on the handling techniques, you are facilitating the student moving this skill into a zone of ability. Figure 3-1 depicts a visual of a student's zones of development in relationship to an evaluation of a complex patient.

The student has knowledge of the diagnosis and is now planning to translate this knowledge from the classroom to the clinic. Figure 3-1 demonstrates what the student can do independently and what they can do with the assistance and guidance of the FWed. The student's zone of independent ability is the occupational profile. The student completed several occupational profiles in the first week of the experience and demonstrated competence. The student is able to verbalize how to assess the patient's bilateral upper extremity function; however, they may need some guidance because this is the first time the skill will be performed on a client with a high-level incomplete SCI. Learning will take place by interactions with you as the FWed. When discussing how to proceed with the functional transfer assessment, the student is somewhat nervous because skills were learned in the classroom and practiced only on classmates. The student has not performed a functional transfer with a patient with this type of injury. With this knowledge, you, the FWed, decide the student will first observe you complete a functional transfer with the patient. This is a skill the student feels they cannot perform independently; however, with practice and guidance the student will be able to learn the skill. The goal will be to move both skills, bilateral upper extremity assessment and handling/transfer skills, into the zone of ability for the student. As the FWed, you assist your student in moving skills into their zone of learning through scaffolding.

Scaffolding is a term utilized when you assist your student to learn through incremental experiences. Understanding where the student is as it relates to their zone of knowledge, for example, an evaluation as we just discussed, allows you to scaffold the student's learning and allows the student to retain a skill and then build upon it. The student has probably already experienced scaffolding of learning as it is often used in occupational therapy didactic curricula. Scaffolding is the process by which support is gradually reduced as the student becomes more competent and confident. Once the scaffolding (support) is totally removed, the student has learned the skill. If the student is able to complete the occupational profile section of an evaluation, and this is where their ability and confidence level starts, then have the student complete this area of the evaluation. Then move to skills where the student needs further guidance from you, such as the bilateral upper extremity assessment. The student can initially complete areas they have practiced and been exposed more to, such as passive range of motion, active range of motion, and goniometer measurements; however, they may need guidance for hand placement and correct techniques. With more reflection and elaboration, the student will build these skills quickly. As the student has the opportunity to work with more patients and ask reflective questions, the student will build clinical reasoning skills and the zone of knowledge will grow in the area of evaluation. As the FWed, you may ask a question, such as "Why did you determine the client has 3-/5 strength with shoulder flexion?" or "Based on your bilateral upper extremity assessment what type of adaptive feeding equipment might you use when you assess your patient's feeding ability?" When you get to the zone in which the student is unable to complete a skill, this does not mean the student cannot learn, it just means they have not yet been provided the opportunity to learn. You will want to take time to work with the student on this skill and in the case of the patient diagnosed with a C5 incomplete SCI there will need to be practice of skills and problem solving. Oftentimes it is helpful for the student to be able to watch you and hear your clinical reasoning as to why you are doing what you are doing; your placement of the patient vs. your position during the functional transfer, the preparation of the environment, and the verbal instructions given to the patient. As the student is able to learn from you, they become more confident in their own ability.

Piaget's theory of cognitive development focuses on the teacher guiding the student through their cognitive learning experiences (Stevens-Fulbrook, 2021). Piaget developed stages of cognitive development, which include (1) sensorimotor stage, (2) preoperational stage, (3) concrete operational stage, and (4) operational stage. Children move through these stages of learning and the teacher facilitates moving the children through the stages; however, the students are engaged actively during each stage of the process (Stevens-Fulbrook, 2021). Piaget's cognitive development theory has inspired research on cognitive development of adult learners and has added to the adult learning knowledge base (Merriman & Bierema, 2014). Using Bloom's Taxonomy can assist in scaffolding tasks to promote the cognitive development of the student and assist with developing a scaffolding plan.

Bloom's Taxonomy

Bloom's Taxonomy is often discussed in the education sector as a framework to understanding learning as a hierarchy and to classify different learning thought processes. Bloom developed three domains of learning: cognitive (knowledge), affective (attitudes), and psychomotor skills (Stevens-Fulbrook, 2021). In the occupational therapy classroom, this taxonomy is often used by faculty to build learning objectives and activities within the curriculum. Figure 3-2 depicts the higher- and lower-level thinking skills.

For example, introductory or foundational occupational therapy coursework might focus more on learning and remembering content knowledge (e.g., origin and insertion of muscles during a human anatomy class), followed by a kinesiology course that challenges students to apply previous knowledge of the human body to understand how the human body works and moves, then a higher-level intervention course might occur that requires students to scaffold to more complex

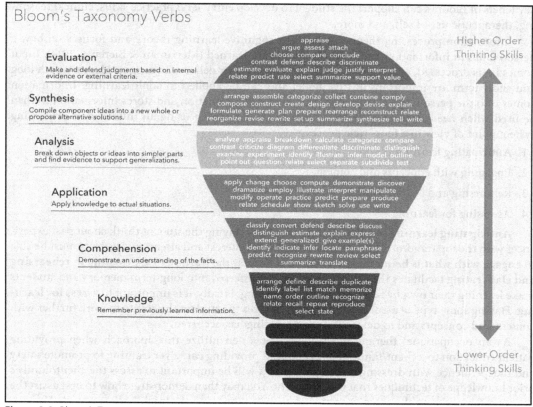

Figure 3-2. Bloom's Taxonomy. ("Bloom's Taxonomy Verbs" from Fractus Learning / used under CC BY-SA 4.0 / desaturated from original.)

skills, such as evaluating and analyzing a client with a musculoskeletal injury and comparing and contrasting intervention techniques to remediate or compensate the known biomechanical impairment. Here is another example of how to use this hierarchical structure using an example of a student working with a client who sustained a right cerebrovascular accident (CVA):

- **Knowledge**: What the student learned in the classroom about a diagnosis of right CVA. They can remember and tell you the definition of a right CVA.

- **Understanding**: The student can explain expected signs and symptoms of a right CVA.

- **Application**: The student will be able to predict how the patient will present because they have knowledge of the definition and understand signs and symptoms.

- **Analysis**: The student is able to process all the information needed to complete a thorough evaluation of the patient and perform the functional transfer safely.

- **Synthesis**: The student can interpret and provide results of the evaluation.

- **Evaluation**: The student is able to then formulate goals and a treatment plan based on the evaluation results.

By using Bloom's Revised Taxonomy (2000) as a guide, the FWed can enable the student to remember, understand, apply, analyze, evaluate, and create to facilitate their own identity as a practitioner. Using the verbs aligned with the different levels of learning according to Bloom's Taxonomy can be helpful to a FWed as they map out site-specific learning objectives, which is a best practice approach you will want to implement. This will be discussed more thoroughly in Chapters 4 and 5. Stepping into the role of educator in a fieldwork setting while implementing the key tenets of Bloom's can support the student to develop entry-level practice skills, clinical reasoning, therapeutic use of self, and more.

Information processing theory stems from cognitive learning theory and focuses on how a person takes in information and retains information learned (Merriman & Bierema, 2014). Input comes in, is processed, and is either stored into memory or delivers an output. Memory both long and short term are important in this model and can be applied to adult learning. Information comes into the person; the person then processes the information and stores information to then be used when needed. Ridgway et al. (2010) describe learning using an information processing system point of view in a four-cycle process:

1. Anticipating learning

2. Engaging with concepts and content

3. Rehearsing and elaborating

4. Assessing for learning

Anticipating learning sets the stage for learning. Having the student think about past experiences with the topic and/or what they know facilitates interest and attention. Students must be able to **engage with what is being taught** in order to process the learning. Participating in **rehearsing and elaborating** facilitates the information to be transferred into long-term memory and students make learning their own by rehearsing and elaborating. Finally, it is important to **assess for learning**. Having some type of assessment for learning gives the student the ability to work further with content and concepts and to determine what learning has occurred.

As an occupational therapy practitioner, you often utilize this approach when providing patient education to a client/family. For example, if providing caregiver training to promote safety and independence with dressing techniques, first it will be important to assess the client/family's prior knowledge of techniques that will be taught. You may then demonstrate how to best assist the patient safely and have the caregiver return demonstration using the teach-back approach. You can assess their performance with the client and provide feedback. To facilitate time for rehearsing and elaborating you may, depending on performance, encourage further training and provide written and picture instructions or short video instructions.

This four-cycle information processing approach can be utilized with your students. For example, a student in their first week of their first Level II fieldwork will be working with a patient recently diagnosed with a right CVA. The student reviews the medical chart and finds the patient is demonstrating left hemiplegia, left visual neglect, and is requiring maximum physical assist with toilet transfers. Upon arrival to the patient's room, the student finds the patient is in bed. In order to implement an occupation-based intervention, the fieldwork student is planning to transfer the patient from the bed to the wheelchair.

1. **Anticipating learning:** Ask the student what type of experience they have had with this type/level of transfer and let the student reflect on the experience and then discuss the process and sequence of what they are planning. This allows the student to think first about how much assist they may require and process the steps of what needs to be done. For example, are there any lines, such as a catheter or oxygen nasal cannula, to be aware of? How will I set up the environment and where will I place the wheelchair for a safe transfer? If you spend the initial time letting the student think through and discuss with you the plan it may be a more successful session.

2. **Engaging with concepts and content:** Give the student the opportunity to take what has been learned in school and apply to practice. The student will complete the toilet transfer with you as the FWed providing direct supervision.

3. **Rehearsing and elaborating:** The student continues to work with the patient, performs bed mobility and functional transfers, and continues to build these skills.

VIGNETTE 3: COGNITIVE LEARNING THEORY

A student is planning a final presentation for the rehabilitation staff at their Level II field-work site. The student has completed a PowerPoint (Microsoft) presentation for a 1-hour presentation and is reviewing with the FWed. The FWed notes that the student has created a presentation based on evidence and it is well organized; however, the student plans to talk through the PowerPoints for the 1-hour session. Understanding principles of adult learning, the FWed facilitates a discussion with the student to reflect on how she educates her clients and their caregivers. The student walks through the process of engaging the client/caregiver by asking familiarity with the task to be taught, the process of actively participating after demonstration, allowing for practice and rehearsal of the skill, and finally having the client and/or caregiver perform again prior to discharge to ensure they have integrated the task in their daily routine. The student then states "Oh, I know why you just asked me that question; I know that I need to apply those same principles to the presentation to engage the audience and promote learning." The student has 1 week to redesign the presentation and the presentation is a success.

---

4. **Assessing for learning:** After the initial session, the student reflects on their performance. Ask the student what went well, and what would they do differently next time, to promote discussion.

Refer to Vignette 3 for an additional illustration of the Cognitive Learning Theory.

Constructivism

Constructivism is about learning. "Rather than behaviors or skills as the goal of instruction, cognitive development and deep understanding are the foci; rather than stages being the result of maturation they are understood as constructions of active learner reorganization" (Fosnot & Perry, 2005, pp. 10-11). Constructivism stems from the field of cognitive science and the works of Piaget and Vygotsky. This theory conceives learning as a mental process as does cognitivism and is considered a branch of cognitivism. Constructivists, however, believe that humans create meaning through their own experiences. Constructivism is a collection of theories, including transitional learning. These theories have a common assumption that people make sense of their learning through their experience and "learning is the construction of meaning from experience" (Merriam & Bierema, 2014, p. 36). Learning occurs by involvement and practice in real-world authentic tasks and contexts, and learners use previous knowledge as a foundation to build or "construct" new knowledge. Fosnot and Perry (2005) suggest a transition to a constructivist approach as learners acquire more knowledge and can deal with more complex problems. As students are faced with more complex clients and situations, they can develop their clinical reasoning. Fosnot and Perry (2005) summarize the overall principles of constructivism as follows:

- Learning is development—allow learners to develop their own questions and test hypothesis
- Disequilibrium facilitates learning—errors discussed and not minimized
- The driving force of learning is allowing time for reflection
- Dialogue within community facilities further thinking

This theory can be applied to educating the fieldwork student. You, as the FWed, can create an environment of collaboration in which you are the facilitator and guide the student through the learning process. You can allow the student to develop their questions for learning. For example, the student can determine an intervention approach with a client based on evidence from the literature. It may not be an approach that you have utilized, but you allow the student to utilize the evidence-based strategy with the client. If there are problems that occur during an interaction with

---

VIGNETTE 4: CONSTRUCTIVISM

A FWed wants to further challenge a student who is demonstrating excellent clinical reasoning and skill development. The student is the only occupational therapy student at the skilled nursing facility, along with a physical therapy student, a speech therapy student, and a nursing student. Over time, the student has demonstrated competency with client evaluations and interventions. There is a client with complex discharge who needs planning to return home to live alone. The student has been working with the client from admission and the client has been at the site for 4 weeks. You challenge your student to take the lead and arrange an interprofessional discharge planning meeting with the other allied health students at the site to develop a safe discharge plan. During the meeting, each student presents their views of the client's discharge needs and plan and give their rationale for the plan with the goal of developing a safe plan for the client to return home. Working together, the students develop a safe discharge plan for the client and within 2 weeks the client returns home. The meeting goes so well the students begin working together each week to review clients and discuss challenges and solutions.

---

a client, this is discussed and learned from. Students learn from experiencing problems or making mistakes, and with discussion and reflection, stronger skills are gained. Critical self-reflection is very important as the student is constructing their skills as an occupational therapist, and this time needs to be built into the fieldwork experience. You can ask the student to journal, you can set aside some time each week to discuss reflections, or you can have the student reflect with other students. The sense of community dialogue is important to learning when utilizing this approach. It is important that the students examine their own beliefs, assumptions, and perspectives related to the learning to build their learning and share with others. See Vignette 4 for a fieldwork scenario aligned with Constructivism. Transformational learning delves further into the ability of the student to engage in learning to transform their perspectives.

Transformative Learning

Transformative adult learning theory has roots in humanism and constructivism. "Transformative learning is a process of making meaning of one's experience" (Merriman & Bierema, 2014, p. 84) and provides a different perspective to other approaches of adult education. "Transformational learning results in new or transformed meaning schemes or, when reflection focuses on premises, transformed meaning perspectives" (Mezirow, 1991, p. 6). An educator assists adult learners to become more critical in assessing their own assumptions and provides discourse so assumptions can foster critical reflection. Mezirow (1991) describes learning to begin with a "disorienting dilemma" that triggers the process of learning to make meaning of one's experience. In transformational learning, reflection is critical. At its core, Mezirow's theory of transformative learning is "a rational, critical, cognitive process that requires thinking, reflection, questioning, and examination of one's assumptions and beliefs" (Merriam & Bierema, 2014, p. 86). An important belief as a FWed is recognizing that you cannot teach your student transformation, but you can foster transformational learning (Santalucia & Johnson, 2010). A student through their learning experience in fieldwork may experience this transformational learning if you as a FWed can provide structured and scheduled experiences that foster critical reflection and examination of their beliefs and assumptions. Refer to Vignette 5 for an illustration of Transformational Learning Theory.

This has just been a brief overview of some influential learning theories. FWeds are encouraged to further research the learning theory that most peaked your interest. You can delve much

---

VIGNETTE 5: TRANSFORMATIONAL LEARNING

A FWed utilizes a collaborative model of supervision. The educator supervises a group of three occupational therapy Level II fieldwork students and each week, added to the normal caseload, a case study is assigned for all students to complete individually. The FWed asks the students to create an intervention plan and provide their clinical reasoning. The fieldwork students meet as a group the next week to discuss each student's rationale for services and plan for this patient. The students have to defend their responses and are encouraged to question each other's clinical reasoning. As the weeks progress, the educator provides more challenging case studies that delve into issues of social injustices and issues of diversity, equity, and inclusion. At the conclusion of the fieldwork, the students stated the case study meetings challenged their thinking and that they learned from each other and transformed the way they will approach their clients in the future.

TABLE 3-3

LEARNING THEORIES: EXAMPLES IN PRACTICE

ORIENTATION TO LEARNING	OVERALL YOU FEEL YOUR ROLE AS A FIELDWORK EDUCATOR IS TO ...	EXAMPLES IN PRACTICE
Behaviorist	Arrange the environment to ensure that the student is producing the desired behavior. Set behavioral goals for student to meet. Ensure that the student learns skills taught through training and competency success.	In an acute hospital setting, you develop a skill-check off or competencies for the student to perform prior to attempting a skill with a patient. Use of the AOTA FWPE for a summative assessment of the student's skills.
Humanist	Provide collaborative and participatory opportunities for learning. Develop the "whole" student, students are different and learn at their own pace and you adjust to that based on the individual student. Facilitate self-actualization and autonomy within the student.	Use role-playing as a way for a student to focus on self-assessment of skills (Mukhalalati & Taylor, 2019). You allow the student to be more self-directed and give more choices to the student. For example, you allow the student to have more input into developing their caseloads and the treatment strategies they feel may be most appropriate for their patients. The student has more power over their pace of learning and their pace to get to the final goal of being competent with an entry-level caseload by the end of the 12 weeks.

(continued)

TABLE 3-3 (CONTINUED)
LEARNING THEORIES: EXAMPLES IN PRACTICE

ORIENTATION TO LEARNING	OVERALL YOU FEEL YOUR ROLE AS A FIELDWORK EDUCATOR IS TO:	EXAMPLES IN PRACTICE
Cognitivist	Facilitate learning of skills through the information processing system. Encourage use of prior knowledge to process new information and skills. Utilize Bloom's six-level cognitive taxonomy when setting goals for student performance.	Have the student develop a learning ePortfolio as a final project. Scaffold your supervision. For example, in an inpatient acute rehabilitation setting when orders are received for an evaluation of a patient diagnosed with a high-level SCI, allow the student to discuss with you their prior experience and knowledge of this diagnosis. Determine together a plan for the evaluation. Provide supervision and support as needed and gradually reduce supervision to allow student to progress with knowledge and engage in the evaluation and intervention.
Constructivist (including transitional learning)	Promote learning by encouraging self-direction so the student can manage their learning. Provide experiential learning to the student to make learning as authentic as possible. Encourage the sharing of student experiences and resources. Assist your student in becoming more self-reflective and able to learn from discourse and critical reflection.	Utilize a collaborative model of supervision (one FWed to two to four students) to facilitate group reflections and sharing of experiences and assumptions. Provide a case example and assign different treatment approaches to the students and have them engage in a critical debate and examination of approaches (Santalucia & Johnson, 2010). Engage students in storytelling when asked to share their own personal experiences (Santalucia & Johnson, 2010). Schedule time for students to share and compare experiences following evaluations and therapy sessions (Santalucia & Johnson, 2010).

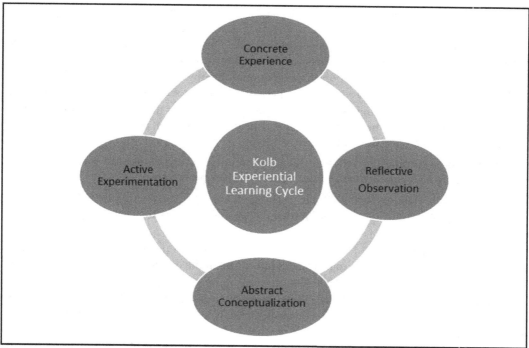

Figure 3-3. Kolb's experiential four-step learning process cycle. (Adapted from Kolb, A. Y., & Kolb, D. A. [2017]. *The experiential educator principles and practices of experiential learning.* EBLS Press.)

deeper into each of the learning theories and focus on those that you feel will benefit you most as a FWed. Refer to Table 3-3 for a summative overview of how educational learning theories can be used in practice.

REFLECTION QUESTION
How do I gather information about the learning preferences of my fieldwork student?

EXPERIENTIAL LEARNING AS A CYCLE AND PROCESS

As noted earlier in this chapter, a key component of adult learning theories is understanding the learner and their motivation, interests, past experiences, and learning preferences. Similar to clinical practice where we implement client-centered approaches and elicit an occupational profile to understand our clients as occupational beings, we can use this same mindset as FWeds to gather information about our fieldwork students. A place to start is to view learning as a process, rather a cycle, which is the basis of Kolb's Experiential Learning Theory. Kolb's experiential learning is a four-step learning process cycle—experience, reflect, think, and act (Kolb & Kolb, 2017). Adult learners continually move through this process.

Learning arises from the resolution of creative tension among these four learning modes. This process is portrayed as an idealized learning cycle or spiral where the learner 'touches all the bases'—experiencing (CE), reflecting (RO), thinking (AC) and acting (AE)—in a recursive process that is sensitive to the learning situation and to what is being learned. (Kolb & Kolb, 2017, p. 32)

Refer to Figure 3-3 for a visual depiction of the cycle. The next paragraph provides an example of how to move your student though this cycle to facilitate learning.

The model of fieldwork education in occupational therapy is very much rooted in the Kolb model of experiential learning. To facilitate experiential learning with your fieldwork student:

- Provide concrete opportunities for the doing at the very start of the experience (if the student is observing on the beginning days of Level II fieldwork with you, have the student transfer a patient rather than just watching you).
- Facilitate opportunities for self-reflection (have student reflect on how an evaluation, treatment session, or other client encounter went from their perspective).
- Engage in conversation to apply their learning and apply concepts that they learned in the classroom (discuss why they are doing what they are doing—why they chose that intervention strategy).
- Apply knowledge to make decisions and solve problems (encourage evidence-based practice and data-driven decision making—what did they find in the literature to support an intervention and how did the overall session go).

As a FWed following an experiential learning model, you will allow your student to engage in concrete experiences—the doing of the treatment, facilitating reflection before and after a session, and engaging in understanding the concepts of what they are doing. Kolb's Experiential Learning Cycle proposes a learner's learning style preference based on four learning phases: accommodator, diverger, converger, and assimilator (Kolb & Kolb, 2017). The Learning Style Inventory (LSI) which takes about 30 to 45 minutes, gives you and the student information on how the student learns but does not evaluate the student's learning ability (Kolb & Kolb, 2017). This will be most beneficial to you as the FWed if you have the student complete the inventory at the beginning of the fieldwork experience. Table 3-4 provides a brief discussion of Kolb's learning style preferences, as well as some strategies of how a Level II FWed can adjust their teaching style to align with the student's learning preferences.

French et al. (2007) found that out of 116 Australian occupational therapy students 30.2% were diverging, 28.4% converging, 22.4% assimilating, and 19% accommodating when tested utilizing the Kolb LSI. D'Amore et al. (2012) found that Australian nursing and midwifery students also demonstrated diverger learning style as the dominant style. Even though these groups of students favor diverging learning it is important for educators to encourage the development of a balanced learning style (D'Amore et al., 2012). As a FWed, you should become aware of your student's learning preference but will work with the student to move through developing other learning styles as based on Table 3-4. If you are interested in other learning inventories, DeIuliis (2017) recommends the following LSIs: the Vark Questionnaire, the National Association of Secondary School Principals Style Profile, the Jackson's Learning Style Profile, or the Grash-Reichmann Learning Style Scale.

REFLECTION QUESTION

Has anyone (a colleague, an AFWC, or fieldwork student) ever asked you for your teaching philosophy as a FWed?

TABLE 3-4
STUDENT LEARNING STYLES

KOLB LEARNING STYLE (KOLB & KOLB, 2017)	LEARNING STYLE PREFERENCE	FIELDWORK STUDENT PREFERENCE
Accommodator: Feel and do—more active	Prefers hands-on experience, using others to assist with problem solving.	As a FWed, you can adjust to this type of learner by providing hands-on experiences. Let the student try out the skill—practice on you first if needed, and then perform on the patient—that is how they will learn best. Having the ability to problem solve with other fieldwork students will be important.
Diverger: Feel and watch—more reflective	Concrete situations through observation and prefers group work, people focused.	May have this student observe you first, provide opportunities for observation. This is the student who will do well in a collaborative model of fieldwork supervision where there is one FWed to two to four students.
Converger: Think and do	Practical problem solving and laboratory experiences are the way they learn best.	This is a practical student—wants to understand the day-to-day problem solving and they use what they learn to solve problems.
Assimilator: Think and watch	Abstract ideas and theories—likes lectures and exploring models.	This student will like to apply theory, read up on all the concepts—will request lots of reading materials, will like to go to any type of lecture-based educational opportunities at the hospital. Will like to explore and discuss their ideas with you and will want to get your thoughts and ideas.

DEVELOPING YOUR TEACHING PHILOSOPHY AS A FIELDWORK EDUCATOR

The *Philosophy of Occupational Therapy Education* (AOTA, 2007) is an important document to review as you embark on your role as a FWed. Understanding the philosophy of our profession in the area of education can assist in linking these principles to fieldwork education. As a FWed, it is important that you begin to understand how to apply these educational theories to develop your own philosophy of teaching. The assumptions of the philosophy of occupational therapy education (AOTA, 2007) are as follows:

- Promotion of competence through experience to improve the student's practice abilities
- Use of active learning to engage the student
- Build on the student's knowledge and experience—integrate knowledge from the classroom, experiential learning, clinical reasoning, and self-reflection

EXAMPLE OF A TEACHING PHILOSOPHY STATEMENT OF A FACULTY MEMBER

My passion for occupational therapy and my desire to develop caring, ethical, and professional occupational therapists puts the student at the core of my teaching philosophy. As a teacher my philosophy is to:

- Facilitate real life experiences for the students
- Convey my passion for occupational therapy
- Respect the student
- Create a variety of interactive learning experiences

I draw from my many years of experience to bring real life case examples to the classroom and strive to engage students with community clients. Case examples bring to life the lectures, books, and labs, enabling the students to integrate information more easily for future practice. Engaging with clients who are experiencing the disease or disorder facilitates the students' understanding of a person as an occupational being and an understanding of their lived experience.

I believe in respecting the student and keeping learning positive. As an occupational therapist, I help clients bring balance to their lives. I respect that my students are graduate students and are trying to balance school, work, and family which can be very stressful, and I try to help students understand the need for balance in their lives. My belief is that if the student learns in a positive environment this will assist them in developing their passion for occupational therapy and life-long learning.

I believe interactive experiences and active learning opportunities are very important to the students' integration of lecture material and I use a variety of student engagement techniques to enhance classroom learning. Analyzing case studies, breakout group discussions, and role playing are all part of my everyday teaching. I use technology as appropriate within lectures to further engage students.

I bring challenges to the classroom that integrate a variety of senses to allow the students to develop positive learning experiences based on their learning styles. In each class I teach, I ensure students are provided with a variety of learning measures including experiential learning activities, quizzes/exams, papers, presentations, self-reflection, and group projects to allow for individual student learning styles. I utilize a student-directed learning approach to empower the student to take the lead in their learning process. I believe teaching in an OTD program requires strong skills as an occupational therapist along with strong skills as a teacher and melding these two is my passion.

REFLECTION QUESTION

Do you have an internal belief system, core values, or a philosophy that informs how you provide supervision and education to your fieldwork students?

Trying to now link educational theories and the philosophy of occupational therapy education will assist you in developing a philosophy for how you would like to provide education to your fieldwork students. This is what is referred to as a *teaching philosophy*, a reflective statement that communicates beliefs and expectations of the teaching-learning process and classroom environment. Most times, if applying for an academic faculty position, you are expected to provide a statement of teaching philosophy (Montell, 2003).

Box 3-2

EXAMPLE OF A FIELDWORK EDUCATOR'S TEACHING PHILOSOPHY

As a FWed, I feel my role is that of a facilitator. I understand that my students are adult learners and come to me with a variety of experiences that will be different from my own. I listen to my students and try to understand their stories. I feel their stories influence who they are as students and how they approach their fieldwork.

As a FWed, I try to create a positive environment for learning and use positive reinforcement as I believe this is the way learning occurs. I come from a positive mindset and always strive to be fair and kind in the feedback I give to my students. The feedback I give promotes improvement and I always provide time for student response and reflection after feedback. Initially I work with students taking a more active role in supervision, but as students are demonstrating learning I always encourage self-direction with learning.

As a FWed, I work with students to provide a variety of learning experiences based on their needs. I encourage self-reflection after clinical experiences to promote learning and allow the student to develop their clinical reasoning skills. I believe being a FWed is a responsibility of being an occupational therapy practitioner and a way to give back.

You **do not need** a teaching philosophy to be a FWed, but it might be a good way for you to synthesize the information in this chapter and further realize your identity as an educator. You may find yourself gravitating toward one singular learning theory approach and integrate this into your philosophy or you may feel drawn to pull principles from several theories. Just like clinical practice, you might develop an eclectic approach to serving as a FWed. What is important is to think about what will ground you in best practice approaches as an educator. Refer to Box 3-1 for an example of a teaching philosophy of an occupational therapy professor. As you read through the example you can probably note components of experiential learning and humanism even though it is not explicitly stated by this educator.

After reading this chapter, you may now have a better idea of what type of FWed you would like to be. Here are some questions you can ask yourself as you begin to develop and articulate your FWed philosophy:

- What is my purpose for becoming a FWed?

- Why do I choose to be a FWed?

- How do I want to share my knowledge with students?

- What values guide me as I work with students?

- What does my student gain from the relationship, and what do I gain from the relationship?

- Is there an educational learning theory that resonates with me, and if so, how does it affect my teaching?

Reread these prompts. What responses do you have? Now, put these responses or ideas down on paper. Just begin writing, as there are no wrong answers when it comes to creating your philosophy of teaching as it relates to your role as a FWed. To start, keep your statement short, you can build upon it as you feel more comfortable in putting your philosophy into words. To get you started, Box 3-2 gives an example of a FWed's teaching philosophy.

After you draft and rework your teaching philosophy statement as a FWed, the most important part is to not keep it to yourself. Share your teaching philosophy! It does not do much good being kept in a file; it is meant to be shared. Share your philosophy with your student during the orientation process. It will provide the student a sense of who you are as an educator and what to expect from you. It can also lead to further discussions about how the student learns and how they best receive feedback. You might also want to share your philosophy statement with AFWCs who might appreciate learning more about your beliefs and core values as a FWed to ensure a more congruent fit with fieldwork students from their program. As you deepen your skillset as a FWed and become more experienced in this role, know that your teaching philosophy will most likely change over time. Iterations are expected and encouraged as you grow as a clinician and as a FWed.

SUMMARY

Returning to the Maya Angelou quote, "*When you learn, teach. When you get, give,*" it becomes important to understand how to best teach your student so they can, in turn, learn to give the best quality of care to clients. Applying best practices of adult learning is of vital importance for the FWed in order to set the stage for student success, establish a trusting rapport, support learning needs, create straightforward site-specific learning objectives, and develop a realistic learning plan. These best practices will be built upon in upcoming chapters. The teaching/learning concepts discussed in this chapter are the essence of responding in a systematic manner to challenging fieldwork scenarios with an underperforming student or to challenge an exemplary student.

LEARNING ACTIVITIES

1. Refer to Table 3-2 and think about what approach are you utilizing and what approaches you may want to utilize to facilitate learning within your student(s).

2. How can you facilitate learning within your student to provide transformational learning? What are some learning prompts you can ask your student?

3. Develop your own philosophy statement that will direct you in your role as a FWed.

4. After reflecting on this chapter, answer the following:

   a. The biggest take away for me is …

   b. I plan to integrate the following concepts when working with my next fieldwork student …

5. Explore continuing education opportunities and create a professional development plan to improve your skills as a FWed. For example, you may want to develop a proposal for your manager/director to support your attendance at the AOTA Fieldwork Educator Certificate Workshop. This is an excellent course and will assist your continued development as a FWed. Another professional development platform is the AOTA Education Summit, which is an annual occupational therapy conference, geared toward educators, FWeds, and the scholarship of teaching and learning in occupational therapy. Create two specific, measurable, attainable, realistic, and timely professional development goals focused on enhancing your own understanding of teaching and learning practices.

REFERENCES

Accreditation Council for Occupational Therapy Education. (2011). Standards and interpretative guide [PDF]. https://www.aota.org/-/media/Corporate/Files/EducationCareers/Accredit/Standards/2011-Standards-and-Interpretive-Guide.pdf

Accreditation Council for Occupational Therapy Education. (2018). Standards and interpretative guide [PDF]. https://acoteonline.org/accreditation-explained/standards/

American Occupational Therapy Association. (2007). Philosophy of occupational therapy education. *American Journal of Occupational Therapy, 61*(6), 678. https://doi.org/10.5014/ajot.61.6.678

American Occupational Therapy Association. (2020a). Guidelines for supervision, roles, and responsibilities during the delivery of occupational therapy services. *American Journal of Occupational Therapy, 74*(Suppl. 3), 1-6. https://doi.org/10.5014/ajot.2020.74S3004

American Occupational Therapy Association. (2020b). Occupational therapy practice framework: Domain and process (4th ed.). *American Journal of Occupational Therapy, 74*(Suppl. 2), 1-87. https://doi.org/10.5014/ajot.2020.74.2001

American Occupational Therapy Association. (2020c). Fieldwork Performance Evaluation (FWPE) Rating Scoring Guide (Revised in 2020) [PDF]. https://www.aota.org/-/media/Corporate/Files/EducationCareers/Fieldwork/Fieldwork-Performance-Evaluation-Rating-Scoring-Guide.pdf

Cole, M. B., & Tufano, R. (2008). Organization of theory in occupational therapy. In M. B. Cole, & R. Tufano, *Applied theories in occupational therapy a practical approach* (pp. 55-70). SLACK Incorporated.

D'Amore, A., James, S., & Mitchell, E. K. L. (2012). Learning styles of first-year undergraduate nursing and midwifery students: A cross-sectional survey utilizing the Kolb Learning Style Inventory. *Nurse Education Today, 32*, 506-515. https://doi.org/10.1016/j.nedt.2011.08.001

DeIuliis, E. D. (2017). *Professionalism across occupational therapy practice.* SLACK Incorporated.

Ertmer, P. A., & Newby, T. J. (2013). Behaviorism, cognitivism, constructivism: Comparing critical features from an instructional design perspective. *Performance Improvement Quarterly, 26*(2), 43-71. https://doi.org/10.1002/piq.21143

Fosnot, C. T. & Perry, R. S. (2005). Constructivism: A psychological theory of learning. In C. T. Fosenot, (Ed.), *Constructivism: Theory, perspectives, and practice* (2nd ed., pp. 8-35). Teachers College Press.

French, G., Cosgriff, T., & Brown, T. (2007). Learning style preferences of Australian occupational therapy students. *Australian Occupational Therapy Journal, 54*, S58-S65. https://doi.org/10.1111/j.1440-1630.2007.00723.x

Knowles, M. S., Holton III, E. F., Swanson, R. A., & Robinson, P. A. (2020). *The adult learner The definitive classic in adult education and human resource development.* Routledge.

Kolb, A. Y., & Kolb, D. A. (2017). *The experiential educator principles and practices of experiential learning.* EBLS Press.

Merriam, S. B., & Bierema, L. L. (2014). *Adult learning linking theory and practice.* Jossey-Bass.

Mezirow, J. (1991). *Transformative dimensions of adult learning.* Jossey-Bass.

Montell, G. A. (2003, March 27). What's your philosophy on teaching, and does it matter? *The Chronicle of Higher Education.* https://www.chronicle.com/article/whats-your-philosophy-on-teaching-and-does-it-matter

Mukhalalati, B., & Taylor, A. (2019). Adult learning theories in context: A quick guide for healthcare professional educators. *Journal of Medical Education and Curricular Development, 6*, 1-10. https://doi.org/10.1177/2382120519840332

Ridgway, A., Sachs, D., & Stephenson, D. (2010). *14,641 lesson plans a flip-book for designing engaging lessons.* Speaker Fulfillment Services.

Santalucia, S., & Johnson, C. R. (2010). Transformative learning facilitating growth and change through fieldwork. *OT Practice, 15*(19), CE-1-CE-8.

Stevens-Fulbrook, P. (2021). *Vygotsky, Piaget, and Bloom: The definitive guide to their educational theories with examples of how they can be applied.* Teacher of Sci.

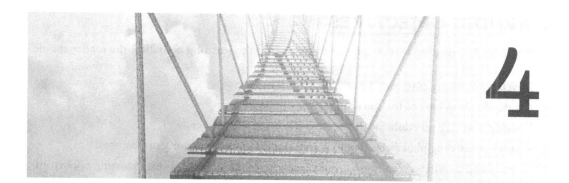

Time to Plan!
Developing a Learning Plan, Site-Specific Objectives, and Schedule for Level II Fieldwork

Rebecca Ozelie, DHS, OTR/L, BCPR

Benjamin Franklin is known for coining the proverb, "If you fail to plan, you are planning to fail." These wise words can be applicable to so many areas of our lives. They are also relevant as we consider fieldwork. Taking the time to establish a plan for an upcoming fieldwork student can facilitate success for both the student and the fieldwork educator (FWed). Time constraints can play a role in the ability of FWeds to provide quality fieldwork supervision (Ryan et al., 2018; Schafer-Clay, 2019). Additionally, FWeds report that they are not adequately trained or prepared to supervise and educate students (Barton et al., 2013; Hanson, 2011; Schafer-Clay, 2019). Lack of preparation can result in inconsistent fieldwork experiences and variability in the development of clinical skills and clinical reasoning among new practitioners (Casares et al., 2003; Haynes, 2011).

To combat these potential inconsistencies and address time constraints, academic fieldwork coordinators (AFWCs) and FWeds should work together to make sure that the necessary resources and tools are in place **prior to** the start of the fieldwork experience. When you decide to begin a fieldwork program at your work setting, it is important to be proactive in developing needed resources and creating a plan for the student and yourself as it will result in a more organized, efficient, and consistent fieldwork experience. This chapter will provide a preparation model for the FWed, including how to create a learning plan, establish site-specific learning objectives (SSLOs), a weekly schedule, and intentional learning opportunities for the experience.

DeIuliis, E. D., & Hanson, D. (Eds.).
Fieldwork Educator's Guide to Level II Fieldwork (pp. 111-136).
© 2023 Taylor & Francis Group.

LEARNING OBJECTIVES

By the end of reading this chapter and completing the learning activities, the reader should be able to:

1. Develop a learning plan for a Level II fieldwork experience.
2. Create SSLOs as part of the learning plan.
3. Develop a weekly schedule for the Level II fieldwork experience.
4. Adapt the learning plan as needed to accommodate student learning preferences.
5. Identify and develop a plan to use available site resources for intentional learning opportunities.
6. Take advantage of unplanned teachable moments.

DEVELOPING THE LEARNING PLAN

This first section of the chapter will outline a process for FWeds to develop a learning plan, which begins with developing SSLOs that will guide all student fieldwork experiences. Next, the FWed should obtain and understand the student's learning preferences. From here, FWeds can deepen their understanding of the student by obtaining their occupational profile, which will help rapport building and ensure future learning experiences are student-centered. Understanding the learning preferences and context of the student will help the FWed design the best possible learning plan so that both the student and the FWed are ultimately successful.

Creating Site-Specific Learning Objectives

The Accreditation Council for Occupational Therapy Education (ACOTE) requires that AFWCs and site FWeds agree on established fieldwork objectives **prior to** the start of the fieldwork experience (ACOTE, 2018). These objectives are often termed site-specific learning objectives or SSLOs. SSLOs are used to measure student performance and entry-level competence in a particular practice setting. The purpose of writing SSLOs is to identify entry-level competencies unique to a specific practice setting. ACOTE (2018) defines "entry-level competency" as being prepared to begin generalist practice as an occupational therapy practitioner with less than 1-year experience (p. 1). Utilization of SSLOs can help guide intentional learning opportunities, assignments, and supervision throughout the fieldwork experience. Use of SSLOs also can allow FWeds to efficiently monitor and evaluate the student's performance for the midterm evaluation, final evaluation, and throughout the fieldwork experience. It is recommended that FWeds routinely refer to these SSLOs as they evaluate a student's performance. FWeds should reflect on the SSLOs and the student's performance as they prepare for weekly review meetings with the student and as part of the midterm and final evaluation process. See Box 4-1 for an example of the utilization of SSLOs during weekly review meetings and for completion of the midterm and final evaluation.

It is critical to have an active partnership between the clinical site and the academic institution in developing objectives. Schafer-Clay (2019) found that 73% of occupational therapy practitioners who currently do not supervise students would want help from the AFWC in establishing SSLOs. Such a partnership may result in an increased willingness to supervise students as clinicians are provided time-saving supports from the academic program and other benefits such as access to educational resources and the development of employee skills. Additionally, this partnership can result in robust benefits to the academic program as the collaboration with clinical sites can help ensure the curriculum content is up to date and representative of practice sites.

BOX 4-1

EXAMPLE OF THE USE OF SITE-SPECIFIC LEARNING OBJECTIVES DURING STUDENT PERFORMANCE EVALUATION

Asia is at week 4 of her Level II fieldwork and her FWed, Mark, has some concerns with her performance. He is having a hard time clearly communicating to Asia his concerns and reaches out to his coworker for advice. Mark's coworker recommends that he bring the SSLOs to their next weekly review meeting and collaboratively review them and reflect on Asia's progress and opportunities for growth as they related to the SSLOs. At the meeting, Asia and Mark identify two main SSLOs of concern:

1. Complete safe functional transfers and functional mobility activities independently by week 12.
2. Produce daily and weekly documentation that meets site and insurance requirements with minimal revisions.

Asia and Mark collaborate and set measurable goals for the upcoming week to help Asia progress in her ability to ultimately meet these SSLOs.

1. Complete functional transfers with known clients with distant supervision and no instances of unsafe behaviors.
2. Independently identify patients and functional transfers that require additional assistance and independently seek assistance from colleagues.
3. Complete and submit daily documentation by end of day for each patient seen with no more than two revisions needed.
4. Develop organizational system to monitor and track patients that need weekly progress notes and initiate progress notes without verbal cues.

Mark identifies some intentional learning opportunities (e.g., videotape Asia completing a transfer and have her watch it and reflect on her skills and then discuss together) that will challenge Asia to make links between these experiences and the identified SSLOs. Mark also plans to re-evaluate the SSLOs as he completes Asia's upcoming midterm evaluation.

While FWeds and the AFWC must agree on the established fieldwork objectives prior to the start of the fieldwork experience, it is also encouraged that they collaborate on the development of these objectives. If you are beginning to develop SSLOs for your fieldwork program and are unsure where to start, see Figure 4-1. First, collaborate with the AFWC at the occupational therapy program. They likely have samples and resources that will help you get started. The AFWC might have a sample set of SSLOs from a similar practice setting that they can share to help begin your process. They can also share their experience with you to help guide your process. You should also sit down and identify what would be considered entry-level competencies at your site. Understanding what is expected of an entry-level clinician will help guide your expectations and thus your SSLOs of a Level II fieldwork student. Examples of competencies that might be considered entry-level could include:

- Independently adhere to COVID-19 precautions
- Fabricate all wrist and hand orthoses requested by physician
- Complete point-of-care documentation that follows site and insurance requirements
- Develop client-centered and evidence-based treatment plans for all patients
- Confidently report patient status at daily interdisciplinary team meetings, etc.

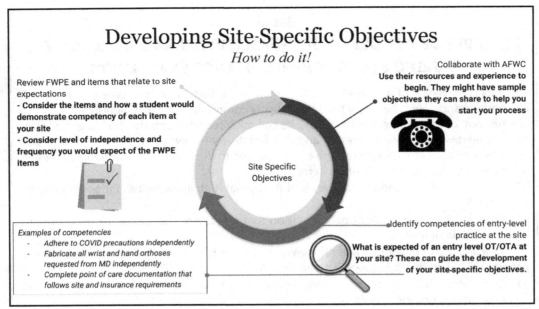

Developing Site-Specific Objectives
How to do it!

Review FWPE and items that relate to site expectations
- Consider the items and how a student would demonstrate competency of each item at your site
- Consider level of independence and frequency you would expect of the FWPE items

Collaborate with AFWC
Use their resources and experience to begin. They might have sample objectives they can share to help you start you process

Site Specific Objectives

Examples of competencies
- *Adhere to COVID precautions independently*
- *Fabricate all wrist and hand orthoses requested from MD independently*
- *Complete point of care documentation that follows site and insurance requirements*

Identify competencies of entry-level practice at the site
What is expected of an entry level OT/OTA at your site? These can guide the development of your site-specific objectives.

Figure 4-1. Developing site-specific objectives.

Note: Be cautious of not confusing entry-level competencies with advanced practice. For example, it is a common pitfall that some sites may identify competence with physical agent modalities or lymphedema to be considered entry level, but often these skills require additional continuing education and should instead be considered advanced practice. Students can certainly have exposure to and expectations of advanced practice skills, but the FWed should consider the expected level of independence and frequency as they develop SSLOs.

Once you have identified expected competencies, you should also review the AOTA Fieldwork Performance Evaluation (FWPE; AOTA, 2020c) subsections and individual items. There are 6 subsections and 37 individual items within the FWPE. The subsections include: Fundamentals of Practice, Basic Tenets, Screening and Evaluation, Intervention, Management of Occupational Therapy Services, and Communication and Professional Behaviors. By choosing specific items or larger subsections from the FWPE, you can then critically think about how that item or subsection is expected to be accomplished at the site, its relation to your expected site competencies, and with what level of independence and frequency the objectives should be completed. For example, if you were to consider the "Management of Occupational Therapy Services" subsection, you might develop an SSLO that is specific to the volume of work expected at your site for students or entry-level clinicians. Utilizing the FWPE subsections and individual items can guide a FWed in the creation of SSLOs. Chapter 12 will go into further detail about evaluation as a key competency of the Level II FWed. See Box 4-2 for sample SSLOs based on items from FWPE.

Wimmer (2004) suggests using the RUMBA framework for writing SSLOs (see Table 4-1). The RUMBA method provides the framework for writing objectives that outline expected levels of independence and frequency. It would be appropriate if the SSLOs have varying levels of independence and frequency based on determined site competencies. Here is an example: An SSLO aligned with AOTA FWPE item number three ("Ensures the safety of self and others during all fieldwork related activities by anticipating potentially unsafe situations and taking steps to prevent accidents" [AOTA, 2020c, p. 1]) at an outpatient hand clinic might be written as *"Student will adhere to all patient precautions and contraindications and fabricate all prescribed wrist and hand*

Box 4-2

USE OF FWPE TO DEVELOP SITE-SPECIFIC LEARNING OBJECTIVES

This diagram specifically uses the four items of the "Management of Occupational Therapy Services" section of the AOTA FWPE (AOTA, 2020c):

25. Demonstrates through practice or discussion the ability to collaborate with and assign appropriate tasks to the occupational therapy assistant, occupational therapy aide, or others to whom responsibilities might be assigned, while remaining responsible for all aspects of treatment.

26. Demonstrates through practice or discussion an understanding of costs and funding systems related to occupational therapy services, such as federal, state, third party, and private payers.

27. Demonstrates knowledge about the organization.

28. Meets productivity standards or volume of work expected of occupational therapy students.

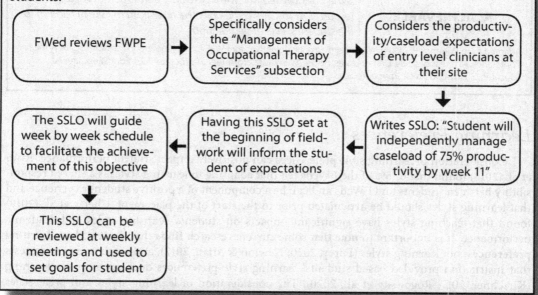

---

orthoses independently by week 10." But the SSLO specific to splinting at an inpatient rehabilitation hospital might be "*Student will adhere to patient precautions and contraindications and fabricate resting hand splints with direct supervision by week 12.*" These differences in frequency and level of independence will be unique to the expectations of the site. Box 4-3 has additional examples across practice settings.

In addition to using the RUMBA method for developing SSLOs, it is recommended that FWeds use official documents endorsed by AOTA to facilitate alignment of SSLOs with the AOTA FWPE items. Table 4-2 provides examples of how each subsection of the AOTA FWPE might be aligned with various AOTA documents. It then provides sample site considerations as it pertains to the FWPE subsections and AOTA documents and sample SSLOs. This can be used as a framework for the development of your own SSLOs.

Additional resources that might be helpful for a FWed to use when brainstorming and fine-tuning SSLOs can be found in Box 4-4.

TABLE 4-1
RUMBA FRAMEWORK FOR DEVELOPING
SITE-SPECIFIC LEARNING OBJECTIVES

R – RELEVANT	*Is this something I would expect of an entry-level occupational therapy practitioner at my site?*
U – UNDERSTANDABLE	*Would a student know what they are supposed to do when they read the objective?*
M – MEASURABLE	*Is there a way that I can clearly identify if the student did or did not successfully meet this objective?*
B – BEHAVIORAL	*Is the objective written in a manner that will allow the expected performance to be clearly observed?*
A- ACHIEVABLE	*Is the objective realistic within the time frame, demands, and resources at my site? Is the objective realistic in my site in relation to the student's level of preparation?*

Adapted from Wimmer, R. (2004). Writing site-specific objectives for FWPE forms [Conference session]. AOTA Annual Conference, Minneapolis, MN, United States. https://www.aota.org//media/Corporate/Files/EducationCareers/Educators/Fieldwork/SiteObj/fwpepre.ppt

Learning Preferences

Consideration of learning style preferences can positively impact student performance. Ryan et al. (2018) found that 67.5% of the FWeds felt that adapting to learning styles is a shared responsibility between students and FWeds and can be a component of a positive student experience and that learning styles should be articulated prior to the start of the placement. Chetty et al. (2019) found that teaching styles have significant impacts on students' learning styles and academic performance. It is important to note that some current research finds that students have learning **preferences**, not learning styles (Furey, 2020; Newton & Miah, 2017), and some research suggests that instruction provided based students' learning style preferences does not improve learning (Kirschner, 2017; Rogowsky et al., 2020). The consideration of learning styles and preferences continues to be common practice in academia, and FWeds should consider the varied research on learning styles and learning preferences as they develop their learning plan for an upcoming fieldwork student.

As each student brings a unique set of experiences, skills, and preferences, the consideration of a student's learning style preference can enable FWeds to develop intentional learning activities and select the best teaching strategies thus contributing to the student's overall success (Viloria et al., 2019). Box 4-5 has select learning style/learning preference inventories that students might complete prior to the start of the fieldwork experience. Having this information can then guide the development of the 8-week (occupational therapy assistant) or 12-week (occupational therapist) Level II fieldwork experience.

> **Box 4-3**
>
> ## Sample Site-Specific Learning Objectives Based on Items From AOTA FWPE (2020c) for the Occupational Therapy Student
>
> **Item #3:** *Ensures the safety of self and others during all fieldwork related activities by anticipating potentially unsafe situations and taking steps to prevent accidents. Examples: body mechanics, medical safety, equipment safety, client-specific precautions, contraindications, community safety.*
>
> - Mental health setting: Able to identify the need for and demonstrates the ability to de-escalate patients with supervision.
> - Inpatient rehabilitation setting: State universal precautions and will adhere to guidelines with 100% of patient encounters.
> - Outpatient hand setting: Responsible for independently identifying and following procedures so that treatment is safe for client, therapist, and related personnel by week 12.
>
> **Item #17:** *Establishes an accurate and appropriate client-centered plan based on the evaluation results, contexts, theories, frames of reference, and/or practice models. Examples: creates relevant and measurable goals in collaboration with the client and/or family/caregivers; recommends additional consultation and referrals.*
>
> - Outpatient pediatrics setting: Using a sensory integration frame of reference student will develop weekly treatment plans that reflect the child's interests and motivations with distant supervision.
> - Acute care setting: With minimal edits, develop long- and short-term goals for each patient using a Person-Environment-Occupation approach by week 12.
> - Subacute rehabilitation setting: with supervision, incorporate results of the Activity Measure for Post-Acute Care into client-centered treatment plans for each patient.
>
> **Item #26:** *Demonstrates through practice or discussion an understanding of costs and funding systems related to occupational therapy services, such as federal, state, third party, and private payers. Examples: billing for occupational therapy services, inventory and ordering of supplies for OT services, and options for client procurement of adaptive equipment.*
>
> - Inpatient rehabilitation: Completes accurate documentation for payment of services with no more than two edits by week 12.
> - School setting: Verbalize the available funding for occupational therapy services in school-based setting (e.g., Medicaid, federal, state, or local allotments) to FWed and other stakeholders by week 12.
> - Outpatient orthopedic setting: Independently makes responsible choices concerning use of physical agent modalities by week 12.

(continued)

Occupational Profile

As part of the FWeds learning plan for an upcoming fieldwork student, the FWed should reset from any prior fieldwork experiences they have had. Each fieldwork experience with a student should be treated uniquely as no two students are alike. This is like the concept of client-centered care. In order to facilitate the best possible fieldwork experience for an upcoming student, the FWed should seek to learn what makes that student unique and to understand the context, past experiences, motivations, and goals that they present with.

BOX 4-3 (CONTINUED)

SAMPLE SITE-SPECIFIC LEARNING OBJECTIVES BASED ON ITEMS FROM AOTA FWPE (2020C) FOR THE OCCUPATIONAL THERAPY STUDENT

Item #6: *Articulates the role of occupational therapy practitioners to clients and other relevant parties clearly, confidently, and accurately. Examples: families, caregivers, colleagues, service providers, administration, the public.*

- School setting: Independently articulates the role of the occupational therapist and occupational therapy assistant in the school environment to FWed, teachers, students, families, etc. by final.
- Inpatient rehabilitation: Confidently and accurately communicate occupational therapist role and focus during family team meetings by final.
- Mental health setting: Articulates the role of the occupational therapist and occupational therapy assistant to patients, families, and the treatment team while incorporating principles of health literacy.

Item #7: *Obtains sufficient and necessary information about factors that support or hinder occupational performance from relevant sources throughout the evaluation process. Examples: record or chart reviews, client, family, caregivers, service providers.*

- School setting: Gathers pertinent information from the student's file, parents, other staff, and community resources, including previous or supplemental services received.
- Outpatient orthopedic setting: Independently complete detailed review of surgical records, physician recommendations and associated protocols prior to each patient encounter.
- Subacute setting: Participate in and obtain necessary information about each assigned patient during interdisciplinary team rounds.

DeIuliis (2011) suggests that FWeds complete an occupational profile with students as they begin the fieldwork experience. It provides an opportunity to discover the occupations, interests, motivations, and goals of the student allowing for optimal engagement in the student's desired occupation. The *Occupational Therapy Practice Framework: Domain and Process, 4th Edition* defines engagement in occupation as "performance of occupations as the result of choice, motivation, and meaning within a supportive context (including environmental and personal factors)" (AOTA, 2020b, p. 5). Understanding the student's choice, motivations, and environmental and personal factors is an important part of developing a successful learning plan for the student. Suggested questions that could be used to guide an occupational profile of a student are in Box 4-6.

BUILDING THE WEEKLY SCHEDULE

Once the SSLOs are completed and you have considered the individual learning needs and goals of your student, a weekly schedule should be developed to help guide the Level II experience and the progression of the expectation to achieve the SSLOs. A weekly schedule that outlines the expectations, responsibilities, intentional learning opportunities, and assignments of a fieldwork student can help both the FWed and student have a successful experience. Often, fieldwork sites create a generic weekly schedule and then simply modify it, as needed, to fit the individual learning needs and goals of the upcoming student. This can be a big time-saving trick.

TABLE 4-2

USING AOTA DOCUMENTS TO ALIGN LEVEL II SITE-SPECIFIC LEARNING OBJECTIVES WITH AOTA FIELDWORK PERFORMANCE EVALUATION ITEMS

AOTA FWPE (2020) SECTIONS FOR OCCUPATIONAL THERAPY STUDENTS	AOTA DOCUMENTS	SITE CONSIDERATIONS	SAMPLE SITE-SPECIFIC LEARNING OBJECTIVES
Fundamentals of Practice	*Occupational Therapy Code of Ethics* (2020a) • Principle 1. Beneficence • Principle 2. Nonmaleficence • Section I: Professional Integrity, Responsibility, and Accountability *Standards of Practice for Occupational Therapy* (AOTA, 2015) *Standards of Continuing Competence* (2015)	List three primary safety risks at setting	Maintain accurate sharps count Demonstrate proper handling techniques Compliance with infection control protocols
Evaluation and Screening	*Occupational Therapy Practice Framework: Domain and Process, Fourth Edition (OTPF-4*; 2020b); Occupational profile and analysis of occupational performance	List three primary occupations addressed List the three most used assessment tools	Competence is assessing occupational performance through standardized and non-standardized tools Complete occupational profile with each client Competent with use of Sensory Profile and Peabody
Intervention	Framework-IV (AOTA, 2020b); Plan, implement, and review, includes approaches of: • Create/promote • Establish/restore • Maintain • Modify • Prevent	Identify three primary approaches used for intervention Identify primary frame of references, practice models, or theories that guide intervention	Competence in planning and executing intervention Competence in altering intervention in response to client and additional issues/concerns from other professionals/staff or significant others Complete daily treatment plans that incorporate evidence to support interventions

(continued)

TABLE 4-2 (CONTINUED)

USING AOTA DOCUMENTS TO ALIGN LEVEL II SITE-SPECIFIC LEARNING OBJECTIVES WITH AOTA FIELDWORK PERFORMANCE EVALUATION ITEMS

AOTA FWPE (2020) SECTIONS FOR OCCUPATIONAL THERAPY STUDENTS	AOTA DOCUMENTS	SITE CONSIDERATIONS	SAMPLE SITE-SPECIFIC LEARNING OBJECTIVES
Managing Occupational Therapy Services	*OTPF-4* (2020b); Outcomes of intervention: Occupational performance, improvement, enhancement, prevention, health and wellness, quality of life, participation, role competence, well-being, occupational justice *Guidelines for Supervision Roles, and Responsibilities During the Delivery of Occupational Therapy Services* (2020c)	Identify three primary outcomes for clients served at setting Identify external constraints of funding and time affecting intervention Identify the role of assistants/aides	Competence in meeting productivity standards Responsible plans that meet constraints of setting Entry-level supervisory skills with assistants/aides
Communication and Professional Behaviors	*OTPF-4* (2020b); *Occupational Therapy Code of Ethics and Standards* (2020a) *Scope of Practice* (2014) *Standards of Practice for Occupational Therapy* (2015) *Standards for Continuing Competence* (2015)	Specify the method and frequency of meetings and written documentation requirements Identify specific professional behaviors expected at the setting Identify expectations for professional growth	Competence with documentation requirements (daily notes, progress notes, and evaluations reports) Skillful use of verbal and nonverbal communication during team meetings Punctual for all scheduled sessions Collaborates with FWed to develop three learning opportunities to maximize the experience

Adapted from Schultz-Krohn, W. (2012). Developing fieldwork experiences; Examples form early intervention and school-based practice. *OT Practice, 17*(1), CE1-CE8.

Box 4-4

OTHER RESOURCES TO HELP DEVELOP
SITE-SPECIFIC LEARNING OBJECTIVES

AOTA Fieldwork Resources: https://www.aota.org/Education-Careers/Fieldwork.aspx
Provides specific examples of SSLOs by practice area
New England Occupational Therapy Education Council: https://neotecouncil.org/
Provides user-friendly templates to assist with the development of SSLOs

---

Box 4-5

LEARNING STYLE/LEARNING PREFERENCES INVENTORIES

AFWCs can encourage students to complete a learning style inventory (LSI) **prior to** the start of the fieldwork experience and share with the FWed. Additionally, FWeds should take a teaching style inventory, so they can understand how that will match with the student's learning style or how they might adapt to their upcoming student.

Examples of Learning Styles

VARK Questionnaire (https://vark-learn.com/wp-content/uploads/2014/08/The-VARK-Questionnaire.pdf)

- The VARK questionnaire categorizes individuals according to the sensory modality preference in learning based on 16 multiple choice questions. The four modes are visual, aural, read/write, and kinesthetic. Research finds that a multimodal approach to teaching is advantageous to fit the diversity of learning preferences of students (Prithishkumar & Michael, 2014). Results of this questionnaire may be helpful for Level I or Level II students to complete prior to the start of the experience so that the FWed can understand the student's preferences and design intentional learning experiences to best match the student's preference.

Kolb Learning Style Inventory (https://experientiallearninginstitute.org/programs/assessments/kolb-learning-style-inventory-4-0/)

- The latest version of the Kolb LSI (4.0) has converted the four original styles of learning—diverging, assimilating, converging, and accommodating—into nine styles: initiating, experiencing, imagining, reflecting, analyzing, thinking, deciding, acting, and balancing. The inventory includes 20 items with the first 12 being similar to the earlier version and the following 8 inquiring about learning in different contexts. This inventory is a practical self-assessment that can help both students and FWeds better understand their preferred approach to learning in everyday life. A conversation about this between the FWed and the student can help avoid any misunderstandings.

Paragon Learning Styles Inventory (https://web.calstatela.edu/faculty/jshindl/plsi/)

- The Paragon LSI is a 48-item questionnaire that assesses learning by examining it in four separate domains: extrovert-introvert, sensate-intuitive, feeler-thinker, and judger-perceiver. It is important for FWeds to assess the learning style of their students so that they can instruct in a way that meets the learning needs of the students. It also helps students realize their own strengths and weaknesses in learning—allowing them to work on weaker areas and capitalize on strengths.

(continued)

> ### Box 4-5 (CONTINUED)
> # LEARNING STYLE/LEARNING PREFERENCES INVENTORIES
>
> **Examples of Teaching Styles**
>
> Grasha-Riechmann Teaching Style Survey (https://www.academia.edu/26515668/Teaching_Style_Survey_Grasha_Riechmann)
>
> - The Grasha-Riechmann Teaching Style Inventory is a 40-item, self-report questionnaire that categorizes and assesses teaching into five different styles: expert, formal authority, personal model, facilitator, and delegator. It is important to use student-centered styles because giving students autonomy and choice in their learning increases their motivation and satisfaction. Flexibility in teaching style is key to success and it is important to assess student satisfaction with an instructor's teaching styles (Arababisarjou et al., 2020).
>
> Reformed Teaching Observation Protocol (RTOP; https://www.physport.org/assessments/assessment.cfm?A=RTOP)
>
> - The RTOP measures reformed teaching, typically in math and science classrooms of all levels, via 25 items. Important measures of reformed teaching include considering preconceptions of students on the subject, active student engagement, learning and working with peers, and presentation and reflection of work for students. With proper training, scores on RTOP predict improved student learning in all levels of math and science classrooms (Piburn et al., 2000). FWeds could translate findings of this assessment to help improve occupational therapy student learning.

> ### Box 4-6
> # FIELDWORK EDUCATOR TIP
>
> The following questions are examples of how to guide interviews to obtain occupational profiles of fieldwork students (Deluliis, 2011):
>
> - What does the student perceive as their strengths and areas of need?
> - What social roles does your student have?
> - What are the student's daily routines, habits, and patterns of performance?
> - What are the student's interests or leisure pursuits?
> - How does the student balance between work, school, and leisure?
> - What motivates the student?
> - How does the student best learn?
> - What are the student's learning priorities?

Preparation and dissemination of a weekly schedule before the start of the fieldwork or within the first few days of the fieldwork experience will provide both the FWed and the student with a guide or checklist to what needs to be accomplished throughout the 12- or 8-week fieldwork experience. ACOTE (2018) requires that Level II fieldwork supervision is direct and then decreases to less direct supervision as appropriate for the setting, the severity of the client's condition, and the ability of the student to support progression toward entry-level competence. Weekly schedules can be developed using incrementally increasing expectations for students to progress toward the goal of competent entry-level practice. A weekly schedule will help ensure that this progression of competence is outlined and can serve as a guide for the student and FWed. FWeds and students can use the weekly schedule as part of a weekly review meeting. They can cross check the weekly schedule and see what has been accomplished, develop goals for the following week, and have an opportunity for dialogue about why some tasks may not have been completed. It is important for both the student and the FWed to note that the established weekly schedule needs to be flexible. Pending the FWed's caseload, the student's strengths, background knowledge, or other contextual or personal factors, the established weekly schedule may need to be modified throughout. An optimal fieldwork experience is modified as the student learns and skills develop throughout the experience (Rodger et al., 2011). The FWed and the student should have open communication about changes to the schedule to ensure transparency about student progress.

Schafer-Clay (2019) surveyed occupational therapy practitioners who have not taken field-work students and found that 66% would want the academic program to help establish a fieldwork schedule of student expectations. Assistance with the development of weekly schedules is another example of time-saving support that academic programs can provide to busy clinicians. Be sure to reach out to the AFWC at the schools that your facility is affiliated with as they might have sample weekly schedules with generic expectations of technical/clinical skills as well as soft skills that are needed for an entry-level clinician in a given practice setting. These schedules might also include best practices such as focus on occupation-based interventions, client-centered practice, evidence-based assignments, and demonstrate a progression of expectations throughout the fieldwork experience with the ultimate goal of entry-level practice. Chapter 6 will provide further exemplars for developing best practice ideals through learning activities and assignments on Level II field-work. Once you have this sample schedule, you can refer to your SSLOs you developed and insert expectations and performance checkpoints that will guide the student's progression to achieve the SSLOs over the fieldwork experience. Be sure to also consider any site competencies that are expected of a student and consider the length of the fieldwork and when these competencies and other expectations should be met to ensure progression to entry-level competence. You may want to use Bloom's Taxonomy as you consider your expectations and the student's progression through the experience. Bloom's Taxonomy, as discussed further in Chapter 3 of this book, involves six cognitive domains used by learners to acquire, retain, and use new information: knowledge, com-prehension, application, analysis, synthesis, and evaluation (Krathwohl, 2002). Bloom's Taxonomy outlines that in order to achieve higher levels of learning such as *synthesis* and *evaluation*, students must first achieve the lower levels of *knowledge* and *comprehension*. Using this taxonomy, you could design expectations and assignments for the first 1 to 2 weeks of a Level II fieldwork that are focused on knowledge and comprehension. For example, you might have the student complete knowledge-based competencies or quizzes about anatomy, universal precautions, vitals, or infec-tion control procedures. In the next few weeks you might focus your expectations and assign-ments on the application of knowledge. Students may be expected to apply anatomy knowledge to fabricate a splint or apply knowledge of universal precautions by donning and doffing personal protective equipment correctly and consistently. And finally, using the taxonomy, the later part of the Level II fieldwork experience may be devoted to higher-level learning domains like *analysis*, *synthesis*, and *evaluation*. Assignments and expectations might be focused on the student's abil-ity to evaluate the effectiveness of interventions, synthesis of ethical dilemmas, or application of evidence in a novel situation.

See Boxes 4-7 through 4-9 for sample weekly schedules for an inpatient rehabilitation setting, a telehealth fieldwork, and a collaborative two-to-one fieldwork supervision model.

Box 4-7
SAMPLE WEEKLY SCHEDULE FOR INPATIENT REHABILITATION

Week 1
- Review student manual and/or review site/role-specific information
- Participate in scavenger hunt/educate self about logistics/location of needed items and places at site/floor
- Observe and assist FWed with treatment sessions
- Observe FWed and learn site-specific practices including:
  - Interdisciplinary rounds, charges, FIM/CARESet Tool and Quality Indicators, daily and progress documentation, discharge documentation, weekend coverage, etc.
- Observe one to two other disciplines and groups
- Demonstrate competence with pulse/blood pressure/pulse O_2 and adherence to safety and patient specific precautions
- Review and develop plan for competence of advanced competencies relevant for site/floor/population
- Identify first patient and work on treatment plan over weekend
- Weekly review meeting (complete self-reflection and review with FWed)

Week 2
- Develop treatment plans for assigned patients (due each morning prior to treatment)
- Review EMR system and demonstrate competence with chart review
- Demonstrate competence with manual muscle testing, range of motion measurements, upper extremity sensation testing
- Observe new evaluations
- Contribute to daily notes
- Attend all staff meetings
- Identify one skill to practice with FWed
- Caseload by end of week 2: Two treatment hours (may include leading group)
- Weekly review meeting (complete self-reflection and review with FWed)

Week 3
- Develop treatment plans for assigned patients (due each morning prior to treatment)
- Evaluate new patient with supervisor
- Administer one standardized assessment with supervision
- Present in staff meetings/rounds on assigned patients
- Caseload by end of week 3: Three to four treatment hours
- Weekly review meeting (complete self-reflection and review with FWed)

Week 4
- Develop treatment plans for assigned patients (due each morning prior to treatment)
- Determine topic for evidence-based inservice/journal club for midterm
- Evaluate new patient with distant supervision
- Caseload by end of week 4: Four to five treatment hours
- Weekly review meeting (complete self-reflection and review with FWed)

(continued)

SAMPLE WEEKLY SCHEDULE FOR INPATIENT REHABILITATION

Week 5
- Develop treatment plans for assigned patients (due each morning prior to treatment)
- Basic competency with patient caseload responsibilities
- Caseload by end of week 5: Six treatment hours
- Weekly review meeting (complete self-reflection and review with FWed)

Week 6
- Midterm review
- Full caseload and associated responsibilities (e.g., scheduling, discharge planning, family training, equipment ordering)
- Discuss/identify student final project
- Weekly review meeting (complete self-reflection and review with FWed)

Week 7
- Competence with standardized assessments used with patient population
- Present evidence-based inservice/journal club
- Full caseload and associated responsibilities (e.g., scheduling, discharge planning, family training, equipment ordering)
- Weekly review meeting (complete self-reflection and review with FWed)

Week 8
- Observe on another unit/population as appropriate
- Full caseload and associated responsibilities (e.g., scheduling, discharge planning, family training, equipment ordering)
- Weekly review meeting (complete self-reflection and review with FWed)

Week 9
- Full caseload and associated responsibilities (e.g., scheduling, discharge planning, family training, equipment ordering)
- Weekly review meeting (complete self-reflection and review with FWed)

Week 10
- Full caseload and associated responsibilities (e.g., scheduling, discharge planning, family training, equipment ordering)
- Weekly review meeting (complete self-reflection and review with FWed)

Week 11
- Full caseload and associated responsibilities (e.g., scheduling, discharge planning, family training, equipment ordering)
- Present student project
- Weekly review meeting (complete self-reflection and review with FWed)

Week 12
- Full caseload and associated responsibilities (e.g., scheduling, discharge planning, family training, equipment ordering)
- Prepare for hand-off of patients currently on caseload
- Final evaluation review

Box 4-8

Sample Weekly Schedule for Telehealth Fieldwork

WEEK 1	WEEK 2	WEEK 3	WEEK 4	WEEK 5	WEEK 6
Observe FWed daily sessions Write one note for identified patient per day Complete observation checklist on three clients per day ID first clients for week 2 Skill practice: feeding and ROM Interdisciplinary observations Review and write summary of one current article relevant to patient population/treatment Weekly review meeting	Primary for one treatment session per day and associated documentation Continue observing other evals/treatments/team conference meetings/family conferences Daily journal: medical terminology, observation notes, questions Skills practice: assessment Review and write summary of one current article relevant to patient population/treatment Weekly review meeting	Primary for two treatment sessions/day and associated documentation Cont. to journal 2 to 3 times/week Interdisciplinary observation #2 Identify midterm assignment and begin work Continue to observe evaluations, discharge procedures, family conferences, and family training sessions. Review FWed evaluations and discharge write-ups Complete one evaluation/re-evaluation Skills practice: TBD Review and write summary of one current article relevant to patient population/treatment Weekly review meeting	Complete journal notebook one to two entries Complete one to two evaluations/re-evaluations Primary for two to three patients/day, including associated documentation Work on midterm assignment Report in team conference meetings/family meetings on primary patients Skills practice: TBD Review and write summary of one current article relevant to patient population/treatment Weekly review meeting	Primary for three to four patients per day and associated documentation Complete all new evaluations/re-evaluations as they are needed Reports in team conference meeting and/or family conference meeting Journal: weekly entry Discuss opportunities to plan/complete family training session Skills practice: TBD Weekly review meeting Complete FWPE midterm self-evaluation	Responsible for four to five sessions/day Daily documentation for all sessions Progress report for identified clients Treatment plans provided to FWed each morning for sessions COTA supervision activity Skills practice: student to identify two interventions to practice/learn Midterm review

(continued)

Box 4-8 (CONTINUED)

SAMPLE WEEKLY SCHEDULE FOR TELEHEALTH FIELDWORK

WEEK 7	WEEK 8	WEEK 9	WEEK 10	WEEK 11	WEEK 12
Primary for 75% of caseload	Between weeks 8 to 10, student primary for full caseload	Primary for full caseload	Primary for full caseload	Primary for full caseload	Final student evaluation meeting
Daily documentation for all sessions	Communicate daily	Daily documentation for all sessions	Complete all associated OT responsibilities	Final project presentation in week 11 or 12	Complete student evaluation of fieldwork site
Progress report for identified clients	Communicate regularly with family members, involve them in treatment discussions, and discharges as assigned	Progress reports	• Scheduling	Prepare patients/ families/and coworkers for transition	Prepare patients/ families and coworkers for transition
Continue covering evaluations and discharges as assigned		Journal club/inservice to therapy team on identified topic	• Equipment ordering	Weekly review meeting	
Discuss ideas for final project with supervisor		Skills practice: TBD	• Discharge planning		
Skills practice: TBD	and answer their questions without hesitation whenever possible	Weekly review meeting	Complete student project		
Weekly review meeting	Skills practice: TBD		Weekly review meeting		
	Weekly review meeting				

Box 4-9
SAMPLE COLLABORATIVE MODEL WEEKLY EXPECTATIONS

Week 1
- Facility orientation: familiarize yourself with facility, programs offered, student binder and documentation system
- Complete occupational profile on co-student to initiate development of working relationship
- Complete trauma-informed care and principles of harm reduction training
- With co-student, complete guided observation forms during evaluation and treatment sessions
- Assist FWed with evaluation and treatment as able
- With co-student, collaboratively complete draft documentation on clients FWed treats
- Observe federal, state, and facility regulations relating to confidentiality
- One-to-one weekly review meeting with FWed
- Group weekly meeting with co-student
- By end of week 1: Identify first client for caseload

Week 2
- With co-student, observe two other health professionals at facility and complete guided observation form
- Competently perform chart reviews of all clients seen by FWed
- Clearly communicate the role of the occupational therapist to clients and other health care professionals
- Participate in occupational therapy groups and groups led by others at facility
- Attend team meeting and observe communication styles and role of support teams
- Adhere to all safety regulations and report incident appropriately as per facility protocol
- Complete intervention planning and facilitate one to two treatment session for assigned client (FWed present and assisting)
- Observe one of co-student's treatment sessions and complete guided observations forms and provide feedback to student
- Observe FWed administer standardized assessments
- Complete literature review of standardized assessments used at facility
- One-to-one weekly review meeting with FWed
- Group weekly meeting with co-student
- End of week 2 caseload: Two to three treatment hours

Week 3
- Demonstrate ability to complete daily notes with minimal corrections
- Complete intervention planning and facilitate two to three treatment sessions for assigned clients (FWed present as needed)
- Complete standardized assessment for identified client with FWed supervision
- Observe one of co-student's treatment sessions and complete guided observations forms and provide feedback to student
- Verbalize understanding of Model of Human Occupation and Person-Environment-Occupation and the application of these models to practice in this setting
- One-to-one weekly review meeting with FWed
- Group weekly meeting with co-student
- End of week 3 caseload: Three to four treatment hours

(continued)

BOX 4-9 (CONTINUED)

SAMPLE COLLABORATIVE MODEL WEEKLY EXPECTATIONS

Week 4

- Complete progress notes with minimal corrections
- Complete intervention planning and facilitate three to four treatment sessions for assigned clients (FWed present intermittently)
- Observe co-student's treatment sessions and complete guided observations forms and provide feedback to student
- With co-student, organize schedule and independently demonstrate effective time management skills
- One-to-one weekly review meeting with FWed
- Group weekly meeting with co-student
- End of week 4 caseload: Four to five hours

Week 5

- Complete intervention planning and facilitate four to five treatment sessions for assigned clients (FWed present intermittently)
- Email summary of evidence used to support interventions chosen to FWed
- Complete one to two evaluations with minimal assistance from FWed
- Apply clinical judgement and reasoning for interpretation of evaluation data and development of treatment plans
- Use evidence from research and relevant resources to make informed intervention decisions
- Complete daily notes independently and within 24 hours of session
- One-to-one weekly review meeting with FWed
- Group weekly meeting with co-student
- End of week 5 caseload: Five to six hours

Week 6

- Complete intervention planning and facilitate five to six treatment sessions for assigned clients (FWed present intermittently)
- Complete evaluations with distant supervision
- Complete progress notes independently
- One-to-one midterm meeting with FWed
- End of week 6 caseload: Full to 75% productivity

Week 7

- Responsible for full caseload treatment sessions (FWed present as requested by student or as needed). Student should identify when assistance is needed independently
- One-to-one weekly review meeting with FWed
- Group weekly meeting with co-student
- 75% productivity

(continued)

> ## Box 4-9 (continued)
> ## Sample Collaborative Model Weekly Expectations
>
> **Week 8**
> - Demonstrate ability to revise and adapt intervention plans as needed
> - Continue to take responsibility for own learning and request additional responsibilities as comfort increases
> - Independently incorporate evidence from research and relevant resources to make informed intervention decisions
> - One-to-one weekly review meeting with FWed
> - Group weekly meeting with co-student
> - 75% productivity
>
> **Week 9**
> - Complete evaluations independently and demonstrate skill in interpretation of evaluation data and utilization in the development of treatment plans and goals
> - Take responsibility for attaining professional competence by seeking out learning opportunities and interactions with others around the facility
> - To demonstrate effective time management and management of occupational therapy services, demonstrate competency with point of care documentation during sessions
> - One-to-one weekly review meeting with FWed
> - Group weekly meeting with co-student
> - 75% productivity
>
> **Weeks 10-11**
> - Present EBP project by end of week 11
> - Demonstrate competency with billing requirements and funding systems related to occupational therapy services at facility
> - One-to-one weekly review meeting with FWed
> - Group weekly meeting with co-student
> - 75% productivity
>
> **Week 12**
> - Provide written summary of each client on caseload to FWed to ensure efficient continuation of care
> - One-to-one final meeting with FWed
> - Provide written feedback to FWed, co-student, and fieldwork program
> - 75% productivity

INTENTIONAL LEARNING OPPORTUNITIES TO SUPPORT THE LEARNING PLAN

Intentional learning opportunities can be defined as learning that is motivated by intentions and is goal directed (Blumschein, 2012). Intentional learning opportunities include encouraging curiosity, investigating and problem solving in everyday situations, and challenging learners to make links between ideas and experiences. The Intentional Fieldwork Education Model (Crawford & Hanner, 2019) suggests utilizing intentional learning activities to improve the effectiveness of teaching-learning during the fieldwork experience. Mollman and Bondmass (2020) find that intentional learning may prepare students to competently practice in today's dynamic and complex health care system.

As part of developing intentional learning opportunities, FWeds are encouraged to anticipate and recognize teachable moments that go beyond learning assignments. Teachable moments are defined as "a time that is favorable for teaching something, such as proper behavior" ("Teachable Moments," 2020). Utilizing informal learning opportunities that occur during day-to-day interactions with the students can provide them with immediate feedback and support the concept of the teachable moment (Coffelt & Gabriel, 2017). Teachable moments can also be opportunities to further support the student's achievement of SSLOs. Engaging in direct experiences with clients, obtaining feedback from multiple sources, and reflection can also support a student's development of competence (King, 2009). If you are looking for them, teachable moments can be found throughout one's day. See Table 4-3 for examples of teachable moments that are common within fieldwork. Box 4-10 outlines the goal of sample intentional learning opportunities.

CASE SCENARIO

Now that we have reviewed the process of how to develop and implement a plan for Level II fieldwork, let's put together the steps and illustrate the planning process from start to finish.

Read the following scenario:

Play and Function is an outpatient pediatric clinic that serves a variety of pediatric diagnoses. They have four full-time occupational therapists, all of them with 0 to 3 years of experience. As the staff is rather new, they have not taken students previously. As the world was dealing with the implications and new realities of COVID-19, Play and Function got several requests to host students from local schools. The staff recognized the need to help and agreed to take one Level II student for the summer. In the month leading up to the start of the fieldwork, the state restrictions related to COVID-19 increased and the staff transitioned the majority of their practice to telehealth. The staff discussed how this might impact the fieldwork experience and ultimately agreed that they would still be willing to host the student with telehealth as their primary delivery method. Ashley was identified to be the primary FWed for the upcoming Level II. Ashley had 2 years of experience working at Play and Function. Ashley was excited about supervising her first Level II student because she knew it would be an opportunity to increase her teaching skills, learn new things from the student, and foster professional development. Ashley's clinic manager also thought the student could complete a final project related to telehealth, creating educational modules that could be put on the clinic's website, and was very excited about this benefit.

Ashley's clinic manager worked with the school to execute a memorandum of understanding (i.e., affiliation agreement) and put Ashley in touch with the AFWC at the school. The AFWC and Ashley collaborated to develop SSLOs for the Level II fieldwork experience. Ashley referred to the essential functions and job description for a staff occupational therapist at Play and Function. She also used the AOTA FWPE as a guide in developing the SSLOs. Ashley made two to three SSLOs for each of the categories of the AOTA FWPE (Fundamentals of Practice, Basic Tenets of Occupational Therapy, Evaluation and Screening, Intervention, Managing Occupational Therapy Services, Communication and Professional Behaviors). Some of the SSLOs Ashley developed included: (1) Student will incorporate coaching principles during telehealth interventions, (2) Student will assess the environment at the start of each telehealth session and identify any safety concerns, and (3) Student will confidently and articulately describe occupational therapy and the plan of care to the family or caregiver within each session.

After having collaborated with the AFWC to develop the SSLOs, Ashley wanted to make sure she created weekly expectations that would guide the student's progression with the ultimate goal of entry-level competence. She wanted the week-by-week guide to include a demonstrated progression of supervision that is direct and then decreases to less direct supervision. Ashley included intentional learning opportunities like observing the speech-language pathologist's and physical therapist's sessions with the student's client. She also created an intentional learning opportunity

TABLE 4-3
EXAMPLES OF TEACHABLE MOMENTS WITHIN FIELDWORK

SITUATION	TEACHABLE MOMENT
FWed is treating a patient and the patient makes a sexually inappropriate comment to the student. The student freezes and does not know how to respond.	Model an appropriate response to the patient. After, reflect on the encounter with the student and discuss how they felt and what the appropriate responses are when this happens. Have the student practice responding in a safe setting with you so they are better prepared to handle such an encounter in the future.
The student is completing a bed-to-wheelchair transfer and you must step in because the patient is about to slip off the bed.	After making sure the patient is safe and in a comfortable position, stop and briefly explain to the student what happened and why. If the patient is agreeable, have the student complete the transfer again incorporating your feedback and using strategies you provide.
Two clinicians engage in a heated disagreement in the staff office and the student witnesses it.	Pull the student aside and reflect on what they heard. Discuss ways of managing conflict in the workplace and share suggestions on how it could have been handled in a more productive manner using conflict management strategies.
The student is having difficulty meeting the SSLO related to productivity expectations.	At the end of the day, identify moments within the day the student can increase efficiency and provide examples of your own strategies to accomplish productivity expectations.
The student is in a role-emerging setting and the occupational therapy supervisor is on-site only 1 day per week. The student complains to another staff member that they do not know what to do most of the time.	Meet with the student and share the feedback you received from the other staff member. Collaboratively develop a list of occupational therapy–specific activities that the student can engage in when there is downtime or when she is feeling like there is nothing to do. Ask the student to make an hourly schedule for each day next week to facilitate increased engagement and productivity.
Student is completing a session focused on cutting via telehealth with a 5-year-old child. The child is engaging in unsafe behaviors with the scissors and the student does not address it.	Intervene and make sure the child is safe and then redirect the session. After the telehealth session, coordinate time as soon as possible to meet virtually with the student to discuss the safety concerns observed and brainstorm with the student other potential safety concerns that may occur during future telehealth sessions and ways to respond. Role play with the student how to stop and redirect a child from engaging in unsafe behaviors and/or involve the family.

Box 4-10

INTENTIONAL LEARNING OPPORTUNITIES

- Observe surgeries/procedures that clients often experience. *This will give the students a more holistic perspective of what the client is experiencing.*
- Have students complete a written reflection of a session you completed. Why do they think you did what you did? *This will give you an opportunity to see their clinical reasoning.* (Additional strategies to develop clinical reasoning in Level II fieldwork can be found in Chapter 7.)
- Have the student shadow their patient during encounters with other disciplines (e.g., speech-language pathology, physical therapy). *This will allow the student to see how other disciplines address the client's needs and provide them with a holistic view of the client's interprofessional care plan.*
- Have the student complete written treatment plans for each assigned patient. *This is a way the FWed can determine the student's level of clinical reasoning.*
- Have the student identify a skill they want to practice one-to-one with you each week. *This will challenge the student to reflect on what they need to learn and develop the skills of a lifelong learner.*
- Coordinate time for students to observe another level of care (e.g., if in outpatient have them observe acute care or if in school system have them observe a pediatric clinic setting). *This will allow for the student to better understand the continuum of care and assist with learning more about discharge recommendations.*
- Have other students on-site observe each other and provide feedback to one another. *Getting feedback from various sources may help reinforce feedback you have already given or provide them with a new perspective or another way to hear feedback.*
- Record the student completing a specific skill or interaction and then have the student watch it and reflect upon it. *Sometimes seeing yourself do something is sometimes the best way to identify your strengths and areas for improvements.*
- Ask the client, caregiver, family, or team member to provide feedback to the student to enhance learning. *Getting feedback from various sources may help reinforce feedback you have already given or provide them with a new perspective or another way to hear feedback.*

---

specific to the use of evidence to support interventions and will have the student lead a virtual journal club for the staff at week 6. Ashley also incorporated her clinic manager's request of having the student make three educational modules that could be posted on the clinic's website as a final project. With the switch to telehealth Ashley knew her caseload sometimes fluctuated. She shared the SSLOs and weekly expectations with her coworkers, and everyone agreed to help build the student's caseload over the 12 weeks as needed.

After preparing her plan for the student, Ashley communicated with the student and shared both the SSLOs and the weekly expectations. She also requested that the student complete a LSI, answer the student occupational profile questions she prepared, and send the information to her 2 weeks prior to the start of the fieldwork. Having this information helped Ashley get to know the student better and adjust some of the intentional learning opportunities she planned to best meet the student's needs and goals. For example, Ashley discovered from the student's occupational profile that she is a certified yoga instructor, and the student identified that her long-term goals are to work with the birth to 3-year-old population. With this information Ashley developed some intentional learning opportunities for the student to design and implement a yoga group for some of the kids at the clinic. Ashley thought this would be a good opportunity for the student to use her personal knowledge and demonstrate her strengths. Additionally, Ashley made sure to connect with some of her coworkers that had primarily birth-to-3-year-old caseloads and scheduled opportunities for the student to work with them. These preplanned intentional learning opportunities will help highlight the student's strengths and provided student-centered opportunities for growth. Ashley was ready!

Having read this scenario, reflect and respond to the following questions:

- In addition to what Ashley did, what other resources might you use to develop your SSLOs? Why would those be helpful?

- How can Ashley use the SSLOs she developed to monitor her student's performance over the 12 weeks? What is one additional intentional learning activity that you would develop to facilitate achievement of SSLOs for a student doing telehealth fieldwork?

SUMMARY

The baseball great Yogi Berra once said, "If you don't know where you are going, you'll end up someplace else." This great wisdom is practical advice for FWeds planning for upcoming fieldwork students. Without preparation and communication of expectations from the FWed, the student and the FWed may not end at the ultimate goal of entry-level competence. This chapter has outlined how to develop a learning plan for Level II fieldwork including the creation of SSLOs, consideration of student learning preferences, completing a student occupational profile, development of a weekly schedule, and leveraging intentional learning opportunities. Taking the time to create this learning plan will help you get the student to the goal of entry-level competence.

LEARNING ACTIVITIES

1. Refer to Table 4-1, and using each of the subsections of the AOTA FWPE, write one SSLO in each of the AOTA fieldwork evaluation categories for a Level II student that is appropriate to your site.

2. Identify entry-level competencies for your site and outline specific activities that would help a student achieve these competencies. Refer back to Boxes 4-7 and 4-8 for some examples.

3. Using the SSLOs, competencies, and activities you identified in the above questions, draft an 8- or 12-week Level II fieldwork week-by-week schedule. Consider the expected level of independence and frequency as you complete this. For example, if you identified proficiency with the use of a certain standardized assessment, what week-by-week learning activities/expectations would help develop that skill?

4. How can you use your weekly expectations and SSLOs to help evaluate a student's performance at midterm?

REFERENCES

Accreditation Council for Occupational Therapy Education. (2018). 2018 Accreditation Council for Occupational Therapy Education (ACOTE) Standards and Interpretive Guide (effective July 31, 2020). *American Journal of Occupational Therapy, 72*, 7212410005p1-7212410005p83. https://doi.org/10.5014/ajot.2018.72S217

American Occupational Therapy Association. (2020a). Occupational therapy code of ethics. *American Journal of Occupational Therapy 74*(Suppl. 3):7413410005. https://doi.org/10.5014/ajot.2020.74S3006

American Occupational Therapy Association. (2020b). Occupational therapy practice framework: Domain and process-fourth edition. *American Journal of Occupational Therapy, 74*(Suppl. 2), 7412410010p1-7412410010p87. https://doi.org/10.5014/ajot.2020.74S2001

American Occupational Therapy Association. (2020c). New fieldwork performance evaluation tool. AOTA. https://www.aota.org/Education-Careers/Fieldwork/performance-evaluations.aspx

Arababisarjou, A., Akbarilakeh, M., Soroush, F., & Payandeh, A. (2020). Validation and normalization of Grasha-Riechmann Teaching Style Inventory in faculty members of Zahedan University of Medical Sciences. *Advances in Medical Education and Practice*, (11), 305-312.

Barton, R., Corban, A., Herrli-Warner, L., McClain, E., Riehle, D., & Tinner, E. (2013). Role strain in occupational therapy fieldwork educators. *Work, 44*(3), 317-328. https://doi.org/10.3233/WOR-121508

Blumschein, P. (2012). Intentional learning. In N. M. Seel (Ed.), *Encyclopedia of the sciences of learning.* SpringerLink. https://doi.org/10.1007/978-1-4419-1428-6_37

Casares, G. S., Bradley, K. P., Jaffe, L. E., & Lee, G. P. (2003). Impact of the changing health care environment on fieldwork education: Perceptions of occupational therapy educators. *Journal of Allied Health, 32*(4), 246-251.

Chetty, N. D. S., Handayani, L., Sahabudin, N. A., Ali, Z., Hamzah, N., Rahman, N. S. A., & Kasim, S. (2019). Learning styles and teaching styles determine students' academic performances. *International Journal of Evaluation and Research in Education, 8*(4), 610-615. http://doi.org/10.11591/ijere.v8i4.20345

Coffelt, K. J., & Gabriel, L. S. (2017). Continuing competence trends of occupational therapy practitioners. *The Open Journal of Occupational Therapy, 5*(1), 4. https://doi.org/10.15453/2168-6408.1268

Crawford, E. J., & Hanner, N. (2019). The intentional fieldwork educator: Applying the Intentional Fieldwork Education Model (IFWEM) [Conference session]. The Annual Conference of the South Carolina Occupational Therapy Association, Charleston, SC, United States.

DeIuliis, E. D. (2011). Using the occupational profile for student-centered fieldwork education. *OT Practice, 16*, 13. https://www.duq.edu/assets/Documents/occupationaltherapy/FieldworkEducation/Suggested%20Readings/using%20the%20occupational%20profile.pdf

Furey, W. (2020). The stubborn myth of "learning styles". *Education Next, 20*(3). https://www.educationnext.org/stubborn-myth-learning-styles-state-teacher-license-prep-materials-debunked-theory/

Hanson, D. J. (2011). The perspectives of fieldwork educators regarding level II fieldwork students. *Occupational Therapy in Health Care, 25*(2-3), 164-177. https://doi-org.authenticate.library.duq.edu/10.3109/07380577.2011.561420

Haynes, C. J. (2011). Active participation in level I fieldwork: Fieldwork educator and student perceptions. *Occupational Therapy In Health Care, 25*(4), 257-269

King, G. (2009). A framework of personal and environmental learning-based strategies to foster therapist expertise. *Learning in Health and Social Care, 8*(3), 185-199. http://dx.doi.org/10.1111/j.1473-6861.2008.00210.x

Kirschner, P. A. (2017). Stop propagating the learning styles myth. *Computers & Education, 106*, 166-171. https://doi.org/10.1016/j.compedu.2016.12.006

Krathwohl, D. R. (2002). A revision of Bloom's taxonomy: An overview. *Theory into practice, 41*(4), 212-218. https://doi.org/10.1207/s15430421tip4104_2

Mollman, S., & Bondmass, M. D. (2020). Intentional learning: A student-centered pedagogy. *International Journal of Nursing Education Scholarship, 17*(1), 20190097. https://doi-org.ezproxy.rush.edu/10.1515/ijnes-2019-0097

Newton, P. M., & Miah, M. (2017). Evidence-based higher education—is the learning styles "myth" important? *Frontiers in Psychology, 8*, 444. https://doi.org/10.3389/fpsyg.2017.00444

Piburn, M., Sawada, D., Turley, J., Falconer, K., Benford, R., Bloom, I., & Judson, E. (2000). Reformed teaching observation protocol (RTOP) reference manual. Arizona Collaborative for Excellence in the Preparation of Teachers.

Prithishkumar, I. J., & Michael, S. A. (2014). Understanding your student: using the VARK model. *Journal of Postgraduate Medicine, 60*(2), 183-186. https://doi.org/10.4103/0022-3859.132337

Rodger, S., Fitzgerald, C., Davila, W., Millar, F., & Allison. (2011). What makes a quality occupational therapy practice placement? Students' and practice educators' perspectives. *Australian Occupational Therapy Journal, 58*(3), 195-202. https://doi.org/10.1111/j.1440-1630.2010.00903.x

Rogowsky, B. A., Calhoun, B. M., & Tallal, P. (2020). Providing instruction based on students' learning style preferences does not improve learning. *Frontiers in Psychology, 11*, 164.http://doi.org/10.3389/fpsyg.2020.00164

Ryan, K., Beck, M., Ungaretta, L., Rooney, M., Dalomba, E., & Kahanov, L. (2018). Pennsylvania occupational therapy fieldwork educator practices and preferences in clinical education. *The Open Journal of Occupational Therapy, 6*(1). https://doi.org/10.15453/2168-6408.1362

Schafer-Clay, J. S. (2019). What stops some occupational therapy practitioners from providing fieldwork education? [Doctoral Capstone Project, Eastern Kentucky University]. ENCOMPASS: A Digital Archive of the Research, Creative Works, and History of Eastern Kentucky University. https://encompass.eku.edu/otdcapstones/49/

Schultz-Krohn, W. (2012). Developing fieldwork experiences: Examples from early intervention and school-based practice. *OT Practice, 17*(1), CE1-8. https://www.duq/edu/assests/Documents/occupationaltherapy/FieldworkEducation/Suggested%20Readings/Developing%20FW%20experiences.pdf

Viloria, A., Gonzalez, I. R. P., & Lezama, O. B. P. (2019). Learning style preferences of college students using big data. *Procedia Computer Science, 160*, 461-466. http://hdl.handle.net/11323/5986

Wimmer, R. (2004). Writing site-specific objectives for FWPE forms [Conference session]. AOTA Annual Conference, Minneapolis, MN, United States. https://www.aota.org//media/Corporate/Files/EducationCareers/Educators/Fieldwork/SiteObj/fwpepre.ppt

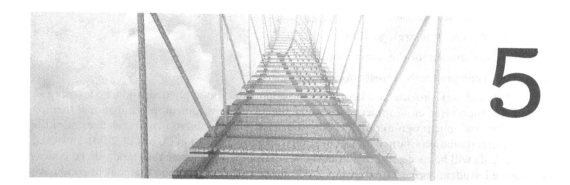

Setting the Student Up for Success

Ranelle Nissen, PhD, OTR/L

Level II fieldwork is an essential step in a student's journey toward becoming an occupational therapy practitioner. Many students identify fieldwork as a pivotal point in their journey that comes with excitement, but it can also come with an equal amount of angst. Students look forward to the opportunity to get real-world experience to apply the skills they have worked so hard to gain in the classroom. Finding the right fit of student to fieldwork educator (FWed) and student to fieldwork site can make the difference between success and failure. Building upon the initial steps of establishing a learning plan in Chapter 4, the FWed can take additional measures to set the Level II fieldwork student up for success. This chapter will provide the FWed with practical tips to establish a positive relationship and start the student on a path to success prior to the Level II fieldwork experience.

LEARNING OBJECTIVES

By the end of reading this chapter and completing the learning activities, the reader should be able to:

1. Conduct a site review process to ensure a successful Level II fieldwork experience.

2. Access resources that support the FWed and site preparation for student arrival.

DeIuliis, E. D., & Hanson, D. (Eds.).
Fieldwork Educator's Guide to Level II Fieldwork (pp. 137-160).
© 2023 Taylor & Francis Group.

3. Create a fieldwork manual.

4. Identify students that are a good fit for the site.

5. Prepare the student for site orientation.

6. Provide a comprehensive on-site orientation.

Level II fieldwork provides students with the opportunity to apply their didactic learning in a structured, supervised environment to advance their skill development in occupational therapy practice. The academic program provides the student with the foundational knowledge and skills to succeed (Accreditation Council for Occupational Therapy Education [ACOTE], 2018). However, not all students will be successful in all fieldwork environments. Despite the standardized education provided, students come with differing levels of ability and preparation that may be conducive in one fieldwork setting but lead to failure in another. The key is to develop a process that sets the student up for success. Ensuring the student has the best chance of success is a collaborative process between the academic fieldwork coordinator (AFWC), student, and FWed. Setting the student up for success also sets the FWed up for success. A student who struggles in fieldwork can add a burden to the FWed that can be minimized by identifying the right steps to finding the right student. The proper steps can also help set up a student to be the right student through planning and preparation. To set the student up for success, the FWed can complete an in-depth site review in advance of the student's arrival at the site.

SITE REVIEW PROCESS

Level II fieldwork education is a professional responsibility that takes planning and preparation. A site that provides high-level fieldwork education has an identified process and structure. One of the first steps to developing a fieldwork program is identifying the site's strengths, weaknesses, and opportunities available to students. Completing a review of the site will help determine what can be changed, what the student must navigate, how the site and student need to prepare for the experience, and how it can offer unique learning opportunities.

A site review process equates to a needs assessment process that is carried out for program development. If the FWed or site has never hosted a fieldwork student before, this may be a process that requires some dedicated time, but it is well worth the investment toward building a strong fieldwork program. If students have been hosted by the occupational therapy department or departments of other disciplines in the past, reviewing current documents and processes will be beneficial in this process. To follow a needs assessment approach, first define the population and environment. Then, check and analyze the data collected to identify the need and desired outcomes (Flecky et al., 2020); see Box 5-1.

An example of this process is **identifying the population** who will be involved in the fieldwork process. This population should include the fieldwork education team: the fieldwork site clinical coordinator, FWed (who may be the same person as the site coordinator), student, AFWC, and other personnel who will interact with the student. It is important to understand each stakeholder's needs, with the student at the center of the process. This is the step where a review of prior student feedback will be helpful. It is also the point where a conversation with the AFWC will help to understand the level of skill and education students from specific programs should be expected to possess before fieldwork. This is also a good step to revisit to review particular needs, learning preferences, and skill levels of a specific student before their start date.

The next step is to **examine the environment**. This encompasses all aspects of the environment, including physical and social. Examine what the facility can provide the student in physical space and what will need to be completed to make the student feel comfortable navigating the facility's entire physical environment. Also, examine the social environment that may benefit or hinder the student's sense of belonging.

BOX 5-1
STEP-BY-STEP PROCESS TO THE SITE REVIEW PROCESS

Step 1: Population
- Describe the student characteristics
  a. Identify differences in students in different fieldwork experience (e.g., first vs. second fieldwork experience)
  b. Different characteristics of occupational therapist and occupational therapy assistant students
  c. Preparation level of students from different academic programs
- Review student feedback from site evaluation forms and/or direct feedback
- Survey or interview students who have completed a fieldwork experience at your site
  a. If your site has not had any students yet, survey prospective students to understand their expectations, concerns, and questions

Step 2: Environment
- Identify weaknesses and barriers in the physical and social environment of the facility
  a. Physical resources available for a student: space, computer, reference materials
  b. Site culture that will support or not support a student's sense of belonging
- Interview other staff about the facility characteristics that may be conducive or prohibitive to a successful student fieldwork experience

Step 3: Outcomes
- Analyze information gathered in steps 1 and 2 to determine the areas of weakness and strengths
- Determine areas to capitalize upon (strengths) and areas to focus on to improve (weaknesses) to develop a strong fieldwork program at the facility
  a. This step should be used to identify characteristics of the site that can be shared with students to help determine the best student to site match

---

The final step is to **review the information collected** on the population and environment to identify strengths, weaknesses, opportunities, and threats (SWOT) to developing a strong fieldwork program.

A SWOT analysis is a framework that is used to gather information, which is used often during strategic or project planning. Identify areas that can be strengthened and how to minimize potential threats to a student's success. This step will be the point to identify what the facility can offer, expectations, and areas of flexibility that can provide modification to a student's specific needs and learning preferences. The needs assessment process should be a continual process that ideally is reviewed or updated after each student. It is also a good project to collaborate with each student to review and refine the site's fieldwork manual. Students and the AFWC are valuable partners (stakeholders) in this process. In the end, the primary goal is to focus on the development of a clear fieldwork program by identifying and addressing the needs of each stakeholder (fieldwork site clinical coordinator, FWed [who may be the same person as the coordinator], student, AFWC, and other personnel); see Boxes 5-1 and 5-2.

Part of the site review process should be to identify the level of preparation the FWed and site have to take a student for a full Level II fieldwork experience. The FWed prepares to take a student by identifying their readiness level to provide fieldwork education. A useful resource in this process is the AFWC. The AFWC can give information about the accreditation standards,

---

Box 5-2
SAMPLE SWOT ANALYSIS PROCESS

1. Interview or survey internal and external stakeholders specifically asking about current strengths, weaknesses, opportunities, and threats to the site's fieldwork program

   a. Examples: Occupational therapists and other health care professionals in the facility, administrative personnel, clients (with administrative approval), fieldwork students, AFWC, academic faculty

2. Review the data collected for common themes in each of the four areas

3. Identify goals that will support the site's fieldwork program and minimize potential weaknesses and threats

EXAMPLE TRADITIONAL FIELDWORK SITE SWOT ANALYSIS RESULTS

	BENEFIT	HARM
INTERNAL	Strengths • Two occupational therapists and two occupational therapy assistants qualified to supervise Level II fieldwork students • Offer services across the life span and in outpatient and inpatient settings for greater student learning opportunities • Administration is supportive of student fieldwork placements • Two extra desks dedicated for occupational therapy students • Dedicated education coordinator to assist with student placement requests and onboarding • Five existing affiliation agreements in place with academic institutions	Weaknesses • One occupational therapist does not have experience as a FWed • No existing fieldwork manual for student policies, procedures, and expectations • Current opening for occupational therapy position—current staff must cover additional caseload
EXTERNAL	Opportunities • Regional university occupational therapy program is offering the AOTA FWed's Certificate Workshop at reduced cost for affiliated fieldwork sites	Threats • Changing reimbursement guidelines may limit level of student participation in client sessions

(continued)

curriculum design and course sequence, fieldwork expectations, and student preparation level. The AFWC should also provide information about resources to enhance the FWed's preparation (ACOTE, 2018; Hanson, 2011). The resources may include assessment tools, reference materials, and educational workshops.

One assessment tool used is the *AOTA Self-Assessment Tool for Fieldwork Educator Competency* (SAFECOM) for novice and experienced occupational therapy and occupational therapy assistant

Box 5-2 (continued)
Sample SWOT Analysis Process

Example Role-Emerging Fieldwork Site SWOT Analysis Results

	BENEFIT	HARM
INTERNAL	Strengths • New full-time occupational therapist position • Plan to hire 5 FTE occupational therapist or occupational therapy assistant within 6 months • Staff support integration of occupational therapy services and student education	Weaknesses • Current occupational therapist has 2 years of practice experience, but no experience supervising students • No students placed in this setting before, so no manual or standard policies and procedures are available
EXTERNAL	Opportunities • Local occupational therapy and occupational therapy assistant programs are open to collaboration on establishing service-learning opportunities for students with plan to expand into Level I fieldwork, Level II fieldwork, and capstone	Threats • Students may not be as open to a nontraditional fieldwork setting • Demand for service may decline if local hospital opens similar programming options

4. Identify goals based upon the SWOT analysis results. The goals must be reasonable and achievable to meet to support the site's fieldwork program.

Example of goals built based upon the *Example Traditional Fieldwork Site SWOT Analysis Results*:

Lack of Fieldwork Education Resources

Goal 1A: All occupational therapy staff who supervise students will attend the AOTA Educator's Certificate Workshop.

Steps to take:

1. Meet with supervisor to discuss funding support to pay for conference registration.

2. Create plan for attendance: all at one time vs. staggered attendance to meet administrative support allowances

Goal 2A: Create a fieldwork student manual.

Steps to take:

1. Meet with AFWCs at partner institutions to review resources and example manual documents.

2. Review sample documents provided on the AOTA website.

3. Send draft manual to partner institutions to review.

4. Assess the manual by requesting student feedback each year.

5. Revise the document as needed when policies and processes change.

(continued)

Box 5-2 (continued)
Sample SWOT Analysis Process

Staffing shortage

Goal 1B: Create a schedule for student rotations to identify capacity for fieldwork education.

    Steps to take:

1. Meet with all occupational therapy staff to identify level of interest for supervising students—identify how many students per year each person wants to supervisor

2. Review the yearly caseload to identify periods of highs and lows

3. Create a plan for the number of students the department can accommodate at a time based upon FWeds available and level of caseload—taking into account added caseload from current staff shortage

4. Re-evaluate this plan after a new occupational therapist is hired

Complex and changing health care environment

Goal 1C: Create a modified approach to a traditional student progression through fieldwork that accommodates students' needs under reimbursement requirements.

    Steps to take:

1. Meet with AFWCs at partner institutions to discuss the new reimbursement guidelines and how this impacts student progression through fieldwork

2. Create a plan that progresses students from direct supervision and support to being able to demonstrate understanding of how to be autonomous while still adhering to the reimbursement requirements—this may include novel approaches to demonstrating autonomy through discussion and role play scenarios

Goal 2C: Develop a process of continual identification of health care policy changes that impact student fieldwork education.

    Steps to take:

1. Schedule an annual meeting with or request information from AFWCs at a partner institution to review changes in policies that impact fieldwork education

2. Sign up for policy alerts through AOTA

3. Review state-level policy updates provided through the state association or other entity that provides policy updates pertinent to student education

FWeds (American Occupational Therapy Association [AOTA], 2009). The FWed can understand their initial level and growth in areas identified as essential competencies for being a FWed. The tool provides flexibility to target those competency areas that apply to the practice setting. It is also a useful tool for developing goals as part of a professional development plan and a means to reassess the FWed's competency. The self-assessment tool has 69 statements to rate oneself on a five-point Likert scale from low to high proficiency. The questions span across five competency categories: professional practice, education, supervision, evaluation, and administration. This tool can be used before and after completing additional training and supervising Level II fieldwork students.

There are workshops and continuing education courses available through AOTA to provide further competency in fieldwork education. There are widely available resources through organizations such as AOTA (www.aota.org), the Occupational Therapy Practice Education Collaborative—Queensland (https://otpecq.group.uq.edu.au/), and fieldwork consortiums such as the New England Occupational Therapy Education Council (https://neotecouncil.org/) to provide

---

Box 5-3

CONTINUING EDUCATION OPPORTUNITIES

Continuing Education Workshops and Courses

American Occupational Therapy Association

- FWed's Certificate Workshop
- Fieldwork Education Module 1: Preparing to Become a FWed
- Fieldwork Education Module 2: Working with occupational therapy and occupational therapy assistant Students During Level I and Level II Fieldwork
- Fieldwork Education Module 3: Fieldwork Career Paths

FWed Resources

- American Occupational Therapy Association: Level II Fieldwork Education
  https://www.aota.org/Education-Careers/Fieldwork/LevelII.aspx
- American Occupational Therapy Association: Student Supervision
  https://www.aota.org/Education-Careers/Fieldwork/StuSuprvsn.aspx
- American Occupational Therapy Association: Resources for Fieldwork Education
  https://www.aota.org/Education-Careers/Fieldwork/Supervisor.aspx
- New England Occupational Therapy Education Council
  https://neotecouncil.org/
- Occupational Therapy Practice Education Collaborative–Queensland: Education for Placements
  https://otpecq.group.uq.edu.au/education-placements
- Occupational Therapy Practice Education Collaborative–Queensland: Resources & Publications
  https://otpecq.group.uq.edu.au/resources-publications

---

a wealth of reference materials about fieldwork education; see Box 5-3. The FWed is also encouraged to reach out directly to their educational partners to identify program-specific resources.

With the wealth of information gained from completing a site review and examining one's own preparation, the FWed can prepare for a student by **developing a fieldwork manual**. The manual should include sections to introduce the site, policies and procedures, fieldwork-specific expectations, and resources; see Appendix A for a sample manual outline. Creating an informative manual can be the product of the needs assessment described in Boxes 5-1 and 5-2. With the manual in place, identifying students that can be a good fit for the site can be initiated. There are three steps to this process: (1) finding the right student, (2) preparing the student, and (3) welcoming the student through a structured orientation.

STEP #1: FINDING THE RIGHT STUDENT

The ACOTE standards designate the fieldwork education requirements (2018). The student should be prepared to apply knowledge learned in the didactic content (AOTA, 2012). All educational programs that are accredited have demonstrated that they meet the minimum standards set forth for the respective education level to equally prepare students to demonstrate entry-level practice skills by the end of the Level II fieldwork experience (ACOTE, 2018). Every student may be prepared the same, but it does not mean every student is the same. Students demonstrate a different level of clinical knowledge and personal skills that impact their ability to succeed in different fieldwork environments (Andonian, 2013; Grenier, 2015; Kemp & Crabtree, 2018; Short et al., 2018). Identifying the student who is the right fit for your practice setting is the first step to setting the student up for success. Four key steps to this process are to:

1. Collaborate with the AFWC

2. Interview the student

3. Host the student for a trial experience

4. Provide site-specific expectations

These four key steps will be discussed in the next section of the chapter.

Collaborate With the Academic Fieldwork Coordinator

ACOTE (2018) standard C.1.11 requires the AFWC to "ensure that the student supervisor is adequately prepared to serve as a fieldwork educator prior to the Level II fieldwork" (p. 42). Part of being prepared for a student is to collaborate with the AFWC to ensure they match the right student with the site and FWed. Developing a collaborative relationship with the AFWC is also the first step to increasing the student to site fit and ensure a successful fieldwork experience. This collaboration may include working together to provide the right preparation to help the student, and the site, be prepared to give the right education level for the student's needs; see Box 5-4. If the site or FWed identifies specific requirements for the student to meet to be successful in that practice setting, collaborating with the AFWC will improve the likelihood that the right student is identified for the specific fieldwork site (Hanson, 2011; Varland et al., 2017).

The AFWC will provide resources that are helpful to determine the level and type of preparation the student should be expected to demonstrate. Reviewing the academic programs curriculum, course content, and types of learning experiences will provide a general understanding of the content the student has already received and their experiences to this point in their program of study. Not all academic programs complete the didactic content before a student's Level II fieldwork experience. Knowing the content that the student has already received and the content that comes after the fieldwork experience will help adapt specific objectives to the student's current needs. Likewise, knowing the types of active learning experiences the student was involved in will help identify what skills the student may be ready or not ready to demonstrate. These skills could be a combination of technical skills such as assessment administration, implementation of diverse interventions, and soft skills such as developing therapeutic rapport. A good working relationship with the AFWC will provide an opportunity to collaborate on a shared understanding of the site, setting expectations for students, and how the program prepares students for fieldwork. This shared understanding allows the AFWC to identify a student who has the necessary skills to meet the practice setting's unique needs. This will result in experiences that are positive for the FWed and student.

Interview the Student

The next step to finding the right student is to request an interview. An interview is an opportunity to meet the student and identify if they will be a good fit for the practice setting. It also allows the student to self-identify if the site's expectations are a good fit for their learning preferences and needs. The FWed and the student should actively participate in the interview process to provide a reciprocal conversation. Focusing the interview on identifying both parties' characteristics and expectations will increase the likelihood of a good fit and successful fieldwork experience (Short et al., 2018).

There are characteristics of the student and site that increase the likelihood of a good fit and successful fieldwork experience. It is important to understand that just because a student is not a

---

Box 5-4

COLLABORATION MEETING DISCUSSION

Sample Meeting Agenda Items

- Introductions
  - a. FWed should provide information about practice experience, special certifications, history of student fieldwork education, and other relevant experience
  - b. AFWC should provide experience in academia
- Overview of fieldwork program (academic program and site program)
- Specific review of the site practice setting and student fieldwork education opportunities
- Specific review of the academic program requirements for Level II fieldwork education
- Discussion of match between fieldwork site offering and academic program requirements
- Preferred dates and number of students per fieldwork experience and year for Level II fieldwork experiences
  - a. Discuss the site's capacity for student fieldwork experience
  - b. Discuss the academic program's desire for number of student placements and identified fieldwork experience dates
- Administrative policies by the academic program and by the site that may impede development of a memorandum of understanding (or affiliation agreement)
  - a. Examples may include
    - i. Background check requirements
    - ii. Minimum student hours per week
    - iii. Liability, malpractice, or worker's compensation insurance
    - iv. Governing law statements (for sites that are not in the same state as the academic program)
    - v. Required student immunizations

---

good fit does not imply the site is a poor fieldwork experience. Discussing the site's expectations and demands that may be an inherent part of the treated population will help the student understand if they have the soft skills to manage at that site (Short et al., 2018). The interview should include questions or a discussion about the student's learning preferences and expectations of the FWed for the amount and type of feedback provided; see Box 5-5. Furthermore, the FWed can provide the student with their teaching style and resources to assist in the student's learning process. The FWed should be prepared to give the student an understanding of the amount of time that is available in a day for feedback, expectations for student progression, level of knowledge that is needed before starting the fieldwork experience, and other site-specific expectations that may be required for a student to be successful (Short et al., 2018). Some of these expectations or the teaching style can be tailored or discussed on how best to match the student's learning preferences. An open discussion during an interview can help the student and FWed understand if there is a common ground for teaching and learning preferences and if the student can be successful with the specific demands of the practice environment that cannot be modified. To maximize success, the FWed may want to focus on four primary areas of questions: the student's learning preferences, professional interest, confidence level, and preferred rate of progression of skills (Grenier, 2015; Kemp & Crabtree, 2018; Patterson & D'Amico, 2020).

Box 5-5
SAMPLE INTERVIEW QUESTIONS

The student is likely to have a level of anxiety about the interview. To ease the student, start the interview with an introduction of those present, overview of the site, and general overview of the interview process.

General Interview Questions

1. What experiences do you have in a health care setting?

2. What excites you most about Level II fieldwork?

3. What makes you most nervous about Level II fieldwork?

Site-Specific Interview Questions

1. How did you learn about (name of site)?

2. What interests you most about a Level II fieldwork experience at (name of site)?

3. What concerns do you have about a Level II fieldwork experience at (name of site)?

4. What experience do you have working with site population?

5. What makes you stand out from other students to be most qualified for a Level II fieldwork experience at (name of site)?

Fieldwork Supervision Model Interview Questions

1. What is your preferred learning preference?

2. What do you need from a FWed to maximize your learning?

3. How often and in what method do you prefer to receive feedback?

Student Opportunity for Questions

1. What questions do you have about (name of site)?

2. What would you like to know to feel confident that this site is a good fit for your Level II fieldwork education?

End the interview by thanking the student for their time and sharing their experiences. Provide the student with an overview of the next steps in the process and expected timeline of when they can expect to know if they are selected to complete a Level II fieldwork experience at (name of site).

Learning Preference

Ask the student if they have taken personality or learning style assessments such as the Myers-Briggs Type Indicator (MBTI; n.d.) or the Kolb's Learning Styles Inventory (Kolb, 1976). Formal assessments of a student's learning preferences and personality style can provide the FWed with a broader understanding of how the student will learn best. The fieldwork experience and education can be tailored to provide the student with the best experience for success. Other tools and inventories were pointed out in Chapters 3 and 4.

Professional Interest

The ACOTE (2018) standards require that students are exposed to a variety of clients across the lifespan in a variety of settings. Academic programs are allowed to establish criteria of how Level II fieldwork experiences are scheduled. These criteria can vary from a collaborative process between the AFWC and student to identify the student's preferred practice areas to established criteria of specific practice areas that must be completed that align with the academic program's mission. For example, a student may elect to complete one Level II fieldwork experience in a pediatric outpatient facility and the other in a skilled nursing facility. Another academic program may require one experience in a skilled nursing facility and allow choice in the other practice area. The student in the first example may have a desire to work in a skilled nursing facility, while the student in the second example may not have a desire to work in a skilled nursing facility. This may impact a student's overall response to that experience (Andonian, 2013). The student who wants to experience fieldwork in a skilled nursing facility may be more motivated and confident. The second student may struggle more in these areas and need a different level of supervision and guidance to support their progression through the fieldwork experience.

Confidence Level

A student's confidence level is multifaceted. Confidence, or perceived self-efficacy, has been shown to have a positive correlation with the "male gender, being on a second or third internship, and the meaningfulness of the fieldwork [i.e., the perception of the educational value associated with the fieldwork]" (Andonian, 2013, p. 209). Another aspect of confidence is the student's perceived competence. Improving a student's competence can come through a process of making the student feel welcome through a sense of belonging to the team (Berg-Poppe et al., 2017).

Progression of Skills

Students will demonstrate a varying level of preferences to advance their fieldwork expectations based upon multiple factors, including their learning preferences, interest in the population, and confidence level. However, the student may need to be challenged to progress their skills based upon the practice area needs and find a just-right challenge for the student to progress when they may lack the self-efficacy to progress independently. Use of a guide of expected student progression and understanding where flexibility is possible will help guide questions to determine if a student can meet those expectations.

Host Students for a Trial Experience

After the interview is complete, an additional step that can solidify a student's fit with the site is to host the student for an experience on-site. The FWed may invite the student to spend a half-day, full-day, or even to complete a Level I fieldwork experience at the site. During the on-site experience, the FWed may dedicate time to meet with the student for an interview. This method will reduce the time needed if both components are preferred. The addition of an on-site experience provides an opportunity for the student and FWed to trial the fit by gaining a better understanding of the expectations of the site and characteristics of the student (Barlow et al., 2020; Evenson et al., 2002).

The option to host a student for a full Level I fieldwork experience prior to accepting the students for a Level II fieldwork is termed the *same-site model*. The same-site model provides an extended experience for a trial over what is observable in a half-day or full-day experience. Through the same-site model, students gain a familiarity with the site that will help to gain confidence and decrease anxiety (Evenson et al., 2002). The same-site model does not require a change in the typical Level I fieldwork structure. The same expectations of a typical Level I fieldwork can be carried out, but with the intent to provide the student and FWed an opportunity to become more familiar with each other, the student to feel more comfortable in the setting and ultimately to determine if it is a good fit for the student's Level II fieldwork experience.

The key to a successful same-site model program is to work collaboratively with the educational program's AFWC. The collaboration will allow the AFWC and FWed to create a plan that outlines clear expectations for the process. The student must be aware that the expectation is to complete one Level I fieldwork experience at the site. Furthermore, expectations to identify a good fit and acceptance or denial of a Level II fieldwork experience will provide a timely and clear response. Many programs confirm Level II fieldwork experiences well before completion of Level I fieldwork experience. The same-site model may be an exception to that typical process but feasible with good planning and collaboration. The same-site model has also been found to be a favorable process, so the AFWC may find it in the student's best interest to forgo the typical timeline for Level II fieldwork confirmation (Barlow et al., 2020).

Provide Site-Specific Expectations

The interview process and same-site model for a trial experience may not prove to be a feasible option at all sites. A less time-consuming option that may be used in place of the interview or same-site model or in conjunction with these methods is to provide a formal and transparent fieldwork expectations document (Short et al., 2018). In collaboration with the AFWC, the site may supply an expectations document that outlines the minimum qualities and skills a student must possess to succeed. These may be general skills that all students must have to be prepared for Level II fieldwork or specific skills that are unique to the site's population and environment. See Chapter 4 for more information on how to create effective learning objectives.

General Skills

The accreditation standards for all occupational therapy programs require a minimum standard of outcomes that all students must meet exclusive of Level II fieldwork, the Baccalaureate Project, and the Doctoral Capstone expectations (ACOTE, 2018). These outcomes are the B Standards and include:

- B.1.0: Foundational content
- B.2.0: Occupational therapy theoretical perspectives
- B.3.0: Basic tenets of occupational therapy
- B.4.0:
  - Doctoral and Master's Degree Level only:
    - Referral, screening, evaluation, and intervention planning
    - Intervention plan: Formulation and implementation
  - Baccalaureate and Associate Degree Level only:
    - Screening, evaluation, and intervention plan
    - Intervention and implementation
- B.5.0: Context of service delivery, leadership, and management of occupational therapy services
- B.6.0: Scholarship
- B.7.0: Professional ethics, values, and responsibilities

Each academic program identifies a method to meet the standards in these seven core areas of occupational therapy education. Each standard requires a different level of skill acquisition that ranges from demonstration of knowledge, demonstration of ability, to application, analysis, and evaluation of the content. The AFWC of the academic program can provide support to synthesize the understanding of these standards and how the students meet the content in their program.

Specific Skills

Each practice setting and facility will have unique requirements that will draw on different accreditation B Standards areas. In collaboration with the AFWC, it may be helpful to examine which standards are the primary skills the student will need. This can be taken a step further to identify if the practice setting or site requires an additional level of skills specific to the patient population's needs and site-specific policies. For example, one core objective that may be of importance at the facility is the occupational therapy student's ability to "B.4.5 select and apply assessment tools, considering client needs, and cultural and contextual factors" (ACOTE, 2018, p. 29). The FWed may identify specific skills by identifying specific assessment tools the student will need to select from to use in relation to specific cultural and contextual factors unique to the patient population in that setting. Additional specific skills may also include advancing the level of demonstration the student may need to be successful in the specific practice setting. For example, the occupational therapy assistant student may need to not only "B.1.1 demonstrate knowledge of the structure and function of the human body" (ACOTE, 2018, p. 25) but also apply that knowledge specific to the hand for outpatient therapy services. This specific skill will be developed during Level II fieldwork through active learning and resources provided by the FWed.

STEP #2: STUDENT PREPARATIONS

After you have agreed to take a student for a Level II fieldwork experience, steps can be taken to help prepare the student before their first day on site. The student can prepare by reviewing materials and meeting with the FWed to introduce the site. This method helps provide the student with a better sense of confidence in their preparation, reducing any concerns or anxiousness about this significant step in their academic journey. A few ways to prepare the student and the FWed are to ask the student to complete the AOTA Personal Data Sheet, provide a list of recommended resources to review, provide a list of responses to commonly asked questions, and schedule a pre-fieldwork meeting.

AOTA Personal Data Sheet

The Personal Data Sheet is provided by AOTA (1999) as a free resource on the website (www.aota.org) under the "Resources for Fieldwork Education" section. The student completes the data sheet to provide the FWed with information about the student's education, health information, past work or volunteer experiences, strengths, areas for growth, learning and supervision preferences, housing and transportation needs, and other fieldwork experiences. The AOTA Personal Data Sheet can be used as an initial introduction to the student. The information provided by the student is a starting point for understanding the student's foundational knowledge and areas to further develop during their fieldwork experience. It is also a valuable tool to begin a conversation with the student before or at the start of their fieldwork experience.

Ask the student to complete this assessment prior to an interview or on-site experience as a means to spark conversation about their past experiences and how they prefer to gain knowledge and receive feedback. It can also be used during orientation to identify areas the student feels more confident and areas where the student may want more experience or support to achieve the desired competency level. The FWed can collaborate with the student to tailor the fieldwork experience to the student's needs. Students may be hesitant to share information at first if they feel overwhelmed. Providing this information in writing before the beginning of the experience may give the FWed a foundation for the initial conversations to help the student feel welcome. Taking a vested interest in the student can facilitate a more positive experience (Grenier, 2015). Occupational therapy

---

Box 5-6

STUDENT RESOURCES FOR GAINING
FOUNDATIONAL KNOWLEDGE

Internet Resources
- Facility website
- National organization website
- Standardized assessment or protocol website

Textbooks or Journal Articles
- Books specific to the site patient population
- Books that provide information about a specific intervention protocol
- Foundational studies for the site's occupational therapy services
- Articles that outline literature to provide greater understanding of the site's occupational therapy services or patient population

Site-Specific Information
- Overview of the site's general procedures and policies
- List of commonly used assessment or evaluation methods
- Description of the site's patient population
- Outline of the occupational therapy services provided
- Site-specific objectives
- Weekly expectations for student progression

---

programs that use a database or online platform to support fieldwork (e.g., EXXAT, e-value) might provide an electronic link to the FWed in advance of the placement containing a student profile.

Provide Recommended Resources List

A second means to prepare the student is to ask them to review specific resources that may provide foundational knowledge that will benefit their learning at the site. These resources may be particular websites, reading materials, commonly used assessments, interventions, or other site-specific protocols or materials; see Box 5-6. Direct the student to your facility's website with specific focus on reviewing your facility's mission and vision, services provided, patient resources that may help provide a picture of the aim and focus of the services, and the links to external resources that the facility has deemed as important resources for clients and health professionals. Directing the student to these specific resources provides the student with a foundational understanding of the primary areas to focus on in their preparation. It also allows the FWed to start the learning process before fieldwork and allows the student a starting point for their learning to develop a more active role earlier in the process. This model of assigning preparatory learning activities is consistent with current teaching pedagogies such as the flipped classroom model, which many occupational therapy students will be familiar with from their didactic preparation. In this approach, the FWed can then build on the knowledge acquired during the preparatory learning activities to bolster understanding of the content in daily practice on fieldwork.

Box 5-7

COMMONLY ASKED STUDENT QUESTIONS

- What time should I arrive each day?
- Where should I park?
- What is the dress code?
- What does a typical workday look like?
- What assessments, interventions, or other protocols should I know?
- Do you require a presentation or other assignments?
- How often do I meet with my FWed?
- Do you know of possible housing options?
- What is the best transportation in the area?
- Do I need to travel to multiple sites?
- What is the expected schedule?
- What are the student requirements or training modules (e.g., medical, security)?

Provide an FAQ Resource

An additional resource that can be helpful to students is a list of commonly asked questions. This list can be derived from necessary information about the site, population receiving occupational therapy services at the site, and from students' questions in the past; see Box 5-7. The list can be organized in many ways but should be specific to the site and what the FWed wants the student to know before the fieldwork experience. One method to organize the list is to start with questions about the site, then questions about what to expect on day 1, and then questions about the fieldwork experience flow. This progression of questions and answers will give the student a good overview of preparing for their fieldwork experience. The questions may also be the foundation for more in-depth questions that allow the student to gain a richer understanding of the site without feeling they are asking too many questions. The questions they ask can be focused on more specific content and of greater depth.

Fieldwork sites can proactively create an FAQ resource to provide to students in advance of the experience. This FAQ document should be a live document and continued to be added to as new questions arise from students.

Schedule a Pre-Fieldwork Meeting

Another means to prepare the student is to schedule a meeting to introduce yourself, get to know the student better, and review the materials you have sent the student. If the meeting is timed to allow the student an opportunity to complete the AOTA Personal Data Sheet (1999) and review the resource list and commonly asked questions beforehand, the meeting should be more productive. The FWed will be ready with specific follow-up questions based upon the student's information. The student will be able to ask questions about what they want to know more about how to prepare. If the student can feel secure about their preparation, it may boost their confidence before the first day. It may also provide the student with the assurance that the FWed is vested in their learning and open to collaborating with the student for an effective supervision style tailored to their learning preferences. If the student feels welcome with a FWed that is open to their needs, it will facilitate a more positive fieldwork experience (Grenier, 2015). A survey completed in 2015 by Grenier found that students valued an experience with a FWed who was open and positive, had a structured method of feedback and learning objectives, accommodated the students' learning preferences, provided a space for students, and valued other personnel who treated the student like they were part of the team. For the students, it made the difference in facilitating a successful experience (Grenier, 2015).

STEP #3: WELCOME TO FIELDWORK!

The student has been prepared up to this point by the processes identified for finding a good fit and providing the student with pre-fieldwork resources. Now it is time to prepare the student for a positive fieldwork experience by planning the first day or days of fieldwork that welcome the student into the site and provide clear expectations of what to expect throughout the experience. This process may be predetermined, but infusing opportunities for collaboration with the student to flex some of the activities that will occur throughout their experience provides a more positive fieldwork (Grenier, 2015). Three ways to initiate the process are (1) providing a structured orientation, (2) weekly expectations document, and (3) establishing a meeting schedule. These components can be the foundational content to create a fieldwork manual supplied to the student on the first day. This process is similar to the onboarding process for a new hire to the facility (Rodger et al., 2011). The student will view a site that facilitates this welcoming environment to bring them into the team as a more positive experience (Grenier, 2015).

Orientation

Students appreciate a scheduled orientation session to provide information about the site, introductions to other staff, and orientation to commonly accessed spaces and equipment. Orientation should be a planned time for an initial introduction to the facility and an ongoing process, especially if it is large or has multiple locations. The process of a continuous orientation allows the student to learn over time and not become overwhelmed with everything all in one day. It may also be more feasible with daily tasks and caseload to spread out the orientation over a period of time than to schedule one solid space of time (Rodger et al., 2011).

The orientation will be best organized by including a list of items to cover as part of the fieldwork manual. At a minimum, plan to orient the student to therapy staff and other health care professionals they will interact with regularly, tour the facility, orient the student to common spaces for equipment and assessments, and educate about the documentation system. One method to create the orientation schedule is to use the AOTA Student Evaluation of the Fieldwork Experience (SEFWE) as a guide (AOTA, 2016). Key topics identified in the SEFWE to cover in orientation are site-specific objectives, student supervision process, requirements/assignments, sample schedule, site policies and procedures, documentation procedures, and safety and emergency procedures (AOTA, 2016). Other categories in the SEFWE may also be helpful to identify areas to cover in orientation and beyond. As the student progresses in their autonomy, additional orientation may be needed to provide the student with a higher-level orientation to the documentation system, standard operating procedures, and other required administrative tasks.

Weekly Expectations

As part of the orientation and as a physical list in the fieldwork manual, the FWed should include an identified list of weekly expectations. As discussed in Chapter 4, these expectations are best identified as a weekly guide to how they should progress in their skills and autonomy. Skills that the student should achieve at key intervals in their fieldwork experience should be specific to the site (Grenier, 2015; Rodger et al., 2011). One method to develop the expectations is to identify the expectations of a student who has met entry, generalist-level skills in that setting. This level of skill would be the expectations for the final week of fieldwork. Then complete what would be expected of the student at midterm time. Next, identify the point which the student would be expected to start to gain skills related to the identified objectives for the fieldwork experience. These may be skills such as session planning, interventions, documentation, evaluations, and billing. The skills should be developed through a graded process of development (Grenier, 2015; Rodger et al., 2011). It is best to align the expectations with the identified objectives and student evaluation form used. This alignment will ensure the student is meeting all expectations determined by the academic program and accreditation requirements.

Establish a Meeting Schedule

A final important component of welcoming the student to fieldwork is to collaborate on a meeting schedule (Grenier, 2015). There may be a minimum expected amount and type of meeting already established, but the student may request additional meetings to meet their learning preferences. This schedule may vary as the fieldwork progresses and includes different discussions based on the meeting's identified purpose. There should be scheduled meetings to review the student evaluations at midterm and final. Additionally, formal meetings regularly to review the student's progress can help the student gauge how they are progressing in their skills development. These meetings should occur on a regular basis that fits the needs of everyone involved. An example could be scheduled meetings every Friday at the end of the workday, Thursdays over lunch, or first thing Monday mornings. The schedule could evolve as the fieldwork progresses. Fewer meetings may be needed as the student becomes more autonomous. Conversely, if the meetings are scheduled every other week, the student may need more frequent meetings to support their learning preferences or need for added support. To help structure the formal meetings, a student progress form can be used to share feedback in writing that the student can review throughout the week. This form should provide areas of strength, areas to improve or focus on in the next week, goals to achieve, and tasks or activities to complete; see Appendix B for an example weekly student progress form. Additional informal meetings may also provide the student with a way to assess their progress. These informal meetings may be scheduled or impromptu as the student needs greater assistance initially or as they progress to a higher-level skill. Developing an agreed-upon time for these impromptu meetings helps the student understand the most appropriate time to ask questions or receive feedback (Grenier, 2015; Kemp & Crabtree, 2018; Patterson & D'Amico, 2020; Rodger et al., 2011).

SUMMARY

Through a seven-step process, found in Appendix C, the success of the student and FWed can lead to long-term benefits that are well worth the time investment. The first three steps involve review of the site, self-analysis, and goal setting. Conducting a reflective analysis of the site and oneself is the foundation of building a program that provides the best outcome potential for the student and the most rewarding experience as a FWed. The analysis identifies the tasks to complete or goals to meet to achieve the desired fieldwork program. The fourth step is to develop a fieldwork manual to guide the experience for the student and the FWed. The final three steps are the process of identifying the right fit based upon the work completed in the first five steps. Promoting the right fit between the student and the site is a three-step process of identifying the right student, preparing the student, and welcoming the student to fieldwork. Utilizing this seven-step process can provide an opportunity for long-term success of student education that benefits the student, site, and FWed.

Level II fieldwork education can be a very rewarding role for any occupational therapy practitioner. It offers the opportunity to give back to the profession, a motivation to maintain one's professional development, and a potential source of recruiting (Hanson, 2011). It can be challenging to supervise a student who is not prepared for Level II fieldwork because it can lead to additional time required and difficulty helping the student navigate a potentially negative fieldwork experience (Hanson, 2011; Varland et al., 2017). Developing a structured fieldwork program at the site through collaboration with the academic program can lead to a more positive experience for the FWed and student. Identifying the necessary skills and level of commitment a student may need to be successful at the site, whether it is a general or specific population treated at the site, sets everyone up for success.

LEARNING ACTIVITIES

1. Use the process outlined in Box 5-1 to develop a needs assessment of your site to identify the areas of strength and weakness currently in your fieldwork program.

2. How can you establish a path for a successful student by outlining the ideal student in the areas of learning preferences, professional interest, confidence level, and preferred rate of progression of skills?

    a. How would you provide structure for a student who does not meet the ideal description in these areas?

3. Develop a plan to establish a protocol of identifying a student who is a good fit for your site. Use the three-step process of finding the right student, preparing the student, and welcoming the student through orientation to identify what techniques will work best for your facility.

    a. Create a step-by-step interview process that fits the needs of your site based upon the SWOT analysis. These steps may include collaborating with the AFWC, interviewing the student, hosting the student for a trial experience, and providing a list site-specific expectations.

    b. Establish a protocol or checklist of items for the student to provide. These items may include the AOTA Personal Data Sheet, a list of recommended resources to review, a list of responses to commonly asked questions, and a scheduled pre-fieldwork meeting.

    c. Create a document or fieldwork binder with details about orientation, weekly expectations, and a meeting schedule to provide the student during the first week of Level II fieldwork.

REFERENCES

Accreditation Council for Occupational Therapy Education [ACOTE]. (2018). 2018 Accreditation Council for Occupational Therapy Education (ACOTE®) Standards and Interpretive Guide. https://acoteonline.org/accreditation-explained/standards/

American Occupational Therapy Association. (1999). Personal data sheet. https://www.aota.org/Education-Careers/Fieldwork/Supervisor.aspx

American Occupational Therapy Association. (2009). The American Occupational Therapy Association self-assessment tool for fieldwork educator competency. https://www.aota.org/Education-Careers/Fieldwork/Supervisor.aspx

American Occupational Therapy Association. (2012). COE guidelines for an occupational therapy fieldwork experience – Level II. https://www.aota.org/Education-Careers/Fieldwork/LevelII.aspx

American Occupational Therapy Association. (2016). Student evaluation of the fieldwork experience. https://www.aota.org/Education-Careers/Fieldwork/StuSuprvsn.aspx

Andonian, L. (2013). Emotional intelligence, self-efficacy, and occupational therapy students' fieldwork performance. Occupational Therapy in Health Care, 27(2), 201-2015. https://doi.org/10.3109/07380577.2012.763199

Barlow, K. G., Salemi, M., & Taylor, C. (2020). Implementing the same site model in occupational therapy fieldwork: Student and fieldwork educator perspectives. *Journal of Occupational Therapy Education, 4*(3). https://doi.org/10.26681/jote.2020.040307

Berg-Poppe, P. J., Karges, J. R., Nissen, R., Deutsch, S., & Webster, K. (2017). Relationship between occupational and physical therapist students' belongingness and perceived competence in the clinic using the Ascent to Competence Scale. *Journal of Occupational Therapy Education, 1*(3). https://doi.org/10.26681/jote.2017.010303

Evenson, M., Barnes, M. A., & Cohn, E. S. (2002). Brief report–Perceptions of Level I and Level II fieldwork in the same site. *American Occupational Therapy Association, 56,* 103-106. https://doi.org/10.5014/ajot.56.1.103

Flecky, K., Doll, J., & Scaffa, M. E. (2020). Community-based and population health program development. In M. E. Scaffa & S. M. Reitz (Eds.), *Occupational therapy in community and population health practice* (3rd ed., pp. 73-93). F.A. Davis.

Grenier, M.-L. (2015). Facilitators and barriers to learning in occupational therapy fieldwork education: Student perspectives. *American Journal of Occupational Therapy, 69*(Suppl. 2), 6912185070. https://doi.org/10.5014/ajot.2015.015180

Hanson, D. J. (2011). The perspectives of fieldwork educators regarding level II fieldwork students. *Occupational Therapy in Health Care, 25*(2-3), 164-177. https://doi.org/10.3109/07380577.2011.561420

Kemp, E. L., & Crabtree, J. L. (2018). Differentiating fieldwork settings: Matching student characteristics to demands. *Occupational Therapy in Health Care, 32*(3), 216-229. https://doi.org/10.1080/07380577.2018.1491084

Kolb, D. A. (1976). *The Learning Style Inventory: Technical Manual.* McBer.

Myers & Briggs Foundation, The [MBTI]. (n.d.). Retrieved February 25, 2021, from https://www.myersbriggs.org/

Patterson, B., & D'Amico, M. (2020). What does the evidence say about student, fieldwork educator, and new occupational therapy practitioner perceptions of successful level II fieldwork and transition to practice? A scoping review. *Journal of Occupational Therapy Education, 4*(2). https://doi.org/10.26681/jote.2020.040210

Rodger, S., Fitzgerald, C., Davila, W., Millar, W., & Allison, H. (2011). What makes a quality occupational therapy practice placement? Students' and practice educators' perspectives. *Australian Occupational Therapy Journal, 58,* 195-2020. https://doi.org/10.1111/j.1440-1630.2010.00903.x

Short, N., Sample, S., Murphy, M., Austin, B., & Glass, J. (2018). Barriers and solutions to fieldwork education in hand therapy. *Journal of Hand Therapy,* 308-314. https://doi.org/10.1016/j.jht.2017.05.013

Varland, J., Cardell, E., Koski, J., & McFadden, M. (2017). Factors influencing occupational therapists' decision to supervise fieldwork students. *Occupational Therapy in Health Care, 31*(3), 238-254. https://doi.org/10.1080/07380577.2017.1328631.

APPENDIX A
Sample Structure for a Fieldwork Site Manual

1. Introduction to the facility mission and vision (and core values as appropriate)
2. Staff resource page: Include staff names, department or unit, specialty areas, years of experience as a practitioner, years of experience as a FWed, and contact information for staff the student will be most commonly interacting with during their experience
3. Important contact information
    a. This may include numbers or codes to the different units, emergency, and facility paging system
4. Policies and procedures
5. Overview of the services (or service lines) provided by the occupational therapy department
    a. Include listing of resources for reference materials
6. Student expectations
    a. Student-specific information about daily schedule, dress code, documentation, etc.
    b. Student requirements, such as background checks, immunization and other requirements, such as CPR training
    c. Assignments or other projects to be completed by students
    d. Weekly expectation for progression
    e. Protocols for scheduled meetings to discuss student progress
    f. Expectations for resolving conflict between student and FWed
7. Appendices for student forms or other documents

APPENDIX B
Sample Weekly Meeting Forms

University of North Dakota
Occupational Therapy Student Weekly Review Form

Student Name _____

Fieldwork Educator Name _____

Date _____ Week # _____

FUNDAMENTAL BASIC TENETS OF PRACTICE	
Areas of Strength	**Areas of Need**
EVALUATION AND SCREENING	
Areas of Strength	**Areas of Need**
INTERVENTION	
Areas of Strength	**Areas of Need**
MANAGEMENT OF OCCUPATIONAL THERAPY SERVICES	
Areas of Strength	**Areas of Need**
COMMUNICATION/PROFESSIONAL BEHAVIORS	
Areas of Strength	**Areas of Need**

PROGRESS SUMMARY

STUDENT LEARNING GOALS

Student Initiated Objectives	Activities to Achieve Goals	Desired Fieldwork Educator Support
1.		
2.		
3.		

FIELDWORK SCHEDULE REVISIONS

ADDITIONAL STUDENT SUPPORT NEEDED

FWed Signature _____   Date _____

Student Signature _____   Date _____

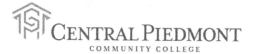

CENTRAL PIEDMONT
COMMUNITY COLLEGE

Fieldwork Weekly Feedback Form

Occupational Therapy Assistant Program – Level II Fieldwork

Student and FWE both complete a form prior to weekly feedback meetings. Use the results to promote dialogue and collaborate on goals for the following week(s).

Student Name	Week #	Date

Strengths and Successes this Week:

Areas for Growth:

Goals:

Signatures

Student Signature:	
FWE Signature:	

Central Piedmont Community College | P.O. Box 35009, Charlotte, NC 28235-5009 | cpcc.edu

APPENDIX C

Sample Fieldwork Program Development Process

- **Step 1:** Conduct a SWOT analysis to identify areas of strength and areas for growth
- **Step 2:** Utilize the results of the SWOT analysis to identify tasks to complete to develop the fieldwork program at the facility
- **Step 3:** Develop personal goal to strengthen your skills as a FWed
- **Step 4:** Create a site-specific fieldwork manual with all required documents and policies and procedures to guide the student fieldwork experience
- **Step 5:** Utilize all available resources and information gained from prior steps to develop a process of finding a student that is a good fit for the site. In this process, consider these steps:
  a. Collaborate with the AFWC
  b. Interview the student
  c. Host the student for a trial experience
  d. Provide site-specific expectations
- **Step 6:** Provide the student with materials to prepare for their Level II fieldwork experience. Consider the following documents to assist with the preparation process for the student and yourself:
  a. Ask the student to complete the AOTA Personal Data Sheet
  b. Provide the student a list of recommended resources
  c. Provide the student a list of frequently asked questions
  d. Schedule a pre-fieldwork meeting to review questions and review recommendations to prepare for the first day of fieldwork
- **Step 7:** Help the student feel welcome on day 1 by providing a structured orientation, weekly expectations document, and establishing a meeting schedule

Unit II

Supporting the Student During a Level II Fieldwork

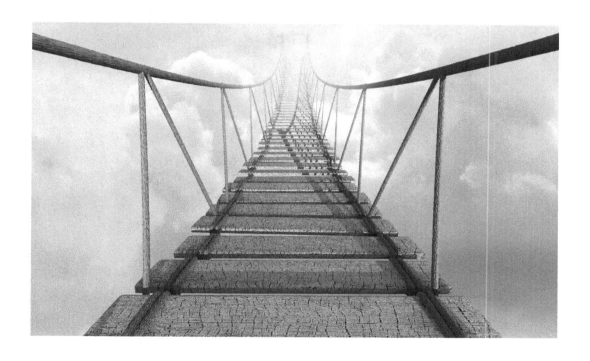

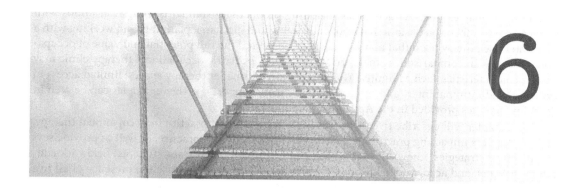

Mentoring in Professional Best Practices During the Level II Fieldwork Experience

Cherie Graves, PhD, OTR/L
and Hannah Oldenburg, EdD, OTR/L, BCPR

The previous chapters have led you through the process of getting ready to host a Level II field-work student. Now that you have thought about the pieces leading up to student arrival, you may be asking yourself, "*What do I do next?*" This chapter will provide practical strategies to mentor students in the professional best practices throughout the Level II fieldwork experience. The *Occupational Therapy Practice Framework: Domain and Process, Fourth Edition* (*OTPF-4*; American Occupational Therapy Association [AOTA], 2020a) identifies the "cornerstones" of occupational therapy practice as "something of great importance on which everything else depends" (p. 6). Further, "contributors" in occupational therapy practice provide a foundation for practitioners and directly influence each cornerstone (AOTA, 2020a). The five best practice principles woven throughout this chapter are each identified as one of the "contributors" highlighted in the *OTPF-4*. These include (1) client-centered practice, (2) cultural humility, (3) ethics, (4) evidence-informed practice, and (5) occupation-based practice. The integration of these five principles ensures the provision of professional best practice in the field of occupational therapy.

As mentioned in the Level I fieldwork text (Oldenburg & Graves, 2022) occupational therapy students often report discrepancy between what was observed in practice and the best practice principles learned during coursework (Clarke et al., 2014, 2015; Ripat et al., 2013; Towns & Ashby, 2014). Level II fieldwork provides a more in-depth experience and students quickly observe and personally encounter the day-to-day demands occupational therapy practitioners face when providing services to clients. Each practice context presents unique characteristics contributing to the challenge of providing services that integrate the five principles of best practice. For example, a large acute

DeIuliis, E. D., & Hanson, D. (Eds.).
Fieldwork Educator's Guide to Level II Fieldwork (pp. 163-201).
© 2023 Taylor & Francis Group.

care hospital may exhibit characteristics including productivity standards, time restrictions with patients, narrow focus on basic activities of daily living and discharge planning, and working with a large interdisciplinary team that may or may not understand the full potential and value of occupational therapy. In comparison, a small private outpatient pediatric occupational therapy clinic may exhibit characteristics such as limited available resources, smaller therapy spaces, limited access to evidence, and minimal inter- and intradisciplinary team support. Further examples can be seen in the mini vignettes provided in the Appendices.

This chapter will describe five principles of professional best practice in occupational therapy, identify barriers impacting practitioners' ability to implement best practice, as well as provide several practical strategies, knowledge resources, and learning tools to assist students, fieldwork educators (FWeds), and academic fieldwork coordinators (AFWCs) to increase the presence of all five principles into the day-to-day experience for both practitioners and fieldwork students.

LEARNING OBJECTIVES

By the end of reading this chapter and completing the learning activities, the reader should be able to:

1. Articulate the five best practice principles of the occupational therapy profession.
2. Describe the value of integrating best practice principles into practice and Level II fieldwork experiences.
3. Analyze and reflect on your practice setting's culture and beliefs for best practice in delivering occupational therapy services.
4. Apply strategies to overcome barriers and facilitate best practice principles during Level II fieldwork and practice.
5. Apply teaching and learning methods and activities that foster growth in best practice principles during Level II fieldwork.

BACKGROUND

This first section of the chapter will provide a brief literature review to help the FWed build a strong foundation of the five best practices principles.

Best Practice Principles

The occupational therapy profession has been philosophically guided from the beginning, with a belief in *client-centered practice* (Bing, 1981). While there have been a variety of definitions for client-centered practice in the literature, most share common tenets including establishing an effective partnership and collaboration with clients, encouraging shared decision making, respecting diversity, recognizing power, and identifying strategies to realign and equally distribute power in the therapeutic relationship (Law et al., 1995; Sumsion & Law, 2006).

Like client-centered practice, the focus on occupation has been around since the beginning of the profession when founding members believed in the value of occupation as a treatment modality (Meyer, 1922, 1977). This belief has evolved into the core belief of the profession emphasizing the positive relationship between occupation and health (AOTA, 2020a). *Occupation-based practice* occurs when a practitioner uses evaluation and interventions to engage a client in occupation (Fisher & Marterella, 2019). To practice from an occupation-based perspective, one must first understand the meaning of occupation, specifically to the client they are providing services to.

TABLE 6-1
BARRIERS TO BEST PRACTICE PRINCIPLES

INSTITUTIONAL BARRIERS	Lack of time, space/storage, supplies; philosophical perspective
ORGANIZATIONAL BARRIERS	Lack of support, power differentials, workplace culture
PERSONAL BARRIERS	Lack of skills, lack of creativity, personal mindset

Decades after the founding of occupational therapy, the medical model gained strength increasing the emphasis on scientific evidence. By the 1980s *evidence-based practice* had emerged in the medical field and slowly gained traction in occupational therapy in the late 1990s. Evidence-based practice is described as the process in which practitioners develop a question, search the evidence, evaluate the evidence, and implement the evidence while considering the wishes of the client and their family (Law & MacDermid, 2014).

With practice setting demands and the complexity of serving the health care needs of others, practitioners are posed with making *ethical practice* decisions to ensure occupational therapy services are delivered in a manner that is safe, beneficial, accurate, and true to the occupational therapy profession's core values. The AOTA *Code of Ethics* (2020b) is a guide that occupational therapy practitioners use in their decision making for various scenarios that may occur across practice settings and clientele interactions. The guide highlights Core Values, Ethical Principles, and Standards of Conduct that occupational therapy practitioners are expected to follow in their daily practice. The six ethical principles include beneficence, nonmaleficence, autonomy, justice, veracity, and fidelity (AOTA, 2020b).

There are many times that ethical considerations may dictate the direction the educator, practitioner, or student may make in their decision making to ensure *culturally relevant practice*. The World Federation of Occupational Therapy (WFOT; 2010) acknowledges that each client presents with unique social, cultural, psychological, biological, financial, political, and spiritual elements that practitioners need to consider when assessing a client's performance and participation in occupation. Furthermore, the federation promotes that occupational therapists should practice in regard to their own beliefs, values, and practices (WFOT, 2010).

Despite the prominence of the professional best practice principles in academic training, discrepancies continue to exist between that training and current practice. For example, Ashby et al. (2016) surveyed students internationally and found that 97% of students considered occupation-based practice to be an important factor in being an occupational therapist, and 64% of students identified discrepancies between their expectations of occupation-based practice and what was observed during practice. Although students have the foundational knowledge to provide best practice, they may not anticipate the barriers that naturally exist in practice.

Barriers to Best Practice Principles

Several sources in the literature identify barriers experienced by clinicians, contributing to difficulty implementing the best practice principles into client care. While each of the best practice principles have unique barriers, they often share some of the same barriers and can be grouped into institutional barriers, organizational barriers, and personal barriers. See Table 6-1 for common barriers experienced in practice and identified in the literature. Activities to facilitate

TABLE 6-2
SIGNIFICANCE OF BEST PRACTICE PRINCIPLES

	HOW DO I DO IT?	WHY SHOULD I DO IT?
EVIDENCE-BASED PRACTICE	• Develop a question, search and evaluate the evidence, implement the evidence, while considering the wishes of the client and their family (Law & MacDermid, 2014).	• Improves client outcomes at a quicker rate, ultimately saving health care dollars (Wilkinson et al., 2012).
CLIENT-CENTERED PRACTICE	• Enhance skills in therapeutic use of self, using the Intentional Relationship Model (Taylor, 2020). • Demonstrate professional behaviors and dispositions such as collaboration, empathy, and humility (AOTA, 2020a). • Challenge the status quo or the institutional culture that does not value client-centered practice.	• Greater patient satisfaction; improved patient compliance; improved treatment outcomes (Korner & Modell, 2009; Plewnia et al., 2016; Zimmerman et al., 2014).

(continued)

understanding of site-specific supports and barriers to implementation of best practice principles can be found in Appendices A and B.

Significance of Best Practice Principles

The best practice principles are identified as contributors of occupational therapy practice, meaning they impact the cornerstones and provide a foundation for practitioners (AOTA, 2020a). The presence of these cornerstones and contributors helps distinguish occupational therapy from other professions. At a time when health care costs are highly scrutinized, it is imperative that the value and distinct nature of the occupational therapy profession is evident in the services provided. Table 6-2 provides a brief explanation for how to engage in best practice as well as why it is important to the profession.

INTEGRATING BEST PRACTICE PRINCIPLES DURING LEVEL II FIELDWORK

Now that the FWed has a foundation of knowledge of what the best practice principles are, let's explore approaches of how to integrate these into the Level II fieldwork experience.

TABLE 6-2 (CONTINUED)

SIGNIFICANCE OF BEST PRACTICE PRINCIPLES

	HOW DO I DO IT?	WHY SHOULD I DO IT?
OCCUPATION-BASED PRACTICE	• Gather occupational history and occupations that are of concern (occupational profile). • Identify resources that are available to you (either from yourself, workplace, or the client). • Challenge the status quo or the institutional culture that does not value or use occupation-based practice	• It is our distinct value that advances the understanding of occupational therapy. • It separates us from other members of the interdisciplinary team. • More enjoyable, rewarding, effective, and client- and family-centered (Estes & Pierce, 2012). • Strengthens professional identity (Ashby et al., 2013; Estes & Pierce, 2012).
ETHICAL PRACTICE	• Identify and challenge the ethical scenarios with the principles and values of the occupational therapy profession. • Apply AOTA *Code of Ethics* principles when managing ethical considerations with use of the principles and values in your decision making.	• Upholds occupational therapy values and trust with delivering occupational therapy services with clients, groups, and populations. • Supports clinical reasoning to ensure ethical decisions are rooted in principles and values of occupational therapy profession (AOTA, 2020b).
CULTURALLY RELEVANT PRACTICE	• Identify cultural perspectives that support and inhibit occupational engagement across the lifespan. • Reflect on self and environment to be aware of bias that may inhibit occupational engagement. • Demonstrate an attitude and intelligence that is receptive and knowledgeable on cultural aspects at a micro and macro level.	• Strengthen therapeutic relationship with client and optimize client-centered approach. • Ensures individualized care that is inclusive of norms, beliefs, attitudes, and behaviors of different cultural groups (AOTA, 2020a). • Challenges practitioners to be lifelong learners of cultural relevance and knowledge to ensure safety and intelligence that is supportive of the unique needs of the client (AOTA, 2020a).

TABLE 6-3

EXPLORING THE MEANING OF OCCUPATION WITH YOUR CLIENT

INDIVIDUAL	FAMILY	COMMUNITY
What do you do as an individual to occupy your time?	What do you do as a family to occupy time?	What do you do as a community (or in your community) to occupy time?
What do you do as an individual that brings you meaning?	What do you do as a family that brings meaning?	What do you do as a community (or in your community) that brings meaning?
What do you do as an individual that brings purpose to your life?	What do you do as a family that brings purpose to life?	What do you do as a community (or in your community) that brings purpose to life?

Integration of Occupation-Based Practice

Starting the fieldwork with openness to collaboration and viewing the experience as a two-way learning opportunity will set the FWed and students up for a valuable learning experience leading to a win-win situation. Hosting fieldwork students has several perks, one of which is sharing new ideas and resources with the fieldwork site (Evenson et al., 2015; Hanson, 2011; Thomas et al., 2007). Students bring new and creative ways of thinking about situations, which allows fresh perspectives and innovation. Over time it is natural for professionals to settle into a comfortable routine, which may limit creativity with providing occupation-based care. FWeds should view hosting a student as an opportunity to freshen up their ideas and to re-engage with professional best practice and their own professional identity as an occupational therapy practitioner.

The integration of occupation into fieldwork learning can be supported by the FWed, student, and AFWC. The FWed can support occupation by guiding the student to develop an understanding of their client as an occupational being. Some questions that may guide the conversation to identify the personal meaning of occupation can be seen in Table 6-3.

Once the occupational therapy practitioner is aware of the meaningful occupations in their client's lives, they can begin to better understand what concerns are present regarding the client's ability to engage in these occupations. Another tool that can be helpful in establishing a client's occupational history or life experiences is the AOTA Occupational Profile Template, which is located electronically on the AOTA website for members (AOTA, 2020c). Using this template contributes to a client-centered approach to the occupational therapy process.

A FWed can continue to support a student in keeping a focus on occupation by brainstorming with the student after the evaluation process with each client and throughout the intervention process. Following a structured format for the brainstorming will improve ease of incorporating it as part of the normal routine. Appendix G provides a structured format that can be used to be intentional with occupation-based practice. The student could be encouraged to complete the brainstorming activity on their own time and bring it back to discuss with the FWed the following day. Additionally, students can support occupation by thinking creatively about occupation while intervention planning. Students can access and share resources supporting occupation-based

---

Box 6-1

EVIDENCE-BASED LEARNING ACTIVITIES FOR LEVEL II FIELDWORK STUDENTS

- Seek out evidence to support intervention planning.
- Facilitate a journal club to review and discuss evidence relevant to fieldwork site.
- Search for and appraise novel or up-to-date tools or resources.
- Locate and review evidence for common interventions used at fieldwork site.

---

practice obtained through their academic program and state and national associations, while simultaneously advocating for professional membership to support the profession at both state and national levels.

Lastly, AFWCs can support occupation-based practice by providing FWeds with resources, offering on-site or virtual educational sessions, donating textbooks, etc. AFWCs may also connect with students throughout Level II fieldwork to foster student application of occupation-based practice by facilitating student reflection and sharing of ideas with peers.

Integration of Evidence-Based Practice

FWeds can encourage the integration of evidence-based practice by incorporating assignments and learning activities required by students during their Level II fieldwork; see Box 6-1.

Throughout the fieldwork experience, there are many ways that each person involved in the fieldwork experience can contribute to the use of evidence. See Table 6-4 for a list of strategies to strengthen the use of evidence during Level II fieldwork.

Integration of Ethical Practice

Fieldwork experiences provide practice and professional opportunities that pose ethical dilemmas. When faced with ethical considerations during fieldwork, educators and students should apply their knowledge of the AOTA *Code of Ethics* when deciding how to approach the ethical scenario. The AOTA *Code of Ethics* (2020b) is a practice document provided to occupational therapy students during didactic coursework with expectations that they integrate the ethical principles in their daily practice and behaviors during fieldwork. During the fieldwork experience, the FWed may be the first practitioner that the student learns from when acknowledging and addressing ethical considerations within practice; see Box 6-2. For example, if the student encounters the FWed participating in a co-treatment with a physical therapy colleague, they may have questions on why the session warranted two disciplines as well as ethical considerations surrounding billing for services that include two interdisciplinary professionals.

The AFWC, FWed, and student (the fieldwork team) work as a dynamic triad that collaborates to ensure successful development of student knowledge, skills, and resources for handling ethical situations that occur in fieldwork. This collaboration between stakeholders is important as well as challenging to everyone's professional identity. There are times the AFWC, educator, and student work together to address ethical considerations the student is experiencing to ensure the student can accurately and confidently articulate the ethical knowledge and behaviors in the fieldwork setting.

TABLE 6-4

STRATEGIES TO STRENGTHEN USE OF EVIDENCE DURING LEVEL II FIELDWORK

LEVEL II FIELDWORK STUDENT	FIELDWORK EDUCATOR	ACADEMIC FIELDWORK COORDINATOR
• Guide FWed in locating resources for evidence-based practice • Provide an inservice on locating resources for evidence-based practice • Create a cheat sheet for FWeds to reference to locate resources for evidence-based practice • Access and share resources with FWeds (e.g., peer-reviewed articles, practice resources) • Advocate for professional membership to support the profession	• Ask students to locate evidence to support intervention planning • Ask students to facilitate a peer-learning opportunity with an article discussion • Ask students to locate and appraise novel or up-to-date tools or resources • Ask students to locate and review evidence for common interventions used at fieldwork site • Ask students to lead a journal club with occupational therapy staff	Directed at students • Encourage students to use evidence • Ask students to share an article with peers that was used to guide an intervention • Facilitate discussion on how to incorporate evidence-based practice, barriers experienced, strategies to overcome barriers, impact of evidence-based practice on client outcomes Directed at FWed • Share resources • Provide tutorials • Provide access to academic databases • Connect them with academic librarian for additional support

---

BOX 6-2

INCORPORATING ETHICAL CONSIDERATIONS IN PRACTICES

During a Level II fieldwork placement in an outpatient pediatric clinic, Jose was preparing for an upcoming treatment session with a 4-year-old child diagnosed with autism spectrum disorder. Jose is considering introducing a new sensory intervention but has questions on the intervention effectiveness. He collaborates with his FWed on his questions on whether to incorporate a new sensory intervention into the child's plan for the upcoming session.

The FWed takes the time to discuss, using debriefing concepts, to determine the following ethical considerations when implementing a sensory intervention:
- Child and family/caregiver goals
- Feasibility of implementing the sensory intervention at home or school
- Cost of the sensory intervention tool or resource
- Effectiveness of sensory intervention for child's specific signs and symptoms

---

Box 6-3

ACTIVITIES TO FOSTER CULTURALLY RELEVANT PRACTICE

AFWCs and FWeds can use the following teaching activities to help students recognize and identify methods to incorporate cultural aspects of a person, group, or population:

- Journaling
- Discussion board
- Debriefing
- Treatment planning
- Professional association resources

Ethical considerations may arise through practice, administration, and education situations specific to patient scheduling, caseload prioritization, billing, policy implementation, safety procedures and processes, education and training, and discipline scope of practice. See the Learning Activities at the end of the chapter for facilitating ethical considerations in practice. Each of these situations provide opportunities for FWeds and students to navigate, using best practice principles. Additionally, this provides an opportunity for the student to collaborate with the FWed to provide updated resources to fieldwork sites regarding suggestions for change while understanding the culture of their fieldwork setting.

Integration of Culturally Relevant Practice

It is important for occupational therapy practitioners to address cultural aspects of our clientele to optimize meaningful occupational performance. Some indicate that culture and client centeredness go hand in hand in optimizing client outcomes (Getty, 2016). Practitioners can implement strategies to assess and accommodate occupational therapy services to ensure the client's sense of culture is treated with dignity and respect. During fieldwork, there are opportunities for educators to help students bridge their knowledge and foster behaviors that promote culturally relevant practice.

There are opportunities within practice that allow educators and students to collaborate and address attitudes and interactions that challenge cultural effectiveness while delivering occupational therapy services. The *OTPF-4* (AOTA, 2020a) supports that practitioners, educators, and students be deliberate in addressing cultural aspects of our clients during the first encounter, which requires occupational therapists to gather, assess, and document client factors specific to culture. There are many methods to help students be deliberate in their ability to be culturally aware of the fieldwork environment in conjunction with clients' cultural needs; refer to Box 6-3 for examples.

It is important for practitioners, educators, and students to be deliberate in identifying and removing beliefs that may cause discord in the ability to support client centeredness (Montgomery, 2020). Educators can help students recognize their own beliefs and methods to optimize therapeutic use of self by tailoring sessions to the populations you are delivering occupational therapy services (Montgomery, 2020). Another consideration for cultural relevance in practice is for educators and students to have an active role in acknowledging and understanding the client's beliefs and health literacy surrounding their health care management. The client's perceived health care management may be influenced by the client's beliefs, experiences, affordances, and barriers. It is important that educators and students utilize therapeutic listening to understand the client's perspective as well as an active participant in educating oneself on the source of those thoughts, beliefs, and values (Montgomery, 2020).

Box 6-4

PROFESSIONAL RESOURCES TO SUPPORT BEST PRACTICE

- AOTA membership: EBP resources, best practice guideline texts, OT Practice Pulse, AOTA Alerts, networking through CommunOT
- AOTA OTPF-4
- AOTA Code of Ethics
- AOTA Cultural Competency Tool Kit
- World Federation of Occupational Therapists (WFOT)—Diversity and Culture document
- State association membership and resources

See Appendix K for further evidence resources that support best practice.

FWeds have a role in helping students bridge classroom knowledge of culture considerations. Educators can use teaching tools or strategies such as reflective journaling, debriefing methods, strategic treatment planning activities, and utilization of network resources through occupational therapy groups to help identify the students' knowledge and awareness of their own beliefs and values as well as strategies to mitigate discord between client and student difference to optimize client goals and outcomes. More specifically, educators or students can implement journaling to identify their beliefs and the impact those beliefs may have on their approach and decision making in delivering occupational therapy services. Refer to Box 6-4 for learning activities that AFWCs and educators may use to foster culturally relevant practice. Learning Activities specific to journaling, debriefing, treatment planning, and network resources can also be found at the end of the chapter.

CAPITALIZING ON THE ROLES OF THOSE INVOLVED

To help integrate the best practice principles during Level II fieldwork, it is important to understand the role of each stakeholder involved in the mentorship of Level II students. By understanding the role of the Level II fieldwork stakeholders in academia and practice, collaboration to ensure occupational therapy students integrate the five best practice principles effectively can be achievable. In Level II fieldwork experiences, there are often three to four key stakeholder roles. These roles are the fieldwork student, the FWed, the AFWC, and in some settings, the site fieldwork coordinator. Each of these individuals play a significant part in the outcome of the experience by tending to the responsibilities required in that role. Occupational therapy best practices can be strengthened by capitalizing on the unique perspectives and skill sets of each person involved. Although introduced in Chapter 1, this next section will dive deeper into how each individual within the fieldwork team plays an integral role regarding promoting these best practice ideals during Level II fieldwork.

Students

Occupational therapy students on Level II fieldwork have many responsibilities to fulfill. While students may be accustomed to similar responsibilities in the classroom setting, students often experience greater challenges in meeting these demands without the day-to-day support of their peers and the structure provided by the academic program. Fieldwork requires a greater level of independence than most students have previously experienced throughout their academic preparation. Students arriving on Level II fieldwork often experience a variety of emotions including excitement, nervousness, and hesitation perhaps second-guessing if they have the skill set to be successful. Although the previously cited literature highlighted the challenge students may experience with integrating best practices during fieldwork, there are some strategies that students can employ to provide services consistent with best practice principles. One learning activity a student can participate in throughout the Level II fieldwork experience can be found in Appendix C. The learning activity guides a student through independent tasks that prompt the student to personally reflect on strengths and areas of growth, analyze the environment, create personal goals and strategies, self-assess on progress, and identify changes needed. The tasks are threaded throughout the Level II fieldwork experience.

Fieldwork Educator

The FWed is the individual responsible for the supervision of a fieldwork student. The role of the FWed requires practitioners to not only think like a practitioner but also to embody the role of an educator, to teach, facilitate, model, and evaluate. While FWeds may demonstrate best practice when providing services to clients, it requires another skill set to verbalize the rationale for their decision making and to connect what is happening in practice with the students' knowledge gained through coursework. It is a significant responsibility to help a student integrate their academic knowledge into practice and continue to foster their development to reach entry-level competency. Table 6-5 outlines strategies that a FWed can employ before the experience starts and throughout the experience. The strategies will assist the FWed with facilitating student learning to include application of best practices throughout the fieldwork experience.

To incorporate the best practice principles throughout the fieldwork experience, the FWed must be intentional from the beginning of the experience to the end of the experience. Implementation of the principles should be monitored as part of a weekly meeting like other areas of competency that are evaluated weekly, such as conducting evaluations, selecting and documenting interventions, demonstrating time management, etc. If a weekly meeting form is utilized, it could be adapted to include self-assessment and feedback on the five areas of best practice. According to Farber and Koenig (2008), increasing opportunities for students to engage in reflective practice during the fieldwork experience is important to improve entry-level competencies. See journal prompts in Appendix D and the weekly meeting form in Appendix E to facilitate reflection on performance.

Clinical Coordinator of Fieldwork

A clinical coordinator of fieldwork, also referred to as a clinical site coordinator, is a representative from the fieldwork site that the AFWC connects with to determine a match regarding a fieldwork placement. This role is essential for bridging learning opportunities in a variety of health care, education, and community settings. The unique role and responsibilities of the site coordinator allows for opportunity to support and foster positive relationships specific to academic programs, practice, and occupational therapy students.

The site coordinator's role and time commitment to fieldwork education can be variable based on the practice setting, department size, clientele, facility mission and values, and management structure. This position can include a variety of responsibilities with a focus on both administrative and educational tasks. Administrative tasks may include contract negotiation between fieldwork site and academic program, organizing processes to support contract and scheduling with a variety of academic programs including immunization processes, background checks, fingerprinting, double indemnity clauses, etc. Educational duties may include development and maintenance

TABLE 6-5

FIELDWORK EDUCATOR PREPARATION FOR GUIDING STUDENTS IN BEST PRACTICE

PRIOR TO STUDENT ARRIVAL	THROUGHOUT EXPERIENCE
1. Reflect on occupational therapy practice at your site and identify how best practice is integrated, including during each stage of the occupational therapy process (evaluation, intervention, discharge).	1. Orient students to how best practice is implemented at your site, specifically addressing each phase of the occupational therapy process (evaluation, intervention, discharge).
2. Reflect on barriers and supports at your site that impact the implementation of best practice into client care.	2. Orient students to SSLOs and weekly learning activities highlighting the application of best practice throughout the experience.
3. Make an action plan to assist occupational therapy practitioners and students overcome previously identified barriers and strategies and to capitalize on support present at your site.	3. Orient students to barriers and supports they may experience at your site, which may impact their ability to implement best practice.
4. Identify strategies to incorporate best practice into student learning experiences such as adding weekly reflection on best practice into the weekly meeting form.	4. Facilitate students' development of a learning plan identifying strategies to overcome barriers and capitalize on support unique to your site.
5. Consider how to balance student performance of demonstrating best practice with performance of entry-level competence and perceived expectation of independently managing a full caseload.	5. During weekly meetings, facilitate students' reflection and self-assessment regarding performance with implementing best practice.
6. Reflect on SSLOs and create ways to incorporate best practice into the students' specific learning objectives, thus naturally adding the focus during the learning experience.	6. Consider brief fieldwork assignments designed to assist the student in implementing best practice.
7. Reflect on weekly learning activities and create ways to incorporate best practice into the students' learning experience. Consider what might be appropriate at week 1 related to best practice in comparison to what might be appropriate at week 9.	7. Regularly evaluate students' ability to implement best practice and adjust students' responsibilities accordingly to positively support continued growth.

Adapted from Graves, C. A. (2019). Integrating best practice into fieldwork: A narrative inquiry in the level II fieldwork experiences of occupational therapy students (Publication No. 22588296) [Doctoral dissertation, University of North Dakota]. ProQuest Dissertations and Theses Global.

of student resources including learning objectives, expectations, student manual, FWed and student relationship management, education, and training to FWeds on site. In addition, individuals in this role advocate for occupational therapy students in practice, foster professional national and regional association resources, and schedule fieldwork placements.

The site coordinator can support best practice within their role. Some best practice strategies the site coordinator can use to support fieldwork across fieldwork settings are:

- Acknowledge and encourage excellence in fieldwork education (Hanson & DeIuliis, 2015).

- Develop and maintain site-specific learning objectives (SSLOs), learning activities, and student expectations in alignment with professional best practices (Hanson & DeIuliis, 2015; refer back to Chapters 4 and 5).

- Facilitate clear and consistent communication between academic and practice stakeholders to help promote knowledge of practice, academic, or management changes.

- Mentor FWeds in best practice principles for student learning in conjunction to practice demands (i.e., encourage completion of AOTA Fieldwork Educator Certificate Course).

- Advocate for student involvement in practice needs (i.e., caseload, projects, research, education).

- Host opportunities for evidence-based practice with collaboration of practice leaders, educators, and academic programs.

- Assist in the evaluation and/or remediation of student performance (Hanson & DeIuliis, 2015).

Academic Fieldwork Coordinator

The role of the AFWC is multidimensional ranging from administrative to educational to mentoring. Stutz-Tanenbaum et al. (2015) identified 10 role clusters that contribute to the complexity of the role. Administratively, the AFWC manages data related to the student, such as ensuring student compliance with fieldwork site requirements and student registration for fieldwork courses. In addition, they manage data related to the fieldwork site, such as negotiating affiliation agreements to scheduling and confirming student placements. Educationally, the AFWC supports FWeds and fieldwork students. For example, the AFWC may collaborate with FWeds to design learning experiences at their site, as well as advise FWeds who are working with a struggling student. The role also involves mentoring students during fieldwork, advising students struggling with fieldwork, and providing opportunities for students to integrate academic coursework during fieldwork. Working with both FWeds and students creates opportunities for the AFWC to support the use of best practices before and during Level II fieldwork. In addition, the AFWC is the representative from the academic program responsible for ensuring that the academic program is in compliance with fieldwork education requirements outlined by the Accreditation Council for Occupational Therapy Education (ACOTE, 2018).

There are numerous strategies that can be explored by AFWCs to support best practice in Level II fieldwork. One example that could occur at any time is providing an on-site or virtual continuing education session on how to better integrate best practices into their own practice and facility. A follow-up session could include how to better integrate best practices into the learning experience for fieldwork students. The following examples would be best suited for the specific time frame in which a FWed is working with a Level II student.

- Provide a template for FWeds/students to complete an environmental analysis of the fieldwork site, to better understand best practices at their site (Appendix A).

- Provide a learning activity to identify barriers to best practice (Appendix B).

TABLE 6-6
SELF-DETERMINATION THEORY

AUTONOMY	COMPETENCE	RELATEDNESS
Need to control the course of their lives	Need to be effective in dealing with environment or task	Need to have a sense of belonging and connectedness with others

Adapted from Orsini, C., Evans, P., & Jerez, O. (2015). How to encourage intrinsic motivation in clinical teaching environment: A systematic review from self-determination theory. *Journal of Educational Evaluation for Health Professions, 12*(8), 1-10 https://doi.org/10.3352/jeehp.2015.12.8

- Provide a template for students to self-assess their progress with implementing best practices (Appendix C).
- Provide a list of questions to facilitate reflection on best practice principles (Appendix D).
- Use a weekly meeting form highlighting best practices (Appendix E).
- Share examples of learning activities highlighting best practices (Appendices F, G, H).
- Provide a sample template for treatment planning that highlights the best practices (Appendix I).
- Provide a template for academia and FWeds to complete a strengths, weaknesses, opportunities, and threats (SWOT) analysis (Appendix J).
- Provide references highlighting best practices in the literature (Appendix K).
- Facilitate a discussion regarding best practice and how those practices are viewed and implemented at the fieldwork site.
- Share examples of SSLOs reflecting best practices (refer back to Chapter 4).
- Provide opportunities for students/FWeds to participate in discussion boards or journal clubs.
- Use social media to create shared space for FWeds.

APPLICATION OF LEARNING THEORIES

Experiential learning through Level II fieldwork experiences allows occupational therapy students to make connections and apply their didactic coursework in a realistic practice context. The Self-Determination Theory is a framework that AFWCs, educators, and students can use to guide learning to foster growth toward entry-level practice. Concepts inherent to the theory can guide occupational therapy educators in helping the student grow in their ability to be autonomous, competent, and relatable within practice. See Table 6-6 for the constructs of the Self-Determination Theory. More specifically, the theory supports an individual's innate desire to be autonomous, competent, and relate well to others to achieve overall wellness (Center for Self Determination Theory, 2020; Ryan & Deci, 2000; Schunk et al., 2014).

During fieldwork experiences, this theory can be applied as the FWed scaffolds the learning experiences provided throughout the 8- or 12-week experience. By being deliberate in grading learning experiences specific to patient care caseload demand, environmental procedures, and feedback process, the FWed can optimize the student's ability to be autonomous, competent, and

---

Box 6-5

SUGGESTIONS FOR FOSTERING STUDENT GROWTH

- Guide the student to identify the connection of the client's beliefs and values.
- Create and sustain a safe and respectful learning environment.
- Allow for choice or autonomy in decision making.
- Facilitate meaningful feedback that is relevant and realistic to accomplish.
- Provide opportunities and time for pattern recognition with similar diagnoses, conditions, or treatment approaches.
- Grade the procedural tasks to provide increased responsibility.

---

relatable in practice. FWeds can introduce experiences that allow the student to experience the just-right challenge in their own performance, which in turn will build competence as well as autonomy in their ability to execute occupational therapy responsibilities (Bolton & Dean, 2018). Allied health students report more positive motivational outcomes when their environment allows them to work toward autonomy in their role and responsibilities (Ballmann & Mueller, 2008; Orsini et al., 2015). For example, in the first week of fieldwork, allow the student to actively participate in therapy sessions and take notes of the session details for documentation. When progressing into the second week, grade up or scaffold the learning activity of how to develop the occupational profile by having the student now facilitate the questions and recording of information from the client. Then, by the third week of fieldwork, allow the student to complete the entire process of the evaluation or treatment session. During this grading process, provide the opportunity for the student to have similar caseload characteristics such as condition or intervention approach in order to help with pattern recognition, which may also help foster autonomy faster.

There are many methods, activities, or behaviors the AFWC and FWed can use to foster student growth. See Box 6-5 for suggestions for fostering student growth as an educator in the field or classroom. From a relatedness standpoint, guiding the student to identify the connection of their client's values, beliefs, and needs to their therapy experience is helpful. Furthermore, the FWed can foster relatedness of the student by ensuring the fieldwork site provides a respectful and safe learning environment for them to assimilate into the culture of the site. From a competence and autonomy standpoint, FWeds can support motivation of the student while growing their clinical reasoning by providing choice, value, structured guidance, and meaningful feedback directed toward performance that is relevant and realistic to accomplish (Orsini et al., 2015).

From a fieldwork environment standpoint, providing learning opportunities that allow students to build strengths by working initially with similar diagnoses or conditions is helpful. Grading the procedural tasks with increased responsibilities on a week-to-week timeframe supports the development of autonomy and competence as well. Additionally, taking the time and being intentional with orientation aspects of the fieldwork site, such as instructing the student during the first week of fieldwork on the safety procedures and processes related to environmental, professional, or administration procedures, helps students build competence as well as relatedness within their given fieldwork environment.

SUMMARY

The integration of these five best practice principles ensures the provision of professional best practice in the field of occupational therapy. As practice demands and contexts evolve with the needs of populations, groups, and individuals, the profession of occupational therapy will continue to lead with innovative methods to sustain best practice principles. Developing skills and habits to support best practice ideals will enable the profession to address the occupational needs of populations, groups, and individuals so that they are able to participate in the occupations they need or want to do in their everyday lives.

Fieldwork provides opportunity for students to bring best practice principles learning in didactic coursework (occupation-based, client-centered, evidence-based, ethical, and culturally relevant care) to the fieldwork environment. AFWCs can help to bring alignment between classroom learning on best practice principles and the opportunities students have during fieldwork. They might also contribute by collaborating with FWeds to design student learning objectives and activities, providing resources to FWeds and students, and facilitating discussions with students during fieldwork to encourage continued growth in clinical and professional reasoning. It is essential that FWeds reflect on facilitators and barriers to implementing best practices in their setting and guide students to acknowledge, reflect, and strategize to incorporate best practices in their delivery of occupational therapy services. Furthermore, it is important that students take ownership of their own learning to develop and implement strategies to support best practice principles in their daily practice responsibilities.

Please review the activities and resources in the Appendices of the chapter to help facilitate best practice principles in the classroom and fieldwork setting. Learning activities such as treatment planning, debriefing, and many more are provided. Additionally, there are vignettes of fieldwork scenarios for student reflection of occupation-based, ethical, and cultural considerations. Learning to incorporate best practices into the occupational therapy process is a journey, supported by daily incorporation of habits of mind and behavior. The benefits achieved are well worth the effort given.

REFERENCES

Accreditation Council for Occupational Therapy Education. (2018). Accreditation council for occupational therapy education standards and interpretive guide. https://www.aota.org/~/media/Corporate/Files/EducationCareers/Accredit/StandardsReview/2018-ACOTE-Standards-Interpretive-Guide.pdf

American Occupational Therapy Association. (2020a). Occupational therapy practice framework: Domain and process (4th ed.). *American Journal of Occupational Therapy, 74*(Suppl. 2), 7412410010. https://doi.org/10.5014/ajot.2020.74S2001

American Occupational Therapy Association. (2020b). AOTA 2020 occupational therapy code of ethics. *American Journal of Occupational Therapy, 74*, 7413410005. https://doi.org/10.5014/ajot.2020.74S3006

American Occupational Therapy Association. (2020c). Improve your documentation with AOTA's updated occupational profile template. https://www.aota.org/Practice/Manage/Reimb/occupational-profile-document-value-ot.aspx

Ashby, S. E., Adler, J., & Herbert, L. (2016). An exploratory international study into occupational therapy students' perceptions of professional identity. *Australian Occupational Therapy Journal, 63*, 233-243. http://dx.doi.org/10.1111/1440-1630.12271

Ashby, S. E., Ryan, S., Gray, M., & James, C. (2013). Factors that influence the professional resilience of occupational therapists in mental health practice. *Australian Occupational Therapy Journal, 60*, 110-119. http://dx.doi.org/10.1111/1440-1630.12012

Ballmann, J. M., & Mueller, J. J. (2008). Using self-determination theory to describe academic motivation of allied health professional-level college students. *Journal of Allied Health, 37*, 90-96.

Bing, R. K. (1981). Occupational therapy revisited: A paraphrastic journey (Eleanor Clarke Slagle Lecture). *American Journal of Occupational Therapy, 35*, 499–518. http://dx.doi.org/10.5014/ ajot.35.8.499

Bolton, T., & Dean, E. (2018). Self-determination theory and professional reasoning in occupational therapy students: A mixed methods study. *Journal of Occupational Therapy Education, 2*(3), 1-22. http://dio.org/10.26681/jote.2018.020304

Center for Self Determination Theory. (2020). The theory. https://selfdeterminationtheory.org/the-theory/

Clarke, C., Martin, M., de Visser, R., & Sadlo, G. (2015). Sustaining professional identity in practice following role-emerging placements: Opportunities and challenges for occupational therapists. *British Journal of Occupational Therapy, 78*(1), 42-50. https://doi.org/10.1177/0308022614561238

Clarke, C., Martin, M., Sadlo, G., & de Visser, R. (2014). The development of an authentic professional identity on role-emerging placements. *British Journal of Occupational Therapy, 77*(5), 222-229. http://dx.doi.org/10.4276/030802214X13990455043368

Estes, J., & Pierce, D. E. (2012). Pediatric therapists' perspectives on occupation-based practice. *Scandinavian Journal of Occupational Therapy, 19*, 17-25. http://dx.doi.org/10.3109/11038128.2010.547598

Evenson, M. E., Roberts, M., Kaldenberg, J., Barnes, M. A., & Ozelie, R. (2015). National survey of fieldwork educators: Implications for occupational therapy education. *American Journal of Occupational Therapy, 69*(Suppl. 2), 6912350020. http://dx.doi.org/10.5014/ajot.2015.019265

Farber, R. S., & Koenig, K. P. (2008). Facilitating clinical reasoning in fieldwork: The relational context of the supervisor and student. In B. A. Boyt-Schell & J. W. Schell (Eds.), *Clinical and professional reasoning in occupational therapy* (pp. 335-367). Lippincott Williams & Wilkins.

Fisher, A. G., & Marterella, A. (2019). *Powerful practice: A model for authentic occupational therapy.* Center for Innovative OT Solutions.

Getty, S. M. (2016). Assessing culture's impact on occupation. *SIS Quarterly Practice Connections, 1*(3), 15-17.

Graves, C. A. (2019). Integrating best practice into fieldwork: A narrative inquiry in the level II fieldwork experiences of occupational therapy students (Publication No. 22588296) [Doctoral dissertation, University of North Dakota]. ProQuest Dissertations and Theses Global.

Hanson, D. J. (2011). The perspectives of fieldwork educators regarding level II fieldwork students. *Occupational Therapy in Health Care, 25*(2-3), 164-177. https://doi-org.ezproxylr.med.und.edu/10.3109/07380577.2011.561420

Hanson, D. J., & DeIuliis, E. D. (2015). The collaborative model of fieldwork education: A blueprint for group supervision of students. *Occupational Therapy in Health Care, 29*(2), 223-239. https://doi.org/10.3109/07380577.2015.1011297

Korner, M., & Modell, E. (2009). A model of shared decision-making in medical rehabilitation. *Rehabilitation, 48,* 160-165.

Law, M., Baptiste, S., & Mills, J. (1995). Client-centered practice: What does it mean and does it make a difference? *Canadian Journal of Occupational Therapy, 62*, 250-257.

Law, M., & MacDermid, J. C. (2014). Introduction to evidence-based practice. In M. Law & J. C. MacDermid (Eds.), *Evidence-based rehabilitation: A guide to practice* (3rd ed., pp. 1-14). SLACK Incorporated.

Mackenzie, L. (2002). Briefing and debriefing of student fieldwork experiences: Exploring concerns and reflecting on practice. *Australian Occupational Therapy Journal, 49*, 82-92. https://doi.org/10.1046/j.1440-1630.2002.00296.x

Meyer, A. (1922, 1977). The philosophy of occupational therapy. *American Journal of Occupational Therapy, 31*, 639-642. (Original work published 1922).

Montgomery, B. (2020). Developing cultural competence in paradise. American Occupational Therapy Association. https://www.aota.org/Education-Careers/Students/Pulse/Archive/fieldwork/Cultural-Competence-Paradise.aspx

Oldenburg, H. Y., & Graves, C. A. (2022). Mentoring in professional best practices during the Level I fieldwork experience. In D. Hanson & E. D. DeIuliis (Eds.), *Fieldwork educator's guide to level I fieldwork* (pp.). SLACK Incorporated.

Orsini, C., Evans, P., & Jerez, O. (2015). How to encourage intrinsic motivation in clinical teaching environment: A systematic review from self-determination theory. *Journal of Educational Evaluation for Health Professions, 12*(8), 1-10. https://doi.org/10.3352/jeehp.2015.12.8

Plewnia, A., Bengel, J., & Korner, M. (2016). Patient-centeredness and its impact on patient satisfaction and treatment outcomes in medical rehabilitation. *Patient Education and Counseling, 99*, 2063-2070. http://dx.doi.org/10.1016/j.pec.2016.07.018

Ripat, J., Wener, P., & Dobinson, K. (2013). The development of client-centeredness in student occupational therapists. *British Journal of Occupational Therapy, 76*(5), 217-224. https://doi.org/10.4276/030802213X13679275042681f

Ryan, R. M., & Deci, E. L. (2000). Self-determination theory and the facilitation of intrinsic motivation, social development, and well-being. *American Psychologist, 55*(1), 68-78. https://doi.org/10.1037///0003-066X.55.1.68

Schunk, D. H., Meece, J. L., & Pintrich, P. R. (2014). *Motivation in education: Theory, research and applications* (4th ed.). Pearson.

Stutz-Tanenbaum, P., Hanson, D. J., Koski, J., & Greene, D. (2015). Exploring the complexity of the academic fieldwork coordinator role. *Occupational Therapy in Health Care, 29*(2), 139-152. https://doi.org/10.3109/07380577.2015.1017897

Sumsion, T., & Law, M. (2006). A review of the evidence on the conceptual elements informing client-centered practice. *Canadian Journal of Occupational Therapy, 73*(3), 153-162.

Taylor, R. R. (2020). *The intentional relationship: Occupational therapy and use of self* (2nd ed.). F. A. Davis.

Thomas, Y., Dickson, D., Broadbridge, J., Hopper, L., Hawkins, R., Edwards, A., & McBryde, C. (2007). Benefits and challenges of supervising occupational therapy fieldwork students: Supervisors' perspectives. *Australian Occupational Therapy Journal, 54*, S2-S12. https://doi.org/10.1111/j.1440-1630.2007.00694.x

Towns, E., & Ashby, S. (2014). The influence of practice educators on occupational therapy students' understanding of the practical applications of theoretical knowledge: A phenomenological study into student experiences of practice education. *Australian Occupational Therapy Journal, 61*, 344-352. https://doi.org/10.1111/1440-1630.12134

Wilkinson, S. A., Hinchliffe, F., Hough, J., & Chang, A. (2012). Baseline evidence-based practice use, knowledge, and attitudes of allied health professionals. *Journal of Allied Health, 41*(4), 177-184.

World Federation of Occupational Therapists. (2010). Position statement: Diversity and culture. https://www.aota.org/Practice/Manage/Multicultural/Cultural-Competency-Tool-Kit.aspx

Zimmerman, L., Michaelis, M., Quaschning, K., Muller, C., & Korner, M. (2014). The significance of internal and external participation for patient satisfaction. *Rehabilitation, 53*, 219-224. https://doi.org/10.1055/s-0033-1357116

APPENDIX A
Environmental Analysis

This learning activity can be done independently by FWeds at any time to increase awareness of the supports and barriers impacting implementation of best practice, that exist within their practice setting. When working with a Level II student, a FWed can assign this activity to the student to complete between weeks 2 and 3 of the fieldwork experience. Once completed, it can be used as a point of discussion between the FWed and student to facilitate implementation of best practice during the fieldwork experience.

Identify supports (S) and barriers (B) present at the site that impact the implementation of best practice principles into client care.				
OCCUPATION BASED	**CLIENT CENTERED**	**EVIDENCE BASED**	**ETHICAL**	**CULTURALLY RELEVANT**
Ex. Time (B)		Ex. Resources (S)		
Reflect on occupational therapy practice at the site and identify how the best practice principles are integrated during evaluation, intervention, and discharge.				
EVALUATION				
INTERVENTION				
DISCHARGE PLANNING				

APPENDIX B

Barriers to Best Practice Principles

The following reflection activity is to assist in identifying different types of barriers that inevitably occur in practice. The mini vignettes depict three different practice contexts, describing the presence (or lack) of best practice principles. Following the mini vignettes, prompts are provided to identify the barriers present and identify strategies to overcome the barriers.

BARRIERS TO BEST PRACTICE PRINCIPLES	
Institutional Barriers	Lack of time, lack of space/storage, lack of supplies, philosophical perspective
Organizational Barriers	Lack of support, power differentials, workplace culture, staff perspective
Personal Barriers	Lack of skills, lack of creativity, personal mindset

ACUTE CARE HOSPITAL	ADULT OUTPATIENT	EARLY INTERVENTION
Context: Metropolitan acute care hospital. The student identified that the role of occupational therapist was occupation-based, primarily safety with activities of daily living for discharge, including toileting, bathroom mobility, donning clothing items, eating, and other self-care tasks. It was difficult to remain client-centered because emphasis was on client independence, discharge, and resources such as appropriate clothing for dressing tasks were lacking, decreasing culturally relevant care.	Context: Outpatient department of a rural hospital. The student identified that most of the interventions were protocol-driven, including rote exercise, modalities, and therapeutic massage. This challenged occupation-based and client-centered practice. The occupational therapy team was up to date with current evidence and actively incorporated evidence-based practice into the interventions they provided.	Context: Early intervention. The student identified working with children and families in their homes supported client-centered and culturally relevant practice. It was challenging to complete online database searches to support evidence-based practice when spending a full day providing in-home services. The transdisciplinary approach led to a better understanding of the team roles and when to refer to a specific team member to ensure safe and ethical practice.
IDENTIFY BARRIERS PRESENT IN MINI VIGNETTES		
1. 2.	1. 2.	1. 2.
IDENTIFY STRATEGIES TO OVERCOME THE BARRIERS		
1. 2.	1. 2.	1. 2.

After reflecting on the mini vignettes, analyze your current fieldwork site. If you have not previously identified barriers impacting implementation of best practice, complete that step next by listing them here. Once a list has been developed, identify strategies to overcome the barriers.

BARRIERS TO BEST PRACTICE	STRATEGIES TO OVERCOME BARRIERS

APPENDIX C

Student Activities for Best Practice in Fieldwork

Reflection in practice is a valuable learning strategy that can be efficient and require little resources to complete. The following activity is created for a student to be used at various points throughout a Level II fieldwork experience to support the use of best practice ideals during the placement.

Before Level II Fieldwork Begins

PERSONAL REFLECTION	IMPACT ON BEST PRACTICE
My personal strengths:	How will my strengths and areas of growth impact my ability to implement best practice?
My personal areas of growth:	Considering common barriers to implementing best practice, how can I capitalize on my strengths to implement best practice?

Early in Level II Fieldwork (Between Weeks 2 and 3)

Identify supports (S) and barriers (B) present at the site that impact the implementation of best practice principles into client care.				
OCCUPATION BASED	CLIENT CENTERED	EVIDENCE BASED	ETHICAL	CULTURALLY RELEVANT
Ex. Time (B)		Ex. Resources (S)		

Reflect on occupational therapy practice at the site and identify how the best practice principles are integrated during evaluation, intervention, and discharge.	
EVALUATION	
INTERVENTION	
DISCHARGE PLANNING	

Review site-specific learning objectives and identify objectives that reflect and encourage implementation of the best practice principles.				
OCCUPATION BASED	CLIENT CENTERED	EVIDENCE BASED	ETHICAL	CULTURALLY RELEVANT

Review weekly learning activities and identify activities that reflect and encourage implementation of the best practice principles.				
OCCUPATION BASED	CLIENT CENTERED	EVIDENCE BASED	ETHICAL	CULTURALLY RELEVANT

Early to Middle of Fieldwork (Between Weeks 4 and 6)

GOALS TO IMPLEMENT BEST PRACTICE	ACTION PLAN TO IMPLEMENT BEST PRACTICE
1.	1.
2.	2.
3.	3.

Middle Through End of Fieldwork (Between Weeks 7 and 12)

SELF-ASSESSMENT	CHANGES GOING FORWARD
What am I doing well?	What changes do I need to make?
What am I struggling with?	What support do I still need to achieve goals?
How is my progress toward my goals?	How will I gain this support?

"Actively challenge yourself, push yourself, take initiative, go above and beyond in pursuit of best practice; it will not come easy."
—Cherie Graves

APPENDIX D

Reflection Questions on the Best Practice Principles

Communication between the AFWC, educator, and student is important to ensure growth in student learning. Perceptions between educators and students for specific client scenarios can be different. One method to help understand a student's perception of a scenario as well as their process to understanding how to address the scenario is through reflective journaling in practice. Many practitioners that transition to fieldwork education in the clinic have many of their own processes established with credible resources and knowledge to help support those processes. As a student, processing scenarios to support best practice can be novel as they are bridging their knowledge from classroom to fieldwork.

The journaling can occur on the students' own time and be reviewed at the beginning or end of the day to help students navigate perceptions and processes to optimize best practice. From a time standpoint, educators and students can use daily or weekly time frames to complete journaling. It is important to address barriers to learning that may be patient care or behavior related quickly to ensure the student has identified the need as well as the strategies on how to approach the situation or learning need to have a successful next session or week with the fieldwork demands and caseload.

Below are some example questions that can be used to discuss or journal with students to help understand their perception and clinical reasoning to help facilitate best practice principles in your practice setting.

Perception of Best Practice Principles

- As your educator, how can I support your learning in the areas you identified as needing growth this next week?
- This past week, what went well with your client caseload?
- This past week, what challenges did you experience with your client caseload?
- What did you learn this week that supported your growth toward becoming an entry-level occupational therapist/occupational therapy assistant? (Provide two to three examples.)
- How will you incorporate best practice into your daily routine this coming week specific to (insert occupation-based practice, evidence-based practice, culturally relevant, client centeredness, ethics)? What resources will help you in this process?

Client-Centered Practice

- If you feel like a patient session was awkward, self-reflect afterward to see if there was something to change, or if after reflection, it went better than what you initially perceived.
- Pick a client on your caseload and write out what you observed with the patient and in the patient's room upon entry.
- Describe what you perceive this patient's learning style to be. How did you educate the patient based on the learning style that you observed?
- How do you accommodate your learning style with that of your patients? Are you different? How do you accommodate between your two learning styles to ensure optimized client centeredness?
- How will you optimize therapeutic use of self to support client centeredness?

Evidence-Based Practice

- Reflect on an intervention you implemented this week with a client. Is there evidence to support your intervention to ensure optimized occupational performance?

- How do you plan to incorporate evidence-based practice in your role and routines as an entry-level occupational therapist?

- How do you see evidence being used in the practice setting of your fieldwork experience? Are there any resources from your didactic coursework that could help support evidence-based resources at your fieldwork site?

- What would be your role in advancing evidence-based practice at your fieldwork site?

- How does your FWed incorporate evidence into their practice?

Occupation-Based Practice

- Reflect on a client that you worked with this week. Identify one of the intervention sessions you provided and provide rationale stating how the intervention was occupation-based.

- Reflect on your current fieldwork experience thus far. What are some strategies you have put into place to incorporate greater use of occupation with clients? What resources did you use to support you?

- Reflect on a client situation in which the value of occupation was evident. Describe the client's response and what you observed that demonstrated the value of occupation.

- What would be your role in advancing occupation-based practice at your fieldwork site? What ideas do you have to support the occupational therapy team in using occupation?

Ethical Practice

- Reflect on a client you provided care to today/this week. How did you ensure you benefitted the client in developing or meeting their occupational therapy goals?

- Reflect on your clientele caseload this week, were there any ethical considerations that were challenging to navigate? If so, what were they? Furthermore, are there specific ethical considerations you can accommodate/not accommodate with your client?

- How did you manage ethical challenges that were presented in practice today or this past week? What professional resources can you use to help you navigate ethical challenges?

- How did you prepare for your client's session today/this past week to ensure you are providing current and relevant care?

- How will you manage your thoughts, values, and beliefs that may be different than your clients?

Culturally Relevant Practice

- Reflect on your own health care beliefs. How do your own thoughts, beliefs, and values facilitate or impede your therapeutic relationship with your clientele?

- Reflect on your client caseload, was there discord between your health care beliefs and your client? How did you handle this discord during your client interaction or sessions?

- What strategies or professional resources can you use to support a therapeutic relationship with a clientele that may have different cultural beliefs than you (e.g., values, routines, roles, thoughts)?

- Are there any cultural affordances or barriers you identified with a particular client in your caseload this week? How will you be mindful of those affordance or barriers during your future intervention sessions?

APPENDIX E
Weekly Meeting Form

Occupational Therapy Student Weekly Review Form

Student Name _____

Fieldwork Educator Name _____

Date _____ Week # _____

FUNDAMENTAL BASIC TENETS OF PRACTICE		
Best Practice Principles	Areas of Strength	Areas of Need

EVALUATION AND SCREENING		
Best Practice Principles	Areas of Strength	Areas of Need

INTERVENTION		
Best Practice Principles	Areas of Strength	Areas of Need

MANAGEMENT OF OCCUPATIONAL THERAPY SERVICES		
Best Practice Principles	Areas of Strength	Areas of Need

COMMUNICATION/PROFESSIONAL BEHAVIORS		
Best Practice Principles	Areas of Strength	Areas of Need

PROGRESS SUMMARY

FIELDWORK SCHEDULE REVISIONS

ADDITIONAL STUDENT SUPPORT NEEDED

STUDENT LEARNING GOALS		
Student Initiated Objectives	**Activities to Achieve Goals**	**Desired Fieldwork Educator Support**
1.		
2.		
3.		

FWed Signature _____   Date _____

Student Signature _____   Date _____

APPENDIX F
Practice Vignettes

Adult: Acute Hospital

A student is beginning their third week of Level II fieldwork in an acute care setting at a large hospital. The student and educator are assigned to a general medicine floor where they are carrying a full caseload and are preparing for an evaluation to determine home safety and discharge planning for a 70-year-old, Black woman, who lives alone in a second-floor apartment. The client was admitted for a standing height fall within their apartment. Additionally, the electronic medical record indicates there was a change in the client's mental status due to dehydration and low glucose upon admission. Images indicate the client did not sustain any broken bones but reports to physicians not remembering the context of the fall. Client's past medical history indicates hypertension, diabetes, and prior falls.

Fieldwork Educator

1. What may be your role in scaffolding the learning to ensure the student can optimize their ability to be autonomous and competent in their evaluation and discharge planning of this client?

2. How will you help the student be client-centered as well as culturally sensitive in their approach when delivering occupational therapy services to the client (i.e., evaluative process and intervention)?

3. How might you support the use of evidence-based practice to support the student's role in acute care and more specifically, with discharge planning?

Student

1. How will you be client-centered when delivering occupational therapy services to this client?

2. How would you integrate cultural elements while ensuring an occupation-based approach in your service delivery?

3. How will you support your evaluation and/or intervention process using an evidence-based approach to optimize client performance and discharge?

Pediatrics: School-Based

An occupational therapy student is beginning their fifth week of Level II fieldwork in a rural school district with occupational therapy coverage for grades K-12. The fieldwork student and educator are providing occupational therapy services to 20 children that qualified for occupational therapy services through their IEPs. The occupational therapist and fieldwork student receive a new evaluation for a first-grade student, 6-year-old Somalian boy. He has recently moved to the district, transitioning from a large metropolitan school, and be screened for autism spectrum disorder (ASD). There was no preschool screening completed and no IEP was developed at the child's previous district. The child's parents, teachers, and counselors have provided evidence the student has difficulty transitioning between academic topics and participating in peer or group activities. The student has been posed with completing the evaluation and selecting the appropriate screening tools for autism spectrum disorder.

Fieldwork Educator

1. What may be your role in scaffolding the learning to ensure the student can optimize their ability to be autonomous and competent in their evaluation and tool selection?

2. How will you help the student be client-centered as well as culturally sensitive in their approach when delivering occupational therapy services to the client (i.e., evaluative process and intervention)?

3. How might you support the use of evidence-based practice to support the selection of valid and reliable screening and/or evaluation tools?

Student

1. How will you be client-centered when delivering occupational therapy services to meet this student's academic needs?

2. How would you integrate cultural elements while ensuring an occupation-based approach in your service delivery?

3. How will you support your evaluation and/or intervention process using an evidence-based approach to optimize the child's academic and play performance?

APPENDIX G
Focusing on Occupation Throughout the Occupational Therapy Process

Reflecting on a current client scenario, complete the worksheet to ensure a focus on occupation is present during the occupational therapy process:

	OCCUPATIONS CLIENT HAS TO DO	OCCUPATIONS CLIENT WANTS TO DO	OCCUPATIONS CLIENT IS EXPECTED TO DO
CLIENT OCCUPATIONS			

CLIENT OCCUPATIONAL CHALLENGES		CLIENT OCCUPATIONAL GOALS	
1.		1.	
2.		2.	
3.		3.	

	ON-SITE	PROVIDED BY CLIENT/FAMILY	PROVIDED BY STUDENT/FWED
RESOURCES FOR OCCUPATION-BASED PRACTICE			

OCCUPATION-BASED INTERVENTION IDEAS		CLIENT FACTORS/PERFORMANCE SKILLS TARGETED	
1.		1.	
2.		2.	
3.		3.	

APPENDIX H

Debriefing Activities

Before and After Client Interaction

Debriefing, also called briefing, can be a meaningful teaching strategy or methodology that is explicit in developing student awareness of clinical reasoning as well as reflective practice during fieldwork. This type of teaching strategy facilitates verbal communication between a FWed and student to optimize reflection of a given situation (e.g., client, environment) as well as opportunity for scaffolding of student learning needs. Furthermore, this teaching strategy may foster opportunities for FWeds and students to explicitly identify and integrate best practice principles in a variety of practice contexts.

Debriefing was first used to military settings but has transitioned to learning in the health care and education setting (Mackenzie, 2002). When using debriefing in the fieldwork setting, it is important to be strategic in the questions you pose to occupational therapy students so they understand the "what," "why," and "how" elements to a given situation to ensure growth for the next client encounter within a given practice setting. FWeds have found debriefing can take 10 to 15 minutes before and after a client encounter. Below are specific questions FWeds can facilitate or students can ask themselves during fieldwork client preparation and encounters.

PRIOR TO CLIENT ENCOUNTER	POST CLIENT ENCOUNTER
1. After chart review, how do you predict the client will present from a performance standpoint? (Be specific.)	1. What was done well or achieved in your session? (Be specific.)
2. What cultural aspects will you have to consider in your session? (Be specific.)	2. What could you improve on or handle differently for the next encounter or similar context? (Be specific.)
3. What environmental considerations will you have to consider in your session?	3. How will you make the improvement or change for next time? (Be specific with action plan.)
4. What safety or precaution elements will you need to consider or address during your session? (Be specific.)	4. Is there anything else you would like to discuss or review from the session?
Note: Understanding the student's perception of how they interpreted their preparation process before the session as well as performance after client interaction is important for clinical development.	

You can use this teaching technique efficiently in a variety of fieldwork settings to optimize identification and implementation of best practice principles. More specifically, FWeds can use debriefing strategies prior to client encounters; it further examines and remediates student unknowns or anxieties, as well as after client encounters, to further reflect on performance and develop strategies for competency or autonomy for future sessions. This process can be facilitated by FWeds mentoring students' traditional or collaborative learning models during terminal fieldwork experiences. Additionally, debriefing has been used by AFWCs and faculty instructors to support clinical reasoning development in didactic coursework.

APPENDIX I

Treatment Planning Activities

Breaking Down the Best Practice Principles

Treatment Template 1 and Treatment Template 2

For many students, additional time and processing is needed to help prepare for current or future client sessions in a variety of fieldwork settings. FWeds can facilitate different learning strategies to help students prepare for their sessions to ensure accuracy and efficiency in their preparation for client interaction and care. One strategy is a structured, self-developed treatment session form that can be tailored for each given practice setting.

FWeds can facilitate opportunities for students to develop learning strategies to support how to navigate clinical systems and clientele aspects to ensure a thorough, accurate, and progressive treatment session. For some medical settings, a more detailed and systematic approach to the evaluation or treatment preparation template forms may be needed whereas educational or community-based fieldwork settings may have a less structured methodology.

Treatment Session Planning

Client Initials _____ Date of Birth/Age _____ Appointment Date/Time _____

Diagnosis/History of Present Illness (HPI) _____

_____

_____

Past Medical History (PMH) _____

_____

_____

Brief Description of Treatment _____

_____

_____

Short- and/ or Long-Term Goals Addressed	Client Performance Deficits Addressed	Tools, Equipment, Space Needed	Precautions/ Considerations	Detailed Description of Planned Treatment (listed in sequence with approximate time allotted for each step)	Rationale
			Cultural		Is there theory to support your intervention?
			Environmental		Is there evidence to support your intervention?
			Personal (i.e., medical, emotional, behavioral)		

Plan B: If original plan does not work out, how can you modify or grade part(s) of the activity?

Plan C: If even Plan B does not work, what other activity can address the specified goal(s)?

Post Treatment Reflection

1. What went well during the session?

2. What could you have done better or differently?

3. If you were to see the client for another treatment, what would be the next logical treatment progression?

4. What feedback did you receive from your FWed(s)?

APPENDIX J
SWOT Analysis

When mentoring a student in Level II fieldwork it is important to examine the personal, environmental, and cultural perspectives of academic and fieldwork stakeholders. Use a SWOT analysis approach to determine strengths, weakness, opportunities, and threats to successfully implement best practice ideals. In review of each of the areas it is important to consider internal and external factors within the analysis. The following table provides questions rooted in the SWOT approach to help you identify areas of strength and needs, to support use of the best practice ideals with a student during Level II fieldwork experiences.

	ACADEMIA	FIELDWORK EDUCATOR
STRENGTHS (S)	• What are facilitators to support the FWed and student in bridging knowledge of best practice ideals into practice?	• What are facilitators to fostering best practice ideals with a Level II fieldwork student at your practice site? • Consider environment, practitioner(s) skill set, clientele, administration, attitudes at site.
WEAKNESSES (W)	• What are the potential barriers to consider when supporting the FWed and/or student in implementing best practice ideals at a given site?	• What are potential barriers to hosting and mentoring a Level II fieldwork student at your practice site? • Consider environment, practitioner skill set, clientele, administration, attitudes at site.
OPPORTUNITIES (O)	• What opportunities are available to you to support your ability to assist the educator and student in implementation of best practice ideals during fieldwork? • Are their opportunities that can come out of your strengths?	• What opportunities are available to you to support your ability to assist the student regarding implementation of best practice ideals during fieldwork? • Are their opportunities that can come out of your strengths at your facility?
THREATS (T)	• What are threats that may hinder your ability to assist the educator and/or student in implementing best practice ideals during fieldwork?	• What are threats that may hinder your ability to assist the student in implementing best practice ideals during fieldwork at your site?

APPENDIX K
Journal Articles on Best Practice Principles

Agner, J. (2020). Moving from cultural competence to cultural humility in occupational therapy: A paradigm shift. *American Journal of Occupational Therapy, 74*(4), 1-7. http://dx.doi.org.ezproxylr.med.und.edu/10.5014/ajot.2020.038067

Ahn, S-N. (2019). Effectiveness of occupation-based interventions on performance's quality for hemiparetic stroke in community-dwelling: A randomized clinical trial study. *NeuroRehabilitation, 44*(2), 275-282. https://doi.org/10.3233/NRE-182429

Aiken, F. E., Fourt, A. M., Cheng, I. K. S., & Polatajko, H. J. (2011). The meaning gap in occupational therapy: Finding meaning in our own occupation. *Canadian Journal of Occupational Therapy, 78*, 294-302. http://doi.org/10.2182/cjot.2011.78.5.4

American Occupational Therapy Association. (2020). Educator's guide for addressing cultural awareness, humility, and dexterity in occupational therapy curricula. *American Journal of Occupational Therapy, 74*, 7413420003. https://doi.org.ezproxylr.med.und.edu/10.5014/ajot.2020.74S3005

Ashby, S. E., Adler, J., & Herbert, L. (2016). An exploratory international study into occupational therapy students' perceptions of professional identity. *Australian Occupational Therapy Journal, 63*, 233-243. http://dx.doi.org/10.1111/1440-1630.12271

Campbell, M. K., Corpus, K., Wussow, T. M., Plummer, T., Gibbs, D., & Hix, S. (2015). Fieldwork educators' perspectives: Professional behavior attributes of level II students. *The Open Journal of Occupational Therapy, 3*(4), 1-13. http://doi.org/10.15453/2168-6408.1146

Clarke, C., Martin, M., de Visser, R., & Sadlo, G. (2015). Sustaining professional identity in practice following role-emerging placements: Opportunities and challenges for occupational therapists. *British Journal of Occupational Therapy, 78*(1), 42-50. https://doi.org/10.1177/0308022614561238

Clarke, C., Martin, M., Sadlo, G., & de Visser, R. (2014). The development of an authentic professional identity on role-emerging placements. *British Journal of Occupational Therapy, 77*(5), 222-229. http://dx.doi.org/10.4276/030802214X13990455043368

Copley, J., & Allen, S. (2009). Using all the available evidence: Perceptions of pediatric occupational therapists about how to increase evidence-based practice. *International Journal of Evidence Based Healthcare, 7*(3), 193-200. http://dx.doi.org/10.1111/j.1744-1609.2009.00137.x

Di Tommaso, A., Isbel, S., Scarvell, J., & Wicks, A. (2016). Occupational therapists' perceptions of occupation in practice: An exploratory study. *Australian Occupational Therapy Journal, 63*, 206-213. http://dx.doi.org/10.1111/1440-1630.12289

Di Tommaso, A., & Wilding, C. (2014). Exploring ways to improve descriptions of occupational therapy. *New Zealand Journal of Occupational Therapy, 61*(1), 27-33.

Dopp, C. M. E., Steultjens, E. M. J., & Radel, J. (2012). A survey of evidence-based practice among Dutch occupational therapists. *Occupational Therapy International, 19*, 17-27. http://dx.doi.org/10.1002/oti.324

Dorocher, E., Kinsella, E. A., Ells, C., & Hunt, M. (2015). Contradictions in client-centered discharge planning: Through the lens of relational autonomy. *Scandinavian Journal of Occupational Therapy, 22*(4), 293-301. http://doi.org/10.3109/11038128.2015.1017531

Dorocher, E., Kinsella, E. A., McCorquodale, L., & Phelan, S. (2016). Ethical tensions related to systemic constraints: Occupational alienation in occupational therapy practice. *OTJR: Occupation, Participation and Health, 36*(4), 216-226. http://dx.doi.org.ezproxylr.med.und.edu/10.1177/1539449216665117

Estes, J., & Pierce, D. E. (2012). Pediatric therapists' perspectives on occupation-based practice. *Scandinavian Journal of Occupational Therapy, 19*, 17-25. http://dx.doi.org/10.3109/11038128.2010.547598

Fange, A., & Ivanoff, S. D. (2009). Integrating research into practice: A challenge for local authority occupational therapy. *Scandinavian Journal of Occupational Therapy, 16*, 40-48. http://dx.doi.org.10.1080/11038120802419357

Finn, C. (2019). An occupation-based approach to management of concussion: Guidelines for practice. *The Open Journal of Occupational Therapy, 7*(2), Article 11. https://doi.org/10.15453/2168-6408.1550

Fisher, A. G. (2014). Occupation-centered, occupation-based, occupation-focused: Same, same or different? *Scandinavian Journal of Occupational Therapy, 21*, 96-107. http://dx.doi.org/10.3109/11038128.2012.754492

Fortune, T., & Kennedy-Jones, M. (2014). Occupation and its relationship with health and wellbeing: The threshold concept for occupational therapy. *Australian Occupational Therapy Journal, 61*, 293-298. http://dx.doi.org/10.1111/1440-1630.12144

Gilman, I. P. (2011). Evidence-based information-seeking behaviors of occupational therapists: A survey of recent graduates. *Journal of the Medical Library Association, 99*(4), 307-310. http://dx.doi.org/10.3163/1536-5050.99.4.009

Graham, F., Robertson, L., & Anderson, J. (2013). New Zealand occupational therapists' views on evidence-based practice: A replicated survey of attitudes, confidence, and behaviors. *Australian Occupational Therapy Journal, 60*, 120-128. http://dx.doi.org/10.1111/1440-1630.12000

Grenier, M. L. (2015). Facilitators and barriers to learning in occupational therapy fieldwork education: Student perspectives. *American Journal of Occupational Therapy, 52*(2), 143-149. http://dx.doi.org/10.5014/ajot.2015.015180

Gupta, J., & Taff, S. D. (2015). The illusion of client-centered practice. *Scandinavian Journal of Occupational Therapy, 22*, 244-251. http://dx.doi.org/10.3109/11038128.2015.1020866

Hazelwood, T., Baker, A., Murray, C. M., & Stanley, M. (2019). New graduate occupational therapists' narratives of ethical tensions encountered in practice. *Australian Occupational Therapy Journal, 66*(3), 283-291. http://doi.org/10.1111/1440-1630.12549

Hitch, D. P. (2016). Attitudes of mental health occupational therapists toward evidence-based practice. *Canadian Journal of Occupational Therapy, 83*(1), 27-32. http://dx.doi.org/10.1177/0008417415583108

Juckett, L. A., Wengerd, L. R., Faieta, J., & Griffin, C. E. (2020). Evidence-based practice implementation in stroke rehabilitation: A scoping review of barriers and facilitators. *American Journal of Occupational Therapy, 74*, 7401205050. https://doi.org/10.5014/ajot.2020.035485

Kessler, D., Walker, I., Sauv e-Schenk, K., & Egan, M. (2019). Goal setting dynamics that facilitate or impede a client-centered approach. *Scandinavian Journal of Occupational Therapy, 26*(5), 315-324. https://doi.org/10.1080/11038128.2018.1465119

Kristensen, H. K., Borg, T., & Hounsgaard, L. (2011). Facilitation of research-based evidence within occupational therapy stroke rehabilitations. *British Journal of Occupational Therapy, 74*(10), 473-483.

Krueger, R. B., Sweetman, M. M., Martin, M., & Cappaert, T. A. (2020). Occupational therapists' implementation of evidence-based practice: A cross sectional survey. *Occupational Therapy in Health Care, 34*(3), 253-276. http://doi.org/10.1080/07380577.2020.1756554

Lavin, K. A. (2018). Use of a journal club during level II fieldwork to facilitate confidence and skills for evidence-based practice. *The Open Journal of Occupational Therapy, 6*(4), Article 11. https://doi.org/10.15453/2168-6408.1475

Lyons, C., Brown, T., Tseng, M. H., Casey, J., & McDonald, R. (2011). Evidence-based practice and research utilization: Perceived research knowledge, attitudes, practices and barriers among Australian pediatric occupational therapists. *Australian Occupational Therapy Journal, 58*, 178-186. http://dx.doi.org/10.1111/j.1440-1630.2010.00900.x

Lyons, C., Casey, J., Brown, T., Tseng, M., & McDonald, R. (2010). Research knowledge, attitudes, practices and barriers among pediatric occupational therapists in the United Kingdom. *British Journal of Occupational Therapy, 73*(5), 200-209. http://dx.doi.org/10.4276/030802210X1234991664147

Marr, D. (2017). Fostering full implementation of evidence-based practice. *American Journal of Occupational Therapy, 71*(1), 1-5. http://dx.doi.org.ezproxylr.med.und.edu/10.5014/ajot.2017.019661

Morrison, T., & Robertson, L. (2016). New graduates' experience of evidence-based practice: An action research study. *British Journal of Occupational Therapy, 79*(1), 42-48. http://dx.doi.org/10.1177/0308022615591019

Mroz, T. M., Pitonyak, J. S., Fogelberg, D., & Leland, N. E. (2015). Health policy perspectives—Client centeredness and health reform: Key issues for occupational therapy. *American Journal of Occupational Therapy, 69*, 6905090010. http://dx.doi.org/10.5014/ajot.2015.695001

Myers, C. T., & Lotz, J. (2017). Practitioner training for use of evidence-based practice in occupational therapy. *Occupational Therapy in Health Care, 31*(3), 214-237. http://dx.doi.org.ezproxylr.med.und.edu/10.1080/07380577.2017.1333183

Nichols, A. (2017). Changes in knowledge, skills, and confidence in fieldwork educators after an evidence-based practice short course. *The Open Journal of Occupational Therapy, 5*(1), 1-14. http://dx.doi.org.ezproxylr.med.und.edu/10.15453/2168-6408.1204

Plewnia, A., Bengel, J., & Korner, M. (2016). Patient-centeredness and its impact on patient satisfaction and treatment outcomes in medical rehabilitation. *Patient Education and Counseling, 99*, 2063-2070. http://dx.doi.org/10.1016/j.pec.2016.07.018

Polatajko, H. J., & Davis, J. A. (2012). Advancing occupation-based practice: Interpreting the rhetoric. *Canadian Journal of Occupational Therapy, 79*, 259-263. http://dx.doi.org/10.2182/cjot.2010.79.5.1

Ripat, J., Wener, P., & Dobinson, K. (2013). The development of client-centeredness in student occupational therapists. *British Journal of Occupational Therapy, 76*(5), 217-224. https://doi.org/10.4276/030802213X13679275042681

Salls, J., Dolhi, C., Silverman, L., & Hansen, M. (2009). The use of evidence-based practice by occupational therapists. *Occupational Therapy in Health Care, 23*(2), 134-145. http://dx.doi.org10.1080/07380570902773305

Shea, C., & Jackson, N. (2015). Client perception of a client-centered and occupation-based intervention for at-risk youth. *Scandinavian Journal of Occupational Therapy, 22*(3), 173-180. http://doi.org/10.3109/11038128.2014.958873

Sonn, I., & Vermeulen, N. (2018). Occupational therapy students' experiences and perceptions of culture during fieldwork education. *South African Journal of Occupational Therapy, 48*(1), 34-39. http://dx.doi.org.ezproxylr.med.und.edu/10.17159/2310-3833/2017/vol48n1a7

Sumsion, T., & Law, M. (2006). A review of the evidence on the conceptual elements informing client-centered practice. *Canadian Journal of Occupational Therapy, 73*(3), 153-162. https://doi.org/10.1177/0008417406073003

Sumsion, T., & Lencucha, R. (2009). Therapists' perceptions of how teamwork influences client-centered practice. *British Journal of Occupational Therapy, 72*(2), 48-54.

Towns, E., & Ashby, S. (2014). The influence of practice educators on occupational therapy students' understanding of the practical applications of theoretical knowledge: A phenomenological study into student experiences of practice education. *Australian Occupational Therapy Journal, 61,* 344-352. https://doi.org/10.1111/1440-1630.12134

VanderKaay, S., Letts, L., Jung, B., Moll, S. E. (2020). Doing what's right: A grounded theory of ethical decision-making in occupational therapy. *Scandinavian Journal of Occupational Therapy, 27*(2), 98-111. http://doi.org/10.1080/1103 8128.2018.1464060

Wilding, C., & Whiteford, G. (2007). Occupation and occupational therapy: Knowledge paradigms and everyday practice. *Australian Occupational Therapy Journal, 54*(3), 185-193, http://dx.doi.org/10.1111/j.1440-1630.2006.00621.x

Wilkins, S., Pollock, N., Rochon, S., & Law, M. (2001). Implementing client-centered practice: Why is it so difficult to do? *Canadian Journal of Occupational Therapy, 68,* 70-79.

Wong, C., Fagan, B., & Leland, N. E. (2018). Occupational therapy practitioners' perspectives on occupation-based interventions for clients with hip fracture. *American Journal of Occupational Therapy, 72,* 7204205050. https://.doi.org/10.5014/ajot.2018.026492

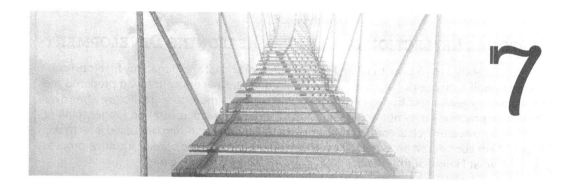

Clinical Reasoning Development During Level II Fieldwork

Amy Mattila, PhD, OTR/L
and Elizabeth LeQuieu, PhD, OTR/L, CLA

Clinical reasoning is a fundamental skill for health care practitioners such as occupational therapy professionals. This skill develops over time beginning in one's educational program and extending into one's professional practice. Since Level II fieldwork is part of the educational process that links the classroom to practice, it becomes quite important to the development of students' clinical reasoning. Therefore, Level II fieldwork educators (FWeds) must be equipped to demonstrate, discuss, and support the continued development of a student's clinical reasoning. The complicating factor is that clinical reasoning becomes more intuitive as one's level of expertise increases, making it more difficult for expert educators to verbalize their intuitive process. The purpose of this chapter is provide the practitioner and FWed with strategies to promote clinical reasoning skills among students during Level II fieldwork. Specifically, the strategies presented in this chapter are aimed to:

- Build a language to describe the intuitive thought processes used by expert practitioners/ FWeds.

- Encourage reflection on how clinical reasoning was developed and when it occurred.

- Provide tools to help students develop clinical reasoning skills.

In this chapter, the authors will define clinical reasoning, discuss how it looks in practice, and explore ways to help students develop their clinical reasoning skills (Box 7-1).

DeIuliis, E. D., & Hanson, D. (Eds.).
Fieldwork Educator's Guide to Level II Fieldwork (pp. 203-226).

> ### Box 7-1
> ## PERSONAL REFLECTION OF CLINICAL REASONING DEVELOPMENT
>
> As I (Elizabeth) think back to when I graduated from school and began my first job, I considered myself a novice or beginner. While I was confident my education had prepared me to be an entry-level practitioner, I knew there was so much more to learn. Today, after over 18 years of practice, I may not be an expert in all areas of practice, but I no longer think of myself as a novice. In fact, according to the novice to expert continuum discussed later in this chapter, I am considered an expert. Clinical reasoning has become a quick intuitive process and I use what I know of the client as well as my experience to guide me.
> - When did it happen?
> - When did I move from a beginner to competent and ultimately to expert?
> - When did I know what I know and how do I help students develop clinical reasoning?

LEARNING OBJECTIVES

By the end of reading this chapter and completing the learning activities, the reader should be able to:

1. Identify types of clinical reasoning and describe how clinical reasoning is used throughout clinical practice in occupational therapy.

2. Reflect on their own use of clinical reasoning.

3. Consider the developmental needs, timing, and context of fieldwork students, particularly from one Level II to the next.

4. Understand the novice to expert continuum and its impact on fieldwork student development.

5. Identify ways to apply problem-solving strategies in clinical reasoning with Level II fieldwork students.

6. Utilize a structured clinical reasoning process to encourage clinical judgment, decision making, and critical thinking in Level II fieldwork students.

7. Identify and describe teaching strategies and self-directed learning to support student clinical reasoning.

AN OVERVIEW OF CLINICAL REASONING

Recognized as one of the foundations of occupational therapy practice, clinical reasoning is comprised of decision-making processes occupational therapists use to guide their approach to client-centered services. It is defined as the "process that practitioners use to plan, direct, perform, and reflect on client care" (Schell, 2019, p. 482). Specifically, occupational therapy practitioners engage in clinical reasoning to analyze activities, occupations, and collaborate with clients throughout the occupational therapy process (American Occupational Therapy Association [AOTA], 2020c).

From the early 1980s to today, approximately 208 original studies and reviews have focused on clinical reasoning (Marquez-Alvarez et al., 2019). The first article investigating clinical reasoning occurred in 1982 by Rogers and Masagatani when they studied how occupational therapists think. In addition to trying to characterize the clinical reasoning process, they found experienced practitioners had difficulty in articulating their reasoning, which was related to skill level. The term clinical reasoning gained more attention the following year with Joan Rogers' AOTA Eleanor Clark Slagle Lecture (Rogers, 1983). In the next few years, AOTA and the American Occupational Therapy Foundation (AOTF) teamed up to fund a research project that became known as the *Clinical Reasoning Study* (Cohn, 1991). Much of the findings from this study were published in a special edition of the *American Journal of Occupational Therapy* (Cohn, 1991). This special edition included an article by Maureen Fleming in which she identified how occupational therapy clinicians used different approaches of reasoning depending on the problem. In doing so, she was the first within occupational therapy to describe the different ways of thinking or aspects of clinical reasoning (Fleming, 1991). Since that time, others have examined clinical reasoning and have named several other aspects used by occupational therapists. However, the clinical reasoning of expert practitioners, by definition, is intuitive. The expert anticipates and recognizes clients' strengths and weaknesses based on experience and does not rely on rules and guidelines for decision making. In fact, experts often find it difficult to explain their multilayered thinking (Dreyfus & Dreyfus, 1986; Neistadt, 1996). However, it is important the FWed "tease out these layers and the associated reasoning for novices" or their students (Unsworth & Baker, 2016, p. 6).

BUILDING A LANGUAGE FOR CLINICAL REASONING

Seasoned practitioners attend to many factors simultaneously and aspects of clinical reasoning become intuitive. Students, however, may become overwhelmed at the number of factors to attend to at once and must learn which are the most important. Thus, students need help in both identifying and verbalizing the clinical reasoning behind their decisions. In order to build a language to assist with communication about clinical reasoning on fieldwork, the following eight aspects of clinical reasoning (scientific, diagnostic, procedural, narrative, pragmatic, interactive, ethical, and conditional reasoning) are defined and demonstrated.

Aspects of Clinical Reasoning

Scientific Reasoning

Scientific reasoning is a systematic approach to making decisions. It allows practitioners to follow a prescribed method to derive conclusions that are reliable and generalizable. It is closely aligned with the use of evidence-based practice. Scientific reasoning may be impersonal as the therapist may be focused on the condition, evidence from research, theory, or the knowledge of typical progression of clients with similar diagnoses. See Box 7-2 for tips to help students with scientific reasoning.

Diagnostic Reasoning

Diagnostic reasoning is a way for clinicians to investigate and analyze the cause of nature of the client's condition. It is often considered a component of scientific reasoning and utilized to justify the need for occupational therapy services. The clinican uses both impersonal (i.e., scientific) information and personal (i.e., client-based) information to guide the therapeutic process. See Box 7-3 for tips to help students with diagnostic reasoning.

BOX 7-2

TIPS TO HELP STUDENTS WITH SCIENTIFIC REASONING

Give students a list of the most common diagnoses in your facility prior to their first day to help prepare them for their Level II experience. The students should complete the following regarding each diagnosis:

1. How does the diagnosis usually present?
2. What is the usual prognosis or long-term potential outcomes?
3. What are typical theories that might be used to guide assessments/interventions with clients with the diagnosis?
4. What evidence-based assessment/interventions might be used? Describe your familiarity with each.
5. Provide research/evidence for each diagnosis.

This activity will help students be prepared for scientific reasoning and the use of evidence.

BOX 7-3

TIPS TO HELP STUDENTS WITH DIAGNOSTIC REASONING

Using the previous exercise (see Box 7-2), the student can build in the client-based information. Students will have information about the diagnosis, usual prognosis, and evidence for the most common diagnoses of the site. Now the student can include information about a specific client. What is the client's current abilities and problems regarding occupational performance? What factors (scientific and client-based) are contributing to the client's problems? Compare the scientific expectations of a person with the client's occupational performance and potential prognosis. What are the similarities and differences when adding the client-specific information?

Procedural Reasoning

Procedural reasoning focuses on the process. Practitioners use procedural reasoning when "thinking about the disease or disability and deciding which intervention activities (procedures) they might employ to remediate the person's functional performance problems" (Fleming, 1991, p. 1008). *How do we get things done to maximize client occupational performance? What is to happen next?* This reasoning addresses the physical diagnosis and treatment techniques. Sometimes this type of reasoning is influenced by a practitioner relying heavily on protocols or routines that may develop within the setting. It is important when using procedural reasoning to acknowledge the origin of the procedures. *Are we as practitioners relying on procedures based in evidence, convenience, or habit?* See Box 7-4 for tips to help students.

Narrative Reasoning

Narrative reasoning uses story making or storytelling as a means to understand the client and their experience. It is a process that can explore where the client is now and where they wish to be in the future. The client begins storytelling during the evaluation and as the occupational therapy practitioner completes an occupational profile. Simultaneously, the practitioner is making sense of the client's story. Mattingly (1991) describes using narrative reasoning not only to understand

> ### Box 7-4
> # TIPS TO HELP STUDENTS WITH PROCEDURAL REASONING
>
> Have the student choose a client with whom they have been working and have the student reflect on the following:
>
> 1. When thinking about the client's disease or disability, what intervention activities did you choose? Why? Are they completed in a specific order?
> 2. How will the activities chosen maximize the client's performance?
> 3. What evidence supports your procedures with this client? Or were the activities supported by the habits/routines of the setting?
> 4. Have you chosen the same activities/procedures with another client with a similar diagnosis or disability? Why?
> 5. Will you continue with the same procedures or change your approach? Why?

> ### Box 7-5
> # TIPS TO HELP STUDENTS WITH NARRATIVE REASONING
>
> Practitioners may consider narrative reasoning as intuitive to the role of occupational therapy. However, it is important to help guide students in verbalizing narrative reasoning in order to ensure its development. The following are some quesitons to generate a discussion regarding the use of narrative reasoning:
>
> 1. Tell me the life story of (a certain client) including what you know about them before injury/illness, about them now, and about their future goals?
> 2. Describe the client's occupations. Which occupations are most important to the client?
> 3. How has their current health status impacted their occupational performance? Will the client be able to return to the same occupations of interest?
> 4. How are you including the client's occupations within the therapy process?
> 5. How have you become part of the client's story/narrative?
> 6. How does the client describe their future/after therapy? How do you see the client in the future/after therapy? What are the similarities and/or differences? Why?

the client's lived experiences of the disability or illness, but also to "structure therapy in a narrative way" (p. 1000). She further describes how the practitioner becomes part of the client's story or narrative through therapy. In clinical practice, practitioners may use narrative reasoning to guide therapy including outcome goals. The practitioner and client create the story of where the client wants to be after discharge. See Box 7-5 for tips to help students.

Pragmatic Reasoning

Pragmatic reasoning encourages therapists to attend to and reflect on practical decisions and realities of providing services. It focuses on the practitioners' personal context and the practical context of therapy itself. The personal context includes one's personal skills and professional skills such as competence and confidence. Some practical context factors that may require this reasoning include scheduling clients, amount of treatment time per client, available supplies, environmental factors, payment/coverage of services, teaming, etc. The practitioner uses pragmatic reasoning to

---

Box 7-6

PRAGMATIC REASONING: A STORY FROM THE FIELD

As a Level II FWed practicing in lymphedema and breast cancer rehabilitation, I teach my students the importance of gathering as much diagnostic criteria as possible. It is also important to gather information from functional assessments, the primary care team, other health care professionals, and of course from the client.

Next, I guide the student to create the client's treatment plan based on all of the information gathered. For instance a client with metastatic breast cancer presents with severe edema in her RUE. Circumference measurements show a difference of 2500 ml (RUE > LUE). The client's RUE shoulder ROM is well below functional limits and her manual muscle testing is 3-/5. The scientific information recommends that I aggressively wrap her arm with multi-layer compression wrapping 5 days/week along with daily manual lymphatic drainage sessions and extensive manual therapy and exercise to improve her ROM, strength, and endurance. However, personal information gathered illustrates a different picture of the client.

Perhaps the client lives quite a long way from therapy, but attends regularly scheduled chemotherapy appointments. The chemotherapy makes her extremely sick and weak leading to safety concerns. Additionally, neuropathic changes related to the chemotherapy make her RUE very sensitive to touch, much less compression.

It is important to help students use pragmatic reasoning attending to and reflecting on practical decisions and realities of providing services. What family or caregiver support does the client have? Do I (the therapist) have the skills to educate the family to perform a home program? How do we create a schedule that will promote regular attendance? What special supplies are available for use? Is there a system the client can donn and doff independently that will also account for the neuropathy?

—James B. Saviers II, MS, OTR/L, CLT-LANA

---

manage portions of the personal and practical contexts. Schell (2018) stated "skilled pragmatic reasoning holds the potential to unleash the power of occupational therapy, as therapists become more effective in negotiation of optimal conditions for practice" (p. 217). Therefore, creating a match between the environment and the client provides the conditions and supports for optimal occupational performance. However, there are times therapists use pragmatic reasoning to solve practical problems. See Box 7-6 for an example of pragmatic reasoning.

Interactive Reasoning

Interactive reasoning explores the relationship between the clinician and the client. Often connected to therapeutic use of self, the clinician can use this form of reasoning to engage with and motivate the client in the therapeutic process. Turpin and Copley (2018) described interactive reasoning as having two distinct aspects: understanding clients as individuals experiencing an injury or illness and developing partnerships with clients. In fact, therapeutic use of self may be one of the most effective tools used by occupational therapists. The relationship is developed through effective communication (verbal and nonverbal), cooperation, empathy, and collaboration. Students can improve interactive reasoning by developing good communication skills and emotional intelligence concepts such as self-awareness, self-regulation, empathy, motivation, and social skills (Goleman, 2005). See Box 7-7 for tips to help students.

> ## Box 7-7
> # Interactive Reasoning: A Story From the Field
>
> I have supervised Level II occupational therapy and occupational therapy assistant fieldwork students at a day center for adults with intellectual and development disabilities. Some clients at this center demonstrate mild to severe behavioral problems that could potentially affect the welfare and safety of themselves and others. This particular setting may be more challenging for students to effectively use interactive reasoning and their therapeutic use of self. However, it is important for the students to perceive each client as an individual, develop partnerships with the clients, and use good verbal and nonverbal communication.
>
> In order to prepare the students, I first use storytelling to describe situations that I have experienced, but could have handled differently. I explain the outcomes and have students give examples of alternative actions that may produce more positive outcomes. Then I allow students to observe my intervention sessions with clients with behavioral issues and follow up with discussion. At times, we may even role play to ensure the students can respond quickly and appropriately to avoid any potential safety issues. We discuss the importance of considering the position of the client, position of the therapist, activities selected, environment, communication, how to relate to the clients, and difficulty of the tasks. The next step is to allow the students to plan and initiate a treatment session with close supervision. As the students demonstrate success, supervision may become more distant.
>
> Throughout these steps, the students learn to be aware of their verbal and non-verbal communication as well as the verbal and non-verbal responses from their clients. Students learn about the environment and actions that may trigger a behavioral outburst. Learning to use interactive reasoning (e.g., students reading the client's signs and adjusting their responses) can be the key to a fun, productive, and safe intervention session.
>
> —*Dr. Tracey Zeiner, OTD, OTR/L*

Ethical Reasoning

Ethical reasoning is the ability of practitioners to make decisions based on ethical principles and actions. It provides a framework for ethical decision making, rooted in ethical theories. There is often tension that accompanies ethical reasoning as the practitioner must determine the "right" thing to do. Ethical reasoning may center around the organization, practice, or the client. The *2020 Occupational Therapy Code of Ethics* of the AOTA outlines core values, ethical principles, and standards of conduct to guide ethical practice (AOTA, 2020a). The core values identified are altruism, equality, freedom, justice, dignity, truth, and prudence. Principles that guide ethical decision making include beneficence, nonmaleficence, autonomy, justice, veracity, and fidelity. Finally, the standards of conduct related to professional integrity, responsibility, and accountability; therapeutic relationships; documentation, reimbursement, and financial matters; service delivery; professional competence, education, supervision, and training; communication; and professional civility (AOTA, 2020a). While Level II students may encounter ethical dilemmas during fieldwork, the code of ethics document provides useful information for FWeds to create ethical questions to explore with students. See Box 7-8 for questions to prompt a student's ethical reasoning.

Conditional Reasoning

Conditional reasoning heavily focuses on context and environment. This context can be where and how the interventions occur, where the client performs occupations, and how to translate the client's needs into adaptations that will facilitate occupational performance. This reasoning may be the most advanced as it blends all the aspects of reasoning and the flexibility of changing

---

Box 7-8

QUESTIONS TO HELP DEVELOP STUDENTS' ETHICAL REASONING

1. Does a client's differing opinion or values influence occupational therapy treatment? If so, how? Should it have any influence?

2. What differences in people do you find most challenging and how do you ensure professional civility?

3. Explain a time when you have demonstrated cultural humility in practice.

4. What are the costs vs. benefits and risks vs. benefits of therapy for a particular client?

5. What should you do if you believe a client needs more therapy, but insurance will not pay for additional intervention?

6. Tell me about an ethical dilemma and how you resolved it.

---

conditions. Practitioners use conditional reasoning to predict how clients will perform in the future and in different contexts such as after discharge. See Box 7-9 for tips to help students with conditional reasoning.

WHERE ARE STUDENTS IN THE CLINICAL REASONING PROCESS?

The occupational therapy process is the client-centered delivery of occupational therapy services. The three-part process includes (1) evaluation and (2) intervention to achieve (3) targeted outcomes and occurs within the purview of the occupational therapy domain. The process is facilitated by the distinct perspective of occupational therapy practitioners engaging in professional reasoning, analyzing occupations and activities, and collaborating with clients. The cornerstones of occupational therapy practice underpin the process of service delivery (AOTA, 2020c). Occupational therapy practitioners use what they know about the profession, themselves, the patient, and the context to guide decisions about practice. Moreover, all of this information and experience is processed efficiently and many times automatically. Students are expected to begin developing clinical reasoning throughout their academic careers. For example, they may use the knowledge gained in anatomy coursework to aid in scientific or diagnostic reasoning within a biomechanical intervention course or apply the therapeutic use of self to engage their clients through interactive reasoning. Level II fieldwork is a continuation of the didactic coursework and is vital to the professional education. It affords students opportunities for learning transfer from the classroom to authentic contexts and clients. Therefore, Level II fieldwork is an optimal setting for students to continue developing clinical reasoning. In fact, one purpose of the fieldwork experience is "to promote clinical reasoning and reflective practice …." (ACOTE, 2018, p. 39). See Box 7-10 for a FWed tip to assess clinical reasoning. In order to do so, FWeds should have a realistic expectation of the students reasoning abilities when beginning Level II fieldwork, the student's goal for the end of the experience, and how to help the student reach that goal.

At the beginning of Level II fieldwork, students will have general didactic knowledge including, but not limited to, theory, research, and the occupational therapy process. They may have had an opportunity to apply this knowledge via Level I fieldwork, simulated patients, case-based learning, etc. However, Level II fieldwork begins the process of bringing everything together for the student allowing them the opportunity to develop into entry-level generalists under the supervision of a qualified practitioner and role model (ACOTE, 2018).

Box 7-9

CONDITIONAL REASONING: A STORY FROM A LEVEL II FIELDWORK STUDENT

Before graduate school, I was not particularly experienced or comfortable playing with small children simply because none of my friends had any! So, when I was a Level II fieldwork student in a pediatric acute care setting, I found myself struggling to identify games and activities that would engage my patients at an age-appropriate level and then adapting these unfamiliar games to match diagnosis-specific needs. Because of the nature of the setting, I could only select a few activities to carry with me from the therapy office to patient rooms, so it was critical to be able to adapt a few activities to fit multiple patients' needs and interests. And if (or when) they decided they did not like the first game, I needed to be able to use these limited materials to create a new activity at a moment's notice.

To help me develop my ability to think in a more conditional way, my FWed encouraged me to create a spreadsheet of all the available resources in the therapy office and in subsequent columns of the same row to list ways each activity could be used to address at least five different functional deficits (fine motor oordination, gross motor coordination, visual scanning, functional cognition, balance, etc). Completing this assignment gave me a great reference tool if I felt a "block" with a particular patient, it helped familiarize me with available activities, and I quickly improved in my ability to adapt the same activity for a variety of diagnoses and ages. It was incredibly helpful and gave me confidence! Eventually, I noticed this process becoming more intuitive and I needed to reference the spreadsheet less and less.

—*Ciara Fleer, OTR/L*

Box 7-10

FIELDWORK EDUCATOR TIP

One way to assess a student's baseline in clinical reasoning and reflection is through the Self-Assessment of Clinical Reflection and Reasoning tool (Royeen et al., 2001). Please see Appendix A for this tool.

TAKING THE TIME FOR DEVELOPING CLINICAL REASONING

Mason et al. (2020) noted clinical reasoning as one of the skills educators spent the most time developing at the beginning of Level II fieldwork. This could be expected since students beginning their Level II experiences should be at a novice status, continuing their education in a real context. In addition to understanding where students are in regard to their clinical reasoning, there are ways to support their clinical reasoning development. First, it is vital to create a safe space for students to communicate with the FWed. A fear of failure can stifle participation and thus learning.

Second, it is important for the FWed to verbalize their clinical reasoning process. Start scaffolding the learning process by choosing one or two aspects of clinical reasoning to discuss following a treatment session. The student will need to not only hear about the reasoning process but also which aspect of clinical reasoning used. Next, the educator might ask the student about the reasoning behind a choice the educator made.

- *"Why do you think I chose that activity?"*
- *"What type of reasoning would that be?"*

As the student becomes more independent with providing care, the FWed could ask similar questions about their clinical reasoning, such as those reflected in Appendix B. The emphasis is verbal communication. Third, students become frustrated with multiple right answers. While this is often innate in occupational therapy practice, students may need to focus on single answer questions at the beginning of their Level II experience when possible. As the student's knowledge expands, so may the possible "correct" answers. Fourth, students need time and repeated practice. Some student will need time to think about the reasoning process and time for reflection. Finally, students need repeated practice. Occupational therapy practitioners must attend to multiple factors within a single treatment session, such as client factors, performance skills, performance patters, contexts, occupations, and anticipated outcomes. This can be overwhelming for Level II students as they try to first understand each of the varying components and then identify those most pertinent (Robertson, 1996). However, by setting the stage and taking the time for developing clinical reasoning skills, FWeds can help student identify the aspects of clinical reasoning and work toward automaticity.

IT IS ABOUT TIMING AND CONTEXT

This next section will consider the importance of timing for the fieldwork student. As the FWed, having an understanding that even the difference between a Level IIA and Level IIB can be significant in terms of clinical reasoning. It is important to have realistic expectations of the student based on their sequence of experiential learning, the context in which they have practiced, as well as prior experiences with FWed. These will be elaborated on further throughout the remainder of the chapter.

The Novice to Expert Continuum Revisited

As discussed in Chapter 5 of the corresponding *Fieldwork Educator's Guide to Level I Fieldwork* (Hanson & Mattila, 2023), it is incredibly important for FWeds to have realistic expectations around the student's abilities to clinically reason. In this chapter, we want to revisit the stages of clinical reasoning that can be graded along a continuum (Neistadt, 1996). What stands out here, even for the Level II fieldwork student, is that post-graduation, new clinicians are entering practice at the novice or advanced beginner at best, emphasizing the need to continue to take a developmental approach for students at the Level II fieldwork stage (Neistadt, 1996). Table 7-1 further elaborates on these stages and key characteristics of the practitioner.

When a FWed receives a Level II student, they will still likely be somewhere in the novice stage. You can expect them to be fairly rigid with their thinking and relying heavily on procedural reasoning or what they remember from the textbook regarding diagnostic and scientific understanding of the client. Some students may come with more experience from Level I, but due to the variety of Level I experiences in practice, others may not have extensive experience to rely on. Table 7-2 presents some potential key differences in the clinical reasoning of a Level I vs. Level II fieldwork student.

Beyond the global skills and abilities of clinical reasoning as shared previously, Mason et al. (2020) found additional technical skills that are reported to be lacking at the start of Level II fieldwork experiences. In their study, the top five technical skills that were insufficient according to 54 Level II FWeds included communication skills, problem-solving skills, initiative, time management, and creativity (Mason et al., 2020). Each of these technical skills are closely aligned with the clinical reasoning process and should be assessed in some way as a baseline for fieldwork students.

TABLE 7-1
STAGES AND KEY CHARACTERISTICS OF CLINICAL REASONING SKILLS

STAGE	YEARS IN PRACTICE	KEY CHARACTERISTICS
Novice	0	Have knowledge of theories, frameworks, and principles around practice; usually rigid in application (textbook knowledge); limited experience to rely on
Advanced beginner	<1	Begins to incorporate context and may practice modification of "rules" to adapt to specific situations; still less flexible in that application and limited ability to prioritize well
Competent	3	Able to adjust therapy to specific needs of client and context; sorts relevant data and prioritizes intervention accordingly; lacks the speed and flexibility of proficient therapist
Proficient	5	Flexible and have the ability to alter both evaluation and treatment plans as needed; has a perception of the case based on experience rather than deliberation; skillful in understanding the narrative of client's needs
Expert	10	Reasoning is a quick and intuitive process; anticipates and recognizes clients' strengths and weakness based on experience; does not rely on rules and guidelines for decision making, but more of intuition (experts often find it difficult to explain this intuition)

Adapted from Dreyfus, S. E., & Dreyfus, H. L. (1980). *A five-stage model of the mental activities involved in directed skill acquisition*. California Univ Berkeley Operations Research Center; and Neistadt, M. E. (1996). Teaching strategies for the development of clinical reasoning. *American Journal of Occupational Therapy, 50*(8), 676-684. https://doi.org/10.5014/ajot.50.8.676

An additional area of importance to remember for the Level II student is that early on, they tend to be less flexible with their application and on-the-spot thinking. Recognizing these traits will be important for the reflexive thinking process elaborated upon later in this chapter. Box 7-11 shares a story of one therapist's journey from novice to expert practitioner whose mentoring experience allowed her to quickly move toward proficiency.

Practitioners who choose to be FWeds devote time to educating future professionals. This professional engagement and commitment is recognized by many including the schools, the academic fieldwork coordinators, and the students. It is assumed that more time would be needed to develop clinical reasoning at the beginning of the Level II experience and decrease over time. There are several suggestions we discuss in this chapter to help weave clinical reasoning development within the usual educational time. As with other aspects of teaching Level II students, some will need instruction during a session and some immediately following while other students have the ability to wait until lunch or even the end of the day for discussions. We feel it optimal for articulation of

TABLE 7-2
NOTABLE DIFFERENCES BETWEEN LEVEL I AND LEVEL II FIELDWORK STUDENTS

LEVEL I FIELDWORK NOVICE	LEVEL II FIELDWORK NOVICE–ADVANCED BEGINNER
Little to no experience	Level I experience to rely on (varied)
Inability to use discretionary judgment	Able to apply some level of discretion in decision making
Limited ability to make predictions for a client's situation	Should be able to apply some diagnostic and scientific reasoning to make sound predictions for client's plan of care
Often struggles to decide priorities in cases	Able to delineate which tasks are most relevant
Focus is on rules and guidelines that have been taught in the classroom	While some clinical knowledge is present, focus is still heavily on rules and guidelines that have been taught in the classroom
Heavier supervision required	Supervision should be graded and reduced, as appropriate, then eventually develop into mentoring as they approach entry-level practice

knowledge to be completed during or at the conclusions of a therapy session. While timing may be important to clinical reasoning development, it may be dictated more by the context.

Therapy occurs within contexts which vary greatly. Some of the causes of variance may include, but are not limited to: caseload, setting, interprofessional relationships, reimbursement, space, time, equipment, etc. One could be working in a traditional setting, such as an inpatient acute psychiatric hospital, school, or outpatient rehabilitation clinic, or perhaps a role-emerging setting, such as a homeless shelter, hospice care, or transition services for college students.

A number of researchers have found that contextual factors may focus or influence the clinical reasoning process (Crepeau, 1991; Holmqvist et al., 2009; Unsworth, 2004). Thus, it is important for the fieldwork student to have a good understanding of the context in which the experience will occur. See Table 7-3 for examples of context and their potential effect on clinical reasoning skills.

THE CLINICAL REASONING PROCESS IN ACTION: INCORPORATING A FIVE-STEP CLINICAL REASONING PROCESS

Once you have established where the student is at by utilizing the Clinical Reasoning Checklist, as a FWed, you can begin to introduce and model the Five-Step Clinical Reasoning Process (Cronin & Graebe, 2018). Having a model for novice students can help facilitate the tools and strategies to organize and enhance their clinical reasoning. This chapter will expand upon the Clinical Reasoning Process introduced by Cronin and Graebe (2018) and share a suggested "roadmap" for Level II fieldwork students.

> ## BOX 7-11
> ## MOVEMENT FROM NOVICE TO EXPERT CONTINUUM
>
> Knowing I always wanted to be in pediatrics, I was excited to get a Level II pediatric placement that had the possibility of both schools and outpatient pediatric clinic experience. I ended up only being placed in the outpatient clinic and had a great experience! They invested in me as a student by providing a weekly seminar that consisted of me preparing with reading articles, watching videos, and reflecting on videos of myself taken during therapy sessions. This meeting was with the Clinic Specialist. I also had another weekly meeting with my FWed to talk about areas to improve and areas of strength from the last week as well as plan for the next week.
>
> I believe my strong experience allowed me to learn and grow into a more competent entry-level therapist. I was offered a position with the same company when I graduated and passed my boards. I began working my first year in both schools and clinics and had 2 paid hours of mentorship every week, one meeting with the clinic specialist and one with the School Specialist. These two meetings consisted of going over documentation for the schools and understanding the processes in school-based therapy as well as diving into client care and problem-solving treatment ideas.
>
> Three years into my career, I was promoted to the role of Programs Manager. I now provide occupational therapy services about 50% of the time and spend the other 50% of my time completing my management and leadership roles to support our school-based staff. I interview, hire, and train new staff as well as complete performance reviews and give regular feedback on job performance. I act as the liaison between the therapist and schools in order to manage workload and caseload expectations and all details with the school contracts. I also hold the title of fieldwork coordinator for our facility, assisting in setting up contracts with schools and continuing our strong fieldwork experience.
>
> —Rebecca Henderson, MOT, OTR/L

Step 1: Client and Referral Information

This stage allows the Level II fieldwork student a first opportunity to apply clinical reasoning. In this stage, the first step is interaction with the referral process and contact with the client. The referral allows the student to reflect upon their diagnostic reasoning.

- *Can the student delineate what client factors might be impacted by this diagnosis? What then is the impact on occupational performance?*

Once they begin interaction with the client, the opportunity for narrative reasoning is present. This step requires consideration of the student's strengths and weaknesses around communication, interaction, and therapeutic use of self. At this point, the student should be gathering information on the occupational profile.

- *How does the student organize their thoughts to compile data around the client's needs, problems, and concerns around occupational performance?*

- *How does the student build rapport with the client? Are they comfortable or at ease with the therapeutic relationship?*

- *Does the student pay attention to any incongruities based on their diagnostic reasoning? For example, did they identify unexpected impairments or comorbidities that were not included in the referral or chart review?*

TABLE 7-3

CONTEXT AND CLINICAL REASONING SKILLS

CASELOAD	Describe the usual client caseload including the types of clients, usual diagnoses, and number of clients. Do you work in teams? If so, who is part of that team? What will be the expectation for the student at stated times during the experience (e.g., 3 weeks, 6 weeks, 9 weeks, 12 weeks)?
SETTING (POLICIES, NORMS, RULES)	Describe the overall setting and expectations. What are the policies? What are the stated and unstated norms/rules for the setting?
TEAMS	Describe how the professions in your setting work together (or do not work together). What are the expectations of the student regarding inter- and/or intra-professional teams?
REIMBURSEMENT	What are the payment systems for services in the setting? Does the payment system determine types of services provided, the length of stay, etc.? If so, how?
SPACE	What is the space in which you usually work? Are there specialized areas for certain treatment, training, privacy, etc.?
TIME	What is the usual treatment time? How is scheduling completed and communicated with others? What is the usual length of therapy for a client?
EQUIPMENT	What equipment and supplies are available for the occupational therapy practitioner and fieldwork student?

Step 2: Clinical Hypotheses

In this stage, the student should use technical skills of clinical reasoning to identify potential approaches to support the client through evaluation and intervention. To develop clinical hypotheses, the student first needs to articulate a working hypothesis and use it to lead their initial data gathering. This step requires a variety of problem-solving strategies and potentially tapping into the scientific reasoning process to consider information from a variety of contexts. For example, students can be prompted to explore:

- *What do I know to be true about the diagnostic information presented in this case?*
- *What are the implications/impact of the performance problems?*
  - *What appears to have contributed to this performance problem?*
  - *What are the domains and occupations of concerns for potential occupational therapy intervention?*
- *Are there findings or principles in this case that might be generalizable to others I have seen in the past?*

Algorithm	Heuristic	Trial and Error	Insight
• Utilizes a formula or step-by-step procedure that will always produce a correct solution • This might get a student "stuck" in the right or wrong of a case • Can be used with well-defined problems, but not efficient for many clinical situations • **Example:** Using an algorithm to explain chronic pain	• A general rule that may or may not work in certain situations • Does not always guarantee a correct solution • Allows students to simplify complex problems and reduce possible solutions to a more manageable outcome • **Example:** Attributing the same chronic pain to the referring diagnosis or past clinical experience	• Trying several solutions and ruling out the ones that do not work • Can be time-consuming, so typically used in a clinical situation after an algorithm or heuristic has been applied • Often used in cases where problem is ill-defined or multiple co-morbid factors are present • **Example:** Trialing a variety of modalities to address the chronic pain to see which works best	• Distinct from other strategies as it is not a structured process, often happens as a sudden awareness or idea to address the problem • Grounded in clinician's knowledge and experience; not often utilized as much by students • **Example:** Applying an emerging practice technique on pain, observed at a workshop or conference

Figure 7-1. Problem-solving strategies to enhance clinical reasoning.

Step 3: Data Collection, Problem Solving, and Hypotheses Evaluation

During this step of the process, objective, measurable occupational performance areas are targeted and data collection procedures are established, allowing the student to trial potential approaches. While sometimes difficult, allowing for reasonable trial and error in this step can be crucial to their development. As much as possible, the student needs to discover, analyze, and resolve their own difficulties to move from novice to advanced beginner in the continuum. Cherry (2020) shares four types of problem-solving strategies that can be facilitated to encourage the Level II fieldwork student's development when appropriate. Figure 7-1 provides an overview of these strategies.

In this step as a FWed, it is equally important to recognize obstacles in problem-solving, particularly for the novice student. One of the most common can be referred to as "functional fixedness" (Cherry, 2020). This refers to the tendency for novice students to view problems only in their most black and white nature. It puts "blinders" on the problem-solving process, as they see a diagnosis and have expectations around what they should do or explore. Utilizing a variety of the approaches discussed in Hanson and Mattila (2023) can help move the student out of their limited critical thinking box including reasoning out loud, chunking information, use of protocols, debriefing, and reflection on practice (all elaborated further in Book One, Chapter 5 of this text series).

Another obstacle for novice students can be the inability to filter irrelevant or misleading information. One strategy that can help in this situation is to encourage the use of a template, such as the AOTA Occupational Profile Template (AOTA, 2020b). Providing a sense of structure to the information gathering phase can help the student to focus, particularly when complex cases are at hand.

Finally, assumptions can get in the way of clear thinking when it comes to problem solving. Allowing the opportunity for students to process any biases or assumptions early on in the fieldwork experience can be helpful to recognize that they exist. Facilitating this process is included in the baseline checklist embedded in this chapter's learning activities.

Moving through steps 2 and 3 require reflection and creative thinking, which will ultimately allow for the testing of any clinical hypotheses.

Step 4: Test and Refine Hypotheses

This step occurs in the occupational therapy process once the client moves toward progress (or lack thereof) in objective, measurable performance targets. The findings of an evaluation should influence what the student will identify as priorities in the case and narrowing of the clinical hypotheses. Following an evaluation of a client, the FWed can prompt the student to articulate the following:

- *What are the possible clinical findings that I might expect in a typical case with these performance deficits?*
  - *How does this client compare?*
- *Are there domain-specific protocols that can be utilized to improve successful outcomes?*
- *Are there psychosocial factors that are limiting or preventing progress? If so, how can I address these needs?*

Once the student reflects on these, the FWed can encourage a return to Step 2, to refine or replace the hypotheses based on the client's data.

Step 5: Appraise the Evidence

This stage, which can feel difficult for the student to arrive at early on in Level II fieldwork, involves a synthesis of information from all sources to produce a plan of care. As a FWed, the most important role in this step is guiding the discussion to allow the student to arrive at a reasonable conclusion. A key factor here is encouraging the student to think beyond just what confirms their hypotheses, but also what might challenge it.

Let's practice using this case example in Box 7-12 about Kate, a scenario that takes place in an outpatient rehabilitation setting. Review the description and use Table 7-4 to identify what reflection questions might be used to encourage the clinical reasoning process.

The next section of this chapter will focus on practical skills for the FWed to facilitate these stages through teaching, modeling, and reflection.

CLINICAL REASONING AND SELF-DIRECTED LEARNING IN THE FIELDWORK II STUDENT

In the 2013 *Commission on Education (COE) Guidelines for a Level II Occupational Therapy Fieldwork Experience*, it is explicitly stated, "By the end of the fieldwork experience, the student should demonstrate the attitudes and skills of an entry-level practitioner, including assumption of responsibility for independent learning" (p. 3). A student's ability to be a self-directed and self-regulated learner will lend to their success in moving from a novice to advanced-beginner clinician. In fieldwork, students are required to be self-directed in their learning, and therefore increase their clinical reasoning, critical thinking, and problem-solving skills (Scaffa & Wooster, 2004). As FWeds, there are key ways we can encourage the "just-right challenge" of autonomy and independent clinical reasoning:

Box 7-12

CASE EXAMPLE: KATE

Reason for referral: Kate was referred to outpatient occupational therapy services by her primary care physician due to persistent pain and reduced range of motion in her shoulder.

General description: Kate is a 57-year-old woman referred for occupational therapy 10 weeks after a right Colles fracture sustained after a fall on an icy sidewalk. Additional diagnoses include chronic fibromyalgia, diverticulitis, and alcohol abuse. Kate has pain with movement of the shoulder in flexion beyond 35 degrees and extension beyond 10 degrees. Her posture and expression suggest that she is in extreme pain. Kate appears overtly anxious and reluctant to participate in any physical assessment.

Medical history: Kate was diagnosed with fibromyalgia 7 years ago. She has a long history of widespread aching, stiffness, and fatigue. She reports multiple tender points bilaterally in her neck, shoulders, and upper back. The pain has intensified since her fall. For the past 4 years Kate has taken various medications to improve her sleep and relax her muscles. There is also a note in her chart that she has previously reported self-medicating with alcohol. Range of motion in Kate's right arm is difficult to assess because of the pain Kate experiences.

- Promote positive self-direction and independence
  - This can be fostered through constructive feedback, open communication, and thoughtful reflection
- Allow the student to develop the ability to take responsibility for learning
  - As Level II fieldwork progresses, shift from a supervision to a mentoring model
  - Utilize questions that promote critical thinking
    - Not just "What did you think?" or "Do you have any questions?", but "*Why did you think that way?*" or "*Tell me more about the approach you took with that client ...*" (refer to Chapter 8 for additional questioning approaches)
- Throughout clinical reasoning, allow the student to develop creativity and promote curiosity
  - The inherent nature of the Level II fieldwork experience can address each of these objectives by design. Emphasize to students that knowing *how* to learn is more important than purely gaining extensive knowledge.

One way to foster self-directed learning and clinical reasoning is through a structured reflective process, such as demonstrated in the examples in Appendices B and C. In addition to these suggestions around self-regulation and clinical reasoning, helpful teaching practices can be found in Chapters 3 and 9 of this text.

TABLE 7-4
FIVE-STEP CLINICAL REASONING PROCESS WITH REFLECTION QUESTIONS

STEPS	APPLICATION OF CLINICAL REASONING	QUESTIONS TO FACILITATE REASONING FOR FIELDWORK STUDENT
Step 1: Client and referral information	Chart review/referral • Procedural reasoning • Diagnostic reasoning • Scientific reasoning	What is the referral for? Diagnosis? What do you know to be true about this diagnosis based on previous knowledge? What do you expect to see?
	Understanding the client • Narrative reasoning • Interactive reasoning	What is Kate's occupational narrative? What activities and roles have been important to Kate in the past? What does Kate want to be able to do following treatment?
Step 2: Clinical hypotheses	Identification of cues • Procedural reasoning • Diagnostic reasoning • Scientific reasoning • Pragmatic reasoning	What information do you know to be true to formulate a plan? What assessments might be available to tell you more about this client and diagnosis? What further information might inform your plan of care? What alternative approaches may be available to create a plan of care for this client?
Step 3: Data collection, problem solving, and hypotheses evaluation	Defining impact on occupational performance • Narrative reasoning • Procedural reasoning • Diagnostic reasoning • Scientific reasoning	Are there specific algorithms or clinical guidelines for Kate's diagnoses? What are the best practice interventions that can support Kate's needs? Have you seen a similar presentation in Level I fieldwork or in the classroom? What was the experience? Does Kate have a social support network that can assist in her recovery? What is the impact of her chronic pain and alcohol use on the referring diagnosis?
	Implications of context on case • Pragmatic reasoning • Ethical reasoning • Conditional reasoning	How might reimbursement impact the outcomes of the client? Does the clinic have the resources to best assist Kate? Does Kate have an accessible environment at home? How will her environment impact her occupational performance?

(continued)

TABLE 7-4 (CONTINUED)
FIVE-STEP CLINICAL REASONING PROCESS WITH REFLECTION QUESTIONS

STEPS	APPLICATION OF CLINICAL REASONING	QUESTIONS TO FACILITATE REASONING FOR FIELDWORK STUDENT
Step 4: Test and refine hypotheses	Understanding the outcomes of assessment on the client • All aspects of clinical reasoning should be considered	What did you identify as the multiple demands for Kate? What are the required skills needed for successful occupational performance? Did Kate demonstrate these skills? What are the potential meanings of Kate's activities and occupations? Were there barriers present? What contextual or environmental factors were present in evaluation that may confirm or challenge your hypotheses?
Step 5: Appraise the evidence	Synthesize the information Create a plan of care Continue the clinical reasoning cycle	Overall, did the evaluation go as expected? Why or why not? Ask the student to summarize Kate's medical and social histories, occupational therapy problems, and current status of those problems, and recommendations for further information or other services.

SUMMARY

Facilitating the development of clinical reasoning and the clinical reasoning process in a Level II fieldwork student is an essential responsibility of the FWed. Having the tools to facilitate not only clinical reasoning but reflection, self-awareness, and self-regulation will be critical to the success of the overall experience. The scenarios and examples presented in this chapter, as well as the additional resources can serve as a "clinical reasoning toolkit" for any FWed.

LEARNING ACTIVITIES

1. **Consider the following scenario:**

   Grace is a 66-year-old woman referred to occupational therapy by her family doctor. Grace is 5 years s/p a CVA with mild residual weakness in her right extremities. She has a 3-year history of progressive behavior changes and difficulty with executive functioning. Language has also been affected. She has been referred to outpatient occupational therapy services to review home safety, explore ongoing support and service needs, and provide education to her husband and daughter.

   Reflect back on the overview of clinical reasoning. Consider each area of clinical reasoning and identify at least two questions per area that can be used to further understand the client's history and presentation.

2. Using Table 7-1, where do you believe you fall, in terms of novice to expert? When you think back to your first occupational therapy position, identify where you believe you started, then where you see yourself today. What behaviors or activities caused you to rank yourself where you did? Were there individuals who supported your development?

3. Using Table 7-3, have your fieldwork student explore each of these areas of context at the start of the experience. Review together how these might impact clinical reasoning.

REFERENCES

Accreditation Council for Occupational Therapy Education. (2018). Standards and interpretative guide [PDF]. https://www.aota.org/~/media/Corporate/Files/EducationCareers/Accredit/StandardsReview/2018-ACOTE-Standards-Interpretive-Guide.pdf

Accreditation Council for Occupational Therapy Education standards and interpretive guide. (n.d.). https://acoteonline.org/accreditation-explained/standards/

American Occupational Therapy Association. (2020a). AOTA 2020 occupational therapy code of ethics. *American Journal of Occupational Therapy, 74*(Suppl. 3), 741341005p1-741341005p13. https://doi:10.5014/ajob.2020.74S3006.

American Occupational Therapy Assocation (2020b). AOTA occupational profile template. https://www.aota.org/~/media/Corporate/Files/Practice/Manage/Documentation/AOTA-Occupational-Profile-Template.pdf

American Occupational Therapy Association. (2020c). Occupational therapy practice framework: Domain and process (4th ed.). *American Journal of Occupational Therapy, 74*(Suppl.2), 7412410010. https://doi.org/105014/ajot.2020.74S2001

Cherry, K. (2020). Problem solving strategies and obstacles. https://www.verywellmind.com/problem-solving-2795008

Cohn, E. S. (1991). Clinical reasoning: Explicating complexity. *American Journal of Occupational Therapy, 45*(11), 969-971. https://doi.org/10.5014/ajot.45.11.969

Commission on Education. (2013). Recommendations for occupational therapy fieldwork experiences. https://www.aota.org/~/media/Corporate/Files/EducationCareers/Educators/Fieldwork/LevelII/COE%20Guidelines%20for%20an%20Occupational%20Therapy%20Fieldwork%20Experience%20--%20Level%20II--Final.pdf

Crepeau, E. B. (1991). Achieving intersubjective understanding examples from an occupational therapy treatment session. *American Journal of Occupational Therapy 45*(11), 1016-1025. https://doi.org/10.5014/ajot.45.11.1016

Cronin, A. & Graebe, G. (2018). *Clinical reasoning in occupational therapy.* AOTA Press.

Dreyfus, S. E., & Dreyfus, H. L. (1980). *A five-stage model of the mental activities involved in directed skill acquisition.* California University Berkeley Operations Research Center.

Fleming, M. H. (1991). The therapist with the three-track mind. *American Journal of Occupational Therapy, 45,* 1007-1014. https://doi.org/10.5014/ajot.45.11.1007

Goleman, D. (2005). *Emotional intelligence.* Bantam.

Hanson, D., & Mattila, A. (2023). Fostering clinical reasoning during level I fieldwork. In E. D. DeIuliis & D. Hanson (Eds.), *Fieldwork educator's guide to level I fieldwork* (pp. 109-142). SLACK Incorporated.

Holmqvist, K., Kamwendo, K., & Ivarsson, A. (2009). Occupational therapists' descriptions of their work with persons suffering from cognitive impairment following acquired brain injury. *Scandinavian Journal of Occupational Therapy, 16,* 13-24. https://doi.org/10.1080/11038120802123520

Marquez-Alverez, L., Calvo-Arenillas, J., Talavera-Valverde, M., & Moruno-Millares, P. (2019). Professional reasoning in occupational therapy: A scoping review. *Occupational Therapy International, 2019*, 1-9. https://doi.org/10.1155/2019/6238245

Mason, J., Haden, C. L. & Causey-Upton, R. (2020). Fieldwork educators' expectations of level II occupational therapy students' professional and techincal skills. *The Open Journal of Occupational Therapy, 8*(3), 1-16. https://doi.org/10.15453/2168-6408.1649

Mattingly, C. (1991). The narrative nature of clinical reasoning. *American Journal of Occupational Therapy, 45*(11), 998-1005. https://doi.org/105014/ajot.45.11.998

Neistadt, M. E. (1996). Teaching strategies for the development of clinical reasoning. *American Journal of Occupational Therapy, 50*(8), 676-684. https://doi.org/10.5014/ajot.50.8.676

Robertson, L. J. (1996). Clinical reasoning, part 2: Novice/expert differences. *British Journal of Occupational Therapy, 59*(5), 212-216. https://doi.org/10.1177/030802269605900507

Rogers, J. C. (1983). Eleanor Clarke Slagle Lectureship – 1983; clinical reasoning: The ethics, science, and art. *American Journal of Occupational Therapy, 37*, 601-616. https://doi.org/10.5014/ajot.37.9.601

Rogers, J. C., & Masagatani, G. (1982). Clinical reasoning of occupational therapists during the initial assessment of physically disabled patient. *The Occupational Journal of Research, 2*(4), 195-219.

Royeen, C. B., Mu, K., Barrett, K., & Luebben, A. J. (2001). Pilot investigation: Evaluation of clinical reflection and reasoning before and after workshop intervention. In P. Crist (Ed.), *Innovations in Occupational Therapy Education* (pp. 107-114). American Occupational Therapy Association.

Scaffa, M. E., & Wooster, D. M. (2004). Effects of problem-based learning on clinical reasoning in occupational therapy. *American Journal of Occupational Therapy, 58*(3), 333-336. https://doi.org/10.5014/ajot.58.3.333

Schell, B. A. B. (2018). Pragmatic reasoning. In B. A. B Schell & J. W. Schell, (Eds.). *Clinical and Professional Reasoning in Occupational Therapy* (2nd ed., pp. 203-243). Wolters Kluwer.

Schell, B. A. B. (2019). Professional reasoning in practice. In B. A. B Schell & G. Gillen (Eds.), *Willard and Spackman's occupational therapy* (13th ed., pp. 483-497). Wolters Kluwer.

Turpin, M. J., & Copley, J. A. (2018). Interactive reasoning. In B. A. B Schell & J. W. Schell (Eds.), *Clinical and professional reasoning in occupational therapy* (2nd ed., pp. 245-260). Wolters Kluwer.

Unsworth, C. A. (2004). Clinical reasoning: How do pragmatic reasoning, worldview and client-centeredness fit? *British Journal of Occupational Therapy 67*(1), 10-19. https://doi.org/10-1177/030802260406700103

Unsworth, C., & Baker, A. (2016). A systematic review of professional reasoning literature in occupational therapy. *British Journal of Occupational Therapy, 79*(1), 5-16. https://doi.org/10.1177/0308022615599994

APPENDIX A

The Self-Assessment of Clinical Reflection and Reasoning

Please rate the following statements on a scale of 1 to 5 with 5 indicating "strongly agree," and 1 indicating "strongly disagree."

1. I question how, what, and why I do things in practice.
2. I ask myself and others questions as a way of learning.
3. I don't make judgments until I have sufficient data.
4. Prior to acting, I seek various solutions.
5. Regarding the outcome of proposed interventions, I try to keep an open mind.
6. I think in terms of comparing and contrasting information about a client's problems and proposed solutions to them.
7. I look to theory for understanding of a client's problems and proposed solutions to them.
8. I look to frames of reference for planning my intervention strategy.
9. I use theory to understand treatment techniques.
10. I try to understand clinical problems by using a variety of frames of reference.
11. When there is conflicting information about a clinical problem, I identify assumptions underlying the differing views.
12. When planning intervention strategies, I ask "what if" for a variety of options.
13. I ask for colleagues' ideas and viewpoints.
14. I ask for the viewpoints of clients' family members.
15. I cope well with change.
16. I can function with uncertainty.
17. I regularly hypothesize about the reasons for my clients' problems.
18. I must validate clinical hypotheses through my own experience.
19. I clearly identify the clinical problems prior to planning intervention.
20. I anticipate the sequence of events likely to result from planned intervention.
21. Regarding a proposed intervention strategy, I think, "What makes it work?"
22. Regarding a particular intervention, I ask, "In what context would it work?"
23. Regarding a particular intervention with a particular client, I determine whether it worked.
24. I use clinical protocols for most of my treatment.
25. I make decisions about practice based on my experience.
26. I use theory to understand intervention strategies.

Royeen, C. B., Mu, K., Barrett, K., & Luebben, A. J. (2001). Pilot investigation: Evaluation of clinical reflection and reasoning before and after workshop intervention. In P. Crist (Ed.), *Innovations in Occupational Therapy Education* (pp. 107-114). American Occupational Therapy Association.

APPENDIX B
Clinical Reasoning Reflection

Aspect of clinical reasoning (procedural, narrative, scientific, etc.):

Define this aspect in your own words:

How you used it:

What was the outcome/decision?

What are the other possible outcomes/decisions?

APPENDIX C
Self-Directed Learning and Reflection Worksheet

Briefly describe the client interaction, intervention, and context:

What did I do well?

What could I have done better?

How can I continue improving my performance in this area? (Be specific! Describe how you make changes to improve your performance including techniques, strategies, etc.)

What do I need to make this happen? (What are the resources/education or support I could access to help me build this skill?)

How will I know I have improved? (What is my measure of success?)

8

Teaching Tips and Strategies for Fieldwork Learning

Elizabeth D. DeIuliis, OTD, MOT, OTR/L, CLA
and Alexandria Raymond, OTD, OTR/L

Experiential learning is a required component within many graduate-level professional degree programs. The origin of several recognized clinical learning approaches can be found within literature outside of occupational therapy and are not typically part of the initial or progressive training as an occupational therapy fieldwork educator (FWed). This chapter will provide an overview of experiential teaching approaches and strategies from clinical learning literature that occupational therapy FWeds can use to further integrate students into the fieldwork experience and guide their journey to achieve entry-level practice status. Although each of the techniques has unique qualities to support student growth and learning, the strategies presented in this chapter are aimed to:

- Foster/deepen critical thinking and problem-solving skills
- Develop progressive independence and autonomy
- Increase self-awareness and self-directness
- Promote technical skill competency
- Build confidence and self-esteem

Occupational therapy practitioners can benefit from studying these techniques to deepen their skill set and craft as a FWed in order to better align their teaching with the student's developmental learning needs and professional growth.

DeIuliis, E. D., & Hanson, D. (Eds.).
Fieldwork Educator's Guide to Level II Fieldwork (pp. 227-254).
© 2023 Taylor & Francis Group.

LEARNING OBJECTIVES

By the end of reading this chapter and completing the learning activities, the reader should be able to:

1. Compare and contrast unique clinical teaching strategies used in experiential learning.
2. Understand different models to approach the feedback exchange process during the implementation of clinical teaching strategies during Level II fieldwork.
3. Recognize indicators that the fieldwork student is learning or at risk for performance issues.

CLINICAL TEACHING AND LEARNING FRAMEWORKS AND STRATEGIES

In general, there is a wide range of teaching strategies used in clinical learning, which can fit into categories of **modeling, observation, case presentations, direct questioning, thinking aloud,** and **coaching** (Burns et al., 2006; Lazarus, 2016). The utilization of these approaches is dependent upon the skill and expertise of the educator as well as the developmental level and expectations of the student. Some approaches are intentionally used to help structure discussion with students, while others are designed to stimulate reflection, role model self-directed learning, and/or help identify gaps in the student's learning. Occupational therapy literature supports FWeds building their capacity to nurture student learning and adapt their teaching styles to meet the needs of their students (Rodger et al., 2011).

MODELING AND OBSERVATION

Modeling is a sequential learning approach that begins with the student directly observing the performance or demonstration of a skill. This is typically followed by the student then demonstrating the skill. This approach is often used during the introductory phases of learning. Modeling can be aligned to David Kolb's Experiential Learning Theory which describes the learning process as a continual cycle: experience, observation, thinking, and action (Kolb, 1984). This experiential learning framework is analogous to the proverb stated by Confucius, a social philosopher, "I hear and I forgot, I see and I remember, I do and I understand." The retention of learning is highest through experience. See Figure 8-1 for the process of Kolb's Learning Theory.

See One, Do One, Teach One

In medical education, modeling is a fundamental component often utilized in preparation for apprenticeship residencies referred to as "see one, do one, teach one" (SODOTO) coined by an American surgeon, William Stewart Halsted, in the early 1900s (Kotsis & Chung, 2013). The concept is centered around that the learner is more likely to learn and remember if there is hands-on learning and then explains it to someone else. During the "see one" phase, the expert, or FWed, performs the activity or procedure. In the "do one" phase, the learner, or fieldwork student, applies the learned procedure into a practical situation, under supervision. In the "teach one" phase, the student uses the achieved accumulative learning and experience and transfers it by teaching another individual. Teaching the skill or task helps reinforce the knowledge learned (retention) and helps the student develop further toward mastery. The teaching phase also helps develop introductory teaching skills within the student that will be of value as they enter practice and

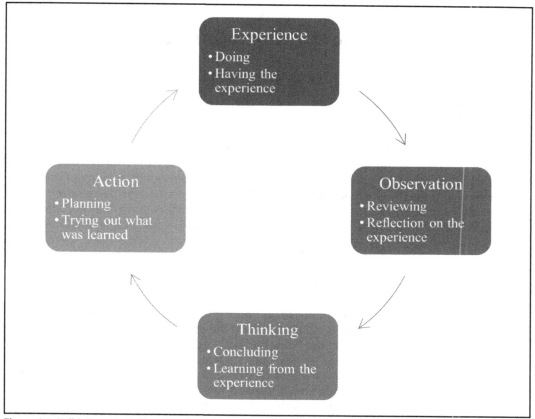

Figure 8-1. Kolb's Experiential Learning Cycle. (Adapted from Kolb, D. A. [1984]. *Experiential learning: Experience as the source of learning and development*. Prentice-Hall.)

eventually undertake the FWed role. This sequential approach for teaching and learning is noted to be preferred by occupational therapy fieldwork students (Grenier, 2015; Rodger et al., 2011). The SODOTO technique can be useful to use within the apprenticeship supervision model or in a collaborative model. In fact, there is emerging research within medical education that indicates that when used in a group format, students may feel more comfortable with the "teaching" aspect and providing feedback within a group of peers vs. with their direct preceptor (Graziano, 2011). See Box 8-1 for an example of SODOTO phase.

FWeds are able to support student learning by giving students the opportunity to observe their techniques and interactions (Furness et al., 2020; Rodger et al., 2011). Students reported that having this opportunity to observe their educator's practice is beneficial to their learning.

MiPlan

MiPlan refers to a learner-centered model that highlights critical preparation needed to ensure a meaningful teaching encounter (Smith & Lane, 2015). This clinical teaching strategy is used to foster bedside teaching and may not be conducive to use during critical and/or acute medical scenarios (Chinai et al., 2018). MiPlan is known to assist learners to become more self-directed (Chinai et al., 2018), which aligns with some of the known needs of the current generation of fieldwork students (DeIuliis & Saylor, 2021). MiPlan recommends that the instructor schedule a meeting with students before engaging in a clinical encounter. The objectives of this meeting include personal introductions, communication goals, discussing the learning environment/teaching

Box 8-1
SEE ONE, DO ONE, TEACH ONE EXAMPLES

APPRENTICESHIP MODEL

Jesse is a Level II fieldwork student in an acute care hospital, who is being supervised by an occupational therapist who primarily works on the burn unit. During the initial weeks of the experience, Jesse is asked to first observe the FWed perform passive range of motion on inpatients who are sedated during dressing changes to avoid joint contractures and promote joint motion. During the observation, the FWed engages Jesse in a dialogue about the appropriate handling and procedures. Next, Jesse has the opportunity to practice the skills on a client, with the direct supervision of the FWed. After several weeks, Jesse now has the opportunity to model the appropriate passive range of motion technique to an occupational therapy assistant student who is starting their Level I fieldwork experience on the same unit.

COLLABORATIVE MODEL

Tom is a FWed in a role-emerging setting in the community who is currently supervising two Level II fieldwork students using the collaborative supervision model. During the first 2 weeks of the experience, Tom directly models for the fieldwork students how to complete intake interviews with the participants at the setting. At the beginning of week 3, Tom requests that Maria, one of the fieldwork students, takes the lead in completing an intake interview, with Javier, the other fieldwork student, being responsible for observing Maria's performance and providing her feedback on how the session went. Maria uses the cumulative learning and experience from observing Tom, and directly applies it to her task of completing the intake interview. After the intake interview is completed, Tom initiates a debriefing session with the two students. Maria is prompted by Tom to reflect and offer self-evaluation of her performance. Javier is prompted to provide constructive feedback on Maria's performance, including strengths as well as specific areas that could be improved next time. The following day, Javier is responsible for leading the intake interviews, with Maria providing feedback.

In this scenario, Tom, the FWed serves more as a facilitator to ensure that the SODOTO model occurs in a peer-to-peer fashion. Facilitating a peer-to-peer learning loop using SODOTO can be an effective approach for students to work towards mastery in particular skills areas, as well as develop competency in giving and accepting feedback.

methods, and overall expectations of the patient encounter (Stickrath et al., 2013). Setting expectations for learning proactively is a perceived support expressed by occupational therapy fieldwork students (Furness et al., 2020). See Figure 8-2 for example of MiPlan in Level II fieldwork.

M—Meeting

The **M** refers to the preparatory meeting between the instructor and the student before engaging in the client encounter. During this meeting, all parties of the team are introduced and communication goals and overall expectations are set. The instructor should facilitate a safe learning environment and collaborate with the student to create learner-centered objectives, which is supported in the occupational therapy literature by Rodger et al. (2011). A learning contract can be a tangible strategy to formalize the objectives and desired goals for this "meeting."

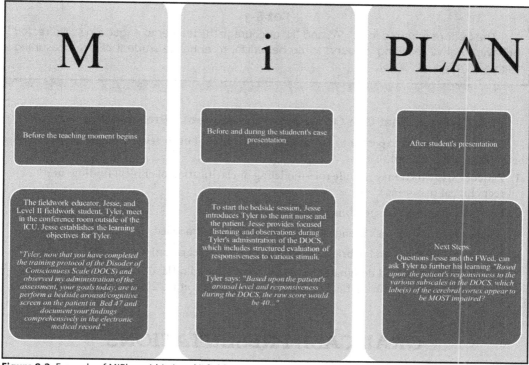

Figure 8-2. Example of MiPlan within Level II fieldwork.

Box 8-2

The five behaviors within "i" advocate the FWed to be "in tune" with their students, which is a proven strategy to enhance the learning and emotional intelligence of allied health students (Gribble et al., 2017b).

i—Behaviors for the Instructor

The **i** encompasses five behaviors for the FWed to adopt during the client encounter with the student, which include (Stickrath et al., 2013):

1. Introductions: The team and the purpose are explained to the patient.

2. In the moment: The instructor stays focused during the student's oral case presentation by being a focused listener, using good eye contact, exhibiting appropriate body language, etc.

3. Inspection: The instructor performs their own clinical observations of the patient so that they can verify the student's findings or offer clarification.

4. Interruptions: The instructor refrains from interrupting the student during their case presentation. This behavior is meaningful as it provides important role-modeling of professional behaviors in front of the student.

5. Independent thought: The instructor encourages an understanding of clinical reasoning. See Box 8-2.

> **Box 8-3**
> The options featured in "P", "A", and "N" encourage the learner to engage in self-directed behavior. Active teaching is found to be beneficial to enhance student clinical reasoning (Naidoo & van Wyk, 2016).

PLAN—Steps That Can Occur After the Student's Presentation

Instructors are not expected to cover all four priorities, but to select a single element as the focus (Stickrath et al., 2013):

1. Patient care (which may include role-modeling or clarification of clinical findings and/or correct clinical reasoning)

2. Learner's questions (responding to student questions)

3. Attending to instructor's agendas (resources to enhance knowledge)

4. Next steps (feedback and debriefs, questions for further learning)

Scheduled debriefs and designated times for feedback and reflection are suggested actions to support student learning during fieldwork education (Furness et al., 2020). See Box 8-3.

ORAL CASE PRESENTATIONS

The ability to obtain and articulate a holistic and thorough client's history (occupational profile) and/or intervention plan is a critical part of the occupational therapy process (American Occupational Therapy Association [AOTA], 2020). One framework to report important findings orally is the use of a communication tool endorsed by the Interprofessional Education Collaborative (2018) called SBAR. SBAR, an acronym that stands for Situation, Background, Assessment, and Recommendation, can be a useful model to teach fieldwork students for organizing and communicating pertinent information to the FWed and other members of the interprofessional team. Case presentations, such as the SBAR, or via other formats can be a powerful teaching tool to identify gaps in student knowledge and drive meaningful discussion between the instructor and learner (Onishi, 2008). Oral case presentations can occur alongside direct client-care or outside of it. FWeds can utilize case presentations as a means to simulate an interprofessional health care team meeting or patient/family caregiver session. A good case presentation requires students to acquire and synthesize relevant information into a concise, coherent oral summary (Melvin & Cavalcanti, 2016). A key component of using case presentations as a teaching tool is for the instructor to provide feedback to the student on the strengths and areas of growth. Key discussion points can be on the sources used to gather pertinent information (e.g., use of medical records, patient/family interviews, tests/measures) and how the data that were gathered was organized. The delivery and flow of information (e.g., was it logical? aligned with safe clinical judgment?) are other areas that a FWed can focus on to provide feedback. Additional strategies of how to provide feedback will be discussed later on in this chapter, however, **probing** and **clarifying** questions are often used within case presentations. A probing question is used to determine the extent of the student's knowledge or understanding. For example, *"What are the normal hematocrit and hemoglobin range for a client who has aplastic anemia and has undergone a bone marrow transplant?"* A clarifying question is used by the FWed to ensure their understanding of what the student communicated. For example, *"Exactly how many degrees of active range of motion was available at the shoulder?"* or *"How did the mother describe the child's food preferences?"* FWeds should be aware of the frequency of use

TABLE 8-1
EXAMPLES OF USING SBAR FOR ORAL CASE PRESENTATIONS

	FIELDWORK STUDENT ORAL REPORT IN A TRADITIONAL MEDICAL MODEL SETTING	PROBING OR CLARIFYING QUESTION FROM FWED
S	"Mr. Adams just finished participating in his morning activities of daily living (ADL) routine. He is sitting at the edge of the bed and complains of dizziness and weakness."	*"What other observations did you make about Mr. Adams's appearance?"*
B	"Mr. Adams is a 67-year-old male with a history of type II diabetes and seizures."	*"How does Mr. Adams's past medical history inform your clinical reasoning?"*
A	"The problem is hypoglycemia."	*"What are the symptoms of hypoglycemia?"*
R	"We should notify the nurse and offer Mr. Adams some approved food choices (e.g., fruit, juice, honey)."	*"How will these food choices help in this situation?"*
	FIELDWORK STUDENT ORAL REPORT IN A ROLE EMERGING SETTING	PROBING OR CLARIFYING QUESTION FROM FWED
S	"The residents have participated in a focus group, completed surveys, and were observed for a group session as part of the needs assessment process."	*"What key themes arose regarding the needs of the stakeholders?"*
B	"Residents live at a halfway house with individuals seeking treatment for alcohol or substance use disorder."	*"What information did you gather on this population, policies, and mission of the site?"*
A	"After directly observing the residents in a group session, the residents lacked social interaction skills due to limited eye contact with one other and minimal conversation initiated."	*"What are two areas for potential program development to address the needs of the residents?"*
R	"The plan is to create group sessions with focus areas in social participation and community engagement."	*"Are there any practical issues with regards to the residents or site that will have any impact on your program plan?"*

in probing and clarifying questions. More frequent probing questions can perplex and fluster the student and negatively impact the ability of the FWed to truly assess the student's knowledge and skill. On the other side of the spectrum, low-frequency questioning during a case presentation can leave the student unguided and a lack of opportunity to get feedback on the quality of their oral summary (Weinholtz, 1983). See examples in Table 8-1 for an illustration of using probing and clarifying questions to support student learning when giving oral case presentations.

DIRECT QUESTIONING

Direct questioning is a complex teaching approach that involves modeling of the process of inquiry (Long et al., 2015). While this instructional tool may appear to be very simple (asking questions), when used skillfully it requires thoughtful, intentionally planned questions from the educator to the learner.

Direct questioning can have several benefits, which include (Lazarus, 2016):

- Assess student knowledge
- Engage students as active participants in the learning process
- Guide understanding of deeper concepts
- Build confidence and self-esteem
- Foster critical thinking skills

The FWed must align the type of questioning to the developmental level of the learner, yet also understand how to evoke a "just-right challenge" to stimulate and scaffold to higher levels of learning. See Table 8-2 for examples of direct questioning. If needed, refer back to Blooms' Taxonomy (Chapter 3) and the Dreyfus Model of Skill Acquisition (Chapter 7).

While direct questioning is designed to be an "on-the-spot" teaching method, instructors should be mindful to not stretch their questioning approaches too far. This may cause embarrassment or discomfort to the learner, particularly if being used in a cohort-learning context, such as the collaborative student supervision model, or within a public setting. Long et al. (2015) recommend that educators allow learners **3 to 5 seconds** to respond to a question and to avoid interrupting learners while they are formulating their response. If a student's response is impartial or not clear, use follow-up probing questions such as *"Can you tell me more about that?"* If the learner is presenting incorrect information, instructors should respond gently and guide them in the right direction, such as *"That's a curious interpretation. If the client had a history of deQuervian's tenosynovitis, how would you explain the absence of protective sensation ..."* Direct questioning may look different depending on the learning preferences or personality of the student. Making adjustments to direct questioning techniques can include providing flexibility in how learning is assessed and how the student expresses their learning. For example, a more introverted student might benefit from having the questions ahead of time. Known direct questioning models and techniques include the One-Minute Preceptor (OMP), Five-Minute Preceptor (5MP), SNAPPS, and MiPlan. Examples of how to use each of these within occupational therapy fieldwork education will be discussed next.

One-Minute Preceptor

The OMP model of clinical teaching was created by Neher et al. (1992) and is widely written about in the training of medical students. A lot of clinical teaching involves the student learning to interview and assess a client, synthesizing the information and data gathered, and presenting the information back to the instructor. This is usually followed by time spent by the instructor questioning and clarifying the information presented by the student. The OMP technique allows the instructor to maximize their teaching effectiveness and more efficiently use direct questioning to stimulate discussion with the student. This direct questioning approach guides the FWed and student encounter via five microskills. The steps of the OMP method include:

TABLE 8-2

EXAMPLES OF DIRECT QUESTIONING

DEVELOPMENTAL STAGE OF LEARNER (DREYFUS)	OBJECTIVES FOR QUESTIONS TO FOCUS ON (BLOOM)	GOAL OF DIRECT QUESTIONING	STEMS TO CONSIDER IN YOUR QUESTIONING	SAMPLE QUESTIONS BASED ON A CLIENT WHO IS DEMONSTRATING SYMPTOMS ALIGNED WITH AUTONOMIC DYSREFLEXIA
Novice	Remember	Build knowledge	List, identify, name	**"Name** two symptoms of autonomic dysreflexia."
Advanced beginner	Understand	Promote understanding of concepts	Explain, describe	**"Explain** the cause of the autonomic dysreflexia."
Competent	Apply	Stimulate application of knowledge into a clinical scenario	Interpret, execute	"Here is the client's BP supine, and here is the BP while seated at the edge of the bed. **Interpret** the cause of the sudden change in blood pressure."
Proficient	Evaluate	Justify a stance or course of action	Compare and contrast, select and critique	**"Compare and contrast** the appropriate course of action when a client experiences autonomic dysreflexia vs. orthostatic hypotension."

Data sources: Dreyfus and Dreyfus, 1980; Anderson and Krathwohl, 2001.

1. Get a Commitment

The first step is to get a commitment from the student to actively participate in the learning process. You, the FWed, are asking the student to think about what is happening during a clinical encounter. For example, after completing a visual oculomotor exam with a patient who recently sustained a head injury and demonstrated inconsistent interaction in the left visual fields, the FWed might say to the student *"Based on the patient's performance with the oculomotor exam, what do you think is going on here?"*

If the student's response is correct (e.g., hemi-visual inattention), this presents the opportunity for the FWed to reinforce a positive skill. If the response is incorrect (e.g., left neglect), this can be a "red flag" that the student may lack didactic or content knowledge, and there is an opportunity to probe for deeper learning. *"What other visual-perceptual conditions could present this way during an oculomotor screen? What standardized assessments should we follow up with?"* Based on the student's response, the FWed can get better insight into the knowledge level of the student to stretch them outside of their comfort zone.

2. Probe for Supporting Evidence

Within this step, the instructor is exploring the basis of the student's clinical reasoning. As a FWed, you want to have a sense of the student's understanding and rationale for clinical decision making, ensuring they did not just have a lucky guess. FWeds should avoid passing judgment but instead use supplicated direct questioning to determine what evidence they used to support their commitment. Prompts may include *"Can you share your rationale behind your choice of that particular assessment?"* or *"What observations from the evaluation support your intervention plan?"*

3. Reinforce What Was Done Well

Praise the student for what they did well. Feedback should be specific to the student's behaviors and performance and not just a simple *"You did a good job"* or *"That is correct."* Examples of how to provide positive reinforcement include *"Your interpretation that the patient has left hemi-visual inattention is well supported as their saccades and smooth pursuits were sporadic and inconsistent in the left visual field."*

4. Give Guidance About Errors and Omissions

These last two microskills in OMP incorporate feedback. Just as it is important for the student to hear what they have done well, it is also important for the educator to tell them areas for growth and improvement. In framing constructive feedback, avoid using words such as "bad" or "poor." Examples include: *"For this patient, due to the area of the brain damaged and performance on the oculomotor screen, a standardized assessment should be administered. Use of the letter cancellation test is an appropriate assessment method to further vet a field cut vs. hemi-attention vs. neglect."* In addition, expressions such as "less successful," "not best," or "not preferred" carry less negative value judgment and may be more palatable to the fieldwork student when indicating areas for improvement.

5. Teach a General Principle

A fundamental outcome of the OMP is that the student can take the information gained from the learning situation and generalize it to other contexts and situations. As a FWed, this is an opportunity for you to share your expertise. Prompts may include *"Recently, there were best practice guidelines published by our profession's national association that include a new protocol to evaluate visual-perceptual disorders in the hospital setting."*

TABLE 8-3
ONE-MINUTE PRECEPTOR MODEL PROMPTS

OMP STEP	FIELDWORK EDUCATOR PROMPT	TIP
Get a commitment	*"What do you think is going on with your client?"*	The goal is to help the student feel responsible and autonomous within their role and engage them in the collaborative learning process.
Probe for supporting evidence	*"What information have you acquired that leads to this hypothesis?"* or *"Have you considered any other hypothesis or conclusions?"*	Use clarifying or probing questions to learn how they arrived at their decision.
Reinforce what was done well	*"I like how you ensured that the client had on safe footwear and locked the bed before you assessed a functional transfer from the bed due to their known fall risk"*	Be specific.
Give guidance about errors and omissions	*"It is essential to ensure that the chair alarm is placed correctly and turned on before leaving the room."* or *"Is there anything else that would be critical to ensure the patient's safety and reduce fall risk after we have finished our session?"*	Use sensitive language (e.g., "not the best" instead of "bad" or "poor"). You can also use this as an opportunity to ask the student what they would do differently next time based upon this discussion to evaluate if the student can correct their "error" on their own. This is a strong indicator of self-awareness and metacognition
Teach a general principle	*"Combined with a known low H/H level, and a sudden drop in their systolic blood pressure greater than 20 mm Hg when in the standing position, we can assume the client is experiencing orthostatic hypotension and you should return the client to a seated and then supine position."*	Teach a brief and focused general rule related to the encounter.

Adapted from Lazarus, 2016; Neher et al., 1992.

Table 8-3 has examples of prompts to guide FWeds to effectively use the OMP model.

Five-Minute Preceptor

Built upon the OMP, nursing education adapted this teaching approach and labeled it as the 5MP model, which includes the following steps:

1. Get the student to take a stand

2. Probe for supporting evidence

3. Teach general rules

4. Reinforce the positives

5. Correct errors or misinterpretations (Bott et al., 2011, p. 38)

The overall rationale of the OMP and 5MP steps are similar, yet the 5MP has slightly different verbiage used to frame the prompts to elicit information from the learner and evaluate clinical decision making. This technique was renamed the 5MP as it is believed that this clinical teaching interaction should take at least 5 minutes (Bott et al., 2011). See Table 8-4.

SNAPPS

Summarize, Narrow differential, Analyze, Probe, Plan, and Select is another established framework used within medical education that can be used as a direct questioning technique after a student has seen or worked with a client. Due to the nature of the questioning, it is well-suited to be used after an initial evaluation with a client and can be an important precursor to the development of diagnostic clinical reasoning (Chiani et al., 2018). In contrast to the OMP model, SNAPPS involves prompting **from both** the teacher and the learner and is designed to engage the student in follow-up learning related to the client encounter/scenario (Pascoe et al., 2015; Wolpaw et al., 2009). As the student's responsibilities are greater using the SNAPPS technique than the OMP, this clinical teaching intervention may be better reserved for more experienced fieldwork students or those who are highly motivated (Lazarus, 2016). Also, due to the inherent collaborative interaction built into the SNAPPS technique, it might be a useful clinical teaching tool within the collaborative student supervision model, and lead to fostering more peer-to-peer questioning.

Summarize

During this first step, **the student initiates** the discussion by summarizing the case based upon the information acquired during the client encounter and presents a **concise oral summary** to the instructor.

Narrow the Differential

Next, the student verbalizes what they think is going on in the case, focusing on two or three relevant possibilities.

Analyze

Third, the student analyzes by comparing and contrasting relevant possibilities or hypotheses. This step forces the student to "think aloud" and is a good opportunity for the instructor to hear the student's clinical reasoning. More discussion about the thinking aloud technique will occur later in this chapter.

TABLE 8-4
EXAMPLE OF FIVE-MINUTE PRECEPTOR

STEP	FIELDWORK EDUCATOR PROMPT	TIP
Get the student to take a stand	*"What do you think is going on with your client?"*	The goal is to help the student feel responsible and autonomous within their role and engages them in the collaborative learning process. (*The instructor should avoid providing correct answers for the student in this step.*)
Probe for evidence	*"Why do you think that is what is going on?"*	The goal is to encourage the student to present their knowledge and clinical reasoning process.
Provide management guidelines	*"Autonomic dysreflexia is a common safety concern in individuals with a spinal cord injury to T6 or above. It is important to distinguish the symptoms of autonomic dysreflexia from orthostatic hypotension as the treatment protocol is different. For example, with orthostatic hypotension, you would want to return the patient to supine, for autonomic dysreflexia you would want to maintain the patient in an upright position."*	The instructor should teach no more than three pieces of information in this stage. Here, the student should be actively listening.
Reinforce what was done well	*"You do a good job of determining that the patient's blood pressure was elevated and did not align with their usual resting blood pressure."*	Provide specific comments on the strengths of the student's clinical reasoning with the intent that the student can generalize to other similar situations.
Correct mistakes	*"Other key clinical observations that are critical to focus on and/or ask your patient if they are experiencing include headache, diaphoresis, and changes in skin color."*	Constructive feedback is provided with specific actions to improve performance.

Adapted from Adapted from Lazarus, J. (2016). Precepting 101: Teaching strategies and tips for successful preceptors. *Journal of Midwifery & Women's Health, 61*(1), S11-S21. https://doi.org/10.1111/jmwh.12520 ; and Pascoe, J. M., Nixon, J., & Lang, V. J. (2015). Maximizing teaching on the wards: Review and application of the One-Minute Preceptor and SNAPPS models. *Journal of Hospital Medicine, 10*(2), 125-130. https://doi.org/10.1002/jhm.2302

Probe

Next, the student probes the instructor for their input by asking questions. In this step, in many ways, the questions that the student asks show a lot of insight to the instructor about any knowledge deficits.

Plan

Here the student starts a dialogue with the instructor and initiates a treatment plan and/or suggests interventions.

Select

In this final step, the learner is responsible for selecting a case-related issue and engaging in self-directed, asynchronous learning related to the client scenario. This step may be challenging for the introductory learner as it requires the student to identify their learning needs and create a plan. For example, they may create a plan to search the literature, review a chapter in a textbook or national practice guidelines to further inform their learning about the encounter (Wolpaw et al., 2015). Because of this last and final step, SNAPPS can be a useful tool for FWeds to use to address knowledge or practice gaps (Chinai et al., 2018). See Table 8-5 for an example of how SNAPPS can be used in occupational therapy fieldwork.

THINK-ALOUD METHOD

Thinking aloud is a teaching-learning concept that makes "clinical reasoning transparent and explicit" (Smith & Lane, 2015, p. 278). Naidoo and Van Wky (2016) discovered that when FWeds verbalized their clinical reasoning to the student it positively impacted the student's professional skills. It is important to make clinical reasoning transparent to easily engage the student in conversation and reassure the student of their own clinical thinking (Naidoo & Van Wky, 2016). FWeds can role model "thinking aloud" as well as encourage their students to do so. Thinking aloud deliberately divulges the steps in the clinical reasoning process and how clinical decisions are made in real time. By inspiring the student to verbalize their thinking within a moment, it also helps to bring awareness to areas of strength as well as areas to further develop. Thinking aloud can be used to require the student to verbalize their thinking as well as stimulate self-reflection in their clinical decision making (Houchens et al., 2017). Thinking aloud is also linked to promoting self-regulated learning, which is derived by higher-level cognitive processes such as metacognition (Pintrich, 2000). In layperson's terms, thinking aloud is asking the student to "walk and talk" or "do and think." Thinking aloud can be used in real time, during a patient-encounter, or afterward to facilitate a debrief. Example prompts for the FWed to gain access to the student's thinking process and promote thinking aloud include:

- "Tell me what you are thinking ..."
- "Go ahead and walk me through how you came to that conclusion ..."
- "Finish this sentence: What I have learned is ...?"
- "Finish this sentence: This client scenario reminded me of ...?"

Based upon the student's verbalizations, FWeds can get an inside glimpse of knowledge and content within the student's working memory. A critical aspect of the think-aloud technique is that the instructor should not judge or critique the outcome of the student's verbalizations, but rather look into the meaning behind what the student said (Lundgren-Laine & Salantera, 2010). FWeds can follow up the think-aloud protocol by reinforcing key knowledge, initiating a dialogue to further stimulate clinical reasoning, or modifying their clinical teaching approach to better align with student learning needs. See Box 8-4 and Table 8-6 for a think-aloud scenario.

Table 8-5
Example of SNAPPS

STEP	STUDENT ROLE	FIELDWORK EDUCATOR ROLE
Summarize	*Mrs. Smith is an 84-year-old woman, who lives alone in a senior high-rise, and was admitted 2 days ago with confusion and unkempt physical presentation. She is currently alert and oriented to person only, and received a score of 22 on the Montreal cognitive assessment. Mrs. Smith is typically continent, yet is currently incontinent and presents with a shuffling gait-like pattern during functional mobility. Vision, perception, and hearing are all intact. She has a past medical history of degenerative joint disease and has limitations of active range of motion in bilateral upper extremities at baseline.*	Provide active listening.
Narrow the differential	*Based upon the bedside evaluation, and chart review, dementia vs. delirium is one possibility as well as a urinary tract infection, due to the elevated white blood cell count noted in the chart review. Normal pressure hydrocephalus is another possibility based upon the confusion, incontinence, and shuffling gait.*	Encourages the student to "think aloud."
Analyze		*"What else could be a reason for XYZ ...?"*
Probe	*"Are there any additional standardized assessments that may be useful in administering?"*	*"Did you notice ...?"*
Plan	*"I would like to look up best practice recommendations surrounding the occupational therapist's role in treating incontinence and bladder management strategies."*	*"Reflect upon your encounter with Mrs. Smith. What knowledge would have helped you to optimize your role as her occupational therapist?"* *"What specific resources will you use to find this information?"*
Select	*"I will spend more time searching the literature on urinary incontinence and symptoms of a UTI."*	*"What do you think the appropriate plan of care for Mrs. Smith is?"*
Debrief to close the loop	*"Here is what I learned about the role of occupational therapy in bowel and bladder management in older adults ..."*	FWed should follow-up and ask the student to present their findings from self-directed learning.

Adapted from Lazarus, J. (2016). Precepting 101: Teaching strategies and tips for successful preceptors. *Journal of Midwifery & Women's Health, 61*(1), S11-S21. https://doi.org/10.1111/jmwh.12520

Box 8-4

THINK-ALOUD SCENARIO

In an orthopedic outpatient setting, a Level II fieldwork student is leading a new patient evaluation for a person with upper extremity limitations. After the student performs a general functional upper extremity screen, the FWed suggests that the student employ some provocative tests such as the Hawkins-Kennedy test and the drop arm test. When the student passively brings the affected extremity into horizontal abduction and requests that the patient holds their arm in that position and activate an isometric contraction to resistive gravity, the patient's arm immediately falls to their side. The FWed prompts the student to think aloud by saying *"Tell me what you are thinking behind the patient's symptoms, impairments, and responses to the provocative tests."* See Table 8-6 for an example of student and FWed dialogue using thinking aloud.

TABLE 8-6

EXAMPLE OF THINKING ALOUD

THINKING ALOUD EXAMPLE FROM THE STUDENT	RESPONSE FROM THE FIELDWORK EDUCATOR
"I believe we can rule out shoulder impingement and should evaluate deeper for a rotator cuff tear."	Response to a student who hits the bull's-eye and comes to the correct response: *"Tell me how you arrived to the hypothesis that the patient most likely presents with a full-thickness rotator cuff tear."*
"Well, I know that the client has normal passive range of motion and moderate pain with external range of motion, yet did not report pain during the Hawkins-Kennedy test. They did seem to have difficulty keeping their arm up during the drop arm test."	Response to a student who is "warm", but not completely on the right path yet: *"Keep talking …" or "Uh-huh,"* which may signal to the student to keep talking and thinking aloud through the scenario.
"The patient has stiffness and pain in their shoulder. I think it could be frozen shoulder, maybe?"	Response to a student who is "cold," or not near target: *"Walk me through how you came to the hypothesis that frozen shoulder is the reason the patient lacks range of motion in the proximal shoulder and had a positive drop arm test."*

COACHING

Coaching is a concept that has gained significant traction throughout the human resource and talent management fields, the private sector, and the foundation of the growing industry of personal development. Within clinical education, coaching can be used to mold a student's (or coachee's) mindset to focus on performance improvement and growth. Instructors as coaches adopt a mindset of emphasizing rapport building and active role-modeling to support the student (DeIuliis & Saylor, 2021). A FWed is a critical role model to a fieldwork student and influences

Table 8-7
Example of Coaching

COACHING USED FOR GOAL SETTING	FIELDWORK EDUCATOR SCRIPT
Initial goal setting (can be done at the beginning of fieldwork, at regular intervals, etc.)	*"What is the goal that you would like to accomplish by midterm week?"*
	"Why is that meaningful to you?" or *"Tell me more about this."*
	"What does being a successful Level II fieldwork student feel like?"
	"In what ways are you committed to stretching yourself to achieve your goal?"
Reflection (used at formative evaluation, such as midterm and final reviews)	*"How did your first 6 weeks go? What went well? What would you have liked to do differently?"*
	"What were barriers that you crossed?"
	"In addition to your strengths, what additional resources or skills do you need to reach the entry-level expectations?"

student learning by demonstrating passion in their roles and responsibilities, implementing professional theory, and empowering students to take responsibility for their own learning (Furness et al., 2020). Coaches motivate the coachee to take ownership of their success and learning and encourage students to engage in frequent reflection on their behaviors and actions. Coaching is similar to the concept of mentoring but employs the essence of transactional and transformational leadership as a foundation (Fletcher & Meyer, 2016). As a clinical coach, a FWed focuses on active listening and observation, facilitating and guiding vs. rote supervision and instruction. Coaching is linked to enhancing well-being, self-esteem, and resilience in addition to enhancing overall performance (Gazelle et al., 2015; Palamara et al., 2015; Wescott, 2016). Strategies that align with the coaching model include:

- Establishing shared goals between the student and the instructor
- Consistent relationship building to develop a strong rapport
- Providing frequent feedback designed to promote growth and development (Orr & Sonnadra, 2019)

Creating a teaching-learning environment and a building a relationship that is open and honest are important attributes that contribute to a quality fieldwork placement (Rodger et al., 2011). The combination of open-ended questions, clarifying questions, and active listening are recommendations to infuse philosophies from coaching models within the educational process (Armson et al., 2019). See Table 8-7 for example prompts a FWed can use to coach their fieldwork student.

A critical aspect of coaching is how feedback is used within the process. Different approaches to provide feedback will be discussed in this next section of the chapter.

TABLE 8-8

FEEDBACK CONSTRUCTS

CONSTRUCTS OF FEEDBACK	EXPLANATION	EXAMPLE
Feedback as information	A message or information directed toward the student. This type of feedback is designed to inform the student.	*"The emergency code to deploy during a psychiatric emergency on this unit is called Dr. Strong."*
Feedback as a reaction	An exchange of information to the student in direct response to observed behavior. The type of feedback informs the student but also includes needs for improvement and may tend to be more corrective in nature.	*"On your next attempt, ensure that you instruct the client to keep their head still during the oculomotor exam."*
Feedback as a cycle	An interactive process of receiving and responding to information between the student and FWed. This inherently includes both *information* and *reaction* and should motivate the student to engage in the exchange.	*"Be sure to directly link how the activity completed during the session is connected to one of the patient's occupational goal areas in your documentation. We will review your next SOAP note together tomorrow afternoon."*

THE IMPORTANCE OF FEEDBACK WITHIN FIELDWORK EDUCATION TEACHING STRATEGIES

Feedback is essential for learning and the required process within many of the clinical education strategies discussed in this chapter. Feedback typically refers to information that is delivered to a learner to correct, reinforce, or influence their knowledge and/or performance (Nottingham & Henning, 2014). Although feedback can be used to address gaps in learning or unsatisfactory performance, the exchange of feedback should not be exclusively punitive. Instead, the feedback exchange should be provided in a personalized manner that also affirms a learner's strengths and the progress they are making toward the goal. Van De Ridder et al. (2008) identify three main constructs to define feedback within medical clinical education (1) feedback as information, (2) feedback as reaction, and (3) feedback as a cycle. See Table 8-8 for examples of feedback constructs.

It is well documented within and outside the occupational therapy profession that feedback is a critical piece during the teaching-learning process, whether in the didactic classroom or clinical practice site (Costa, 2006; Scheerer, 2003). In a 2011 study by Rodger et al., Level II fieldwork students reported timely feedback as the "single most important part of their learning" (p. 199). Koski et al. (2013) determined that both fieldwork students and FWeds ranked constructive feedback as the most valuable behavior to the success of the fieldwork experience. In their recent scoping review, Patterson and D'Amico (2020) reported feedback as an important theme in occupational

---

BOX 8-5

Kritek (2015) and Rodger et al. (2011) list several qualities of effective feedback, which include specificity, a focus on behaviors, timely, honesty, balance, linked to the learner's goal, and nonjudgmental, and is clearly identified as feedback. Here are two example prompts a FWed can use to initiate feedback with their student:

1. *"Would you like me give you some feedback, because I was thinking something a bit different for Mrs. Xu?"*

2. *"Would you mind if I made one or two suggestions of what you have just been talking about here?"*

---

therapy literature that helps shape the student's overall perception of their FWeds and leads to a more positive experience.

As a FWed, providing feedback to a fieldwork student that is both constructive but also designed to help a student grow and be successful is an art and also reported in the literature as a strong facilitator of student learning during fieldwork (Grenier, 2015; Rodger et al., 2011). There are data that discuss various characteristics that impact the outcome of the feedback process including "specificity, timing, tone, and relation to the educational goals" (Nottingham & Henning, 2014, p. 49).

If not used effectively, feedback can negatively impact student learning and performance (Andonian, 2017b; Koski et al., 2013). To be effective, feedback must be given with the intent to improve the student's performance and presented in a way that allows the student to comprehend and accept it so that feedback is applied in practice (Cantillon & Sargant, 2008). In other words, feedback should be provided in an actionable manner. While it is always nice to get a "good job" statement of praise from your educator, this feedback exchange is very general and does not provide specific information that the learner can apply to future performance. *What was good about it?* When feedback is absent, ambiguous, and inconsistent, this is a barrier to student learning (Giles et al., 2014). In addition, insufficient feedback can make the student "feel devalued, directionless, and fearful of change" (Rodger et al., 2011, p. 199). Instead, feedback should be descriptive and specific, based upon direct observation of the learner and a reflection of the student's performance. For example, *"Your intervention session with Mrs. Jones went really well because you responded accurately to her cues of agitation and effectively graded the demands of the task and environment."* Feedback provided by a FWed can emphasize student performance with technical skills related to client care, as well as other aspects of their performance, such as emotional intelligence and professionalism (Gribble et al., 2017a). It is well documented in the occupational therapy literature that emotional intelligence (EI) and aspects of communication skills do play a role in the success of particular aspects of fieldwork. Andonian (2013) found that students with higher emotional intelligence had better intervention skills and communication skills. See Box 8-5 for prompts to initiate feedback.

Effective FWeds should establish the feedback exchange process as a habit, and routinely ask their fieldwork student to provide their own reflection to the feedback exchange process and the delivery method of the educator. Prompts that a FWed can use to encourage their fieldwork student to be interactive with the fieldwork process can include *"Is there a better way for me to provide you feedback on your moving and handling skills?"* or *"What else would be helpful to your learning about how to effectively use this neuromuscular electrotherapeutic modality?"* Feedback is a formative assessment and should be viewed differently from evaluation, which is summative. Although formal feedback typically occurs during formal midterm and final evaluations during Level II fieldwork, effective FWeds provide actionable feedback to their students throughout the learning process, as previously referenced as feedback as a cycle. The context and environment of where the

Box 8-6

Feedback is more than just verbal information provided to a student on their performance. Feedback can also be bidirectional via non-verbal communication. Snyder (2018) claims non-verbal communication, such as attitude, facial expression, body language, and eye contact, can impact the student's interpretation, acceptance, and application of the feedback. When the tone of voice or body language was condescending or accusatory, students were more likely to shut down during the feedback exchange and unlikely to accept the feedback.

FWeds need to be aware of not just what they say, but how they say it and the non-verbal messages that they are sending to their fieldwork students as it can impact future student performance and learning.

feedback exchange process occurs are also relevant to the teaching-learning process. Depending on the developmental level of the learner and the content of the feedback, FWeds should be mindful if a public or private setting is necessary (Costa, 2006).

Feedback should also be bidirectional, meaning that it should be a two-way conversation between the learner and the instructor (Kritek, 2015). A well-known feedback model is the **feedback sandwich** (LeBaron & Jernick, 2000). This involves a three-step process, delivery of positive feedback given before and after constructive feedback. Constructive feedback is never easy to give, but sandwiching criticism between layers of praise can make it more palatable for the receiver.

1. Positive comment (reinforce)
2. Specific constructive suggestion for improvement (inform)
3. Another positive comment (motivate)

Here is an example of the Sandwich Model for feedback used by a Level II FWed in a school-based setting:

1. *"You did a really good job of handling the child's maladaptive behaviors well. I saw you recognize the antecedent and you reacted swiftly."*
2. *"When you move to the second planned activity of the session, I suggest that you first offer a preferred activity to the child to reengage them."*
3. *"You are building a nice rapport with Suzie. Continuing to use and apply the information you gathered in the occupational profile will be beneficial for your developing rapport."*

There is evidence that supports the use of this feedback model with beginner learners or early during the learning experience; however, it can hinder the rapport between the educator and the learner (Lefroy et al., 2015). One reason is that the learner's role within this exchange is passive, and predominately just listens to the comments provided. While this may be a strategy attempting to reinforce what went well and to provide areas of constructive criticism for improvement, it is a unidirectional approach that may not necessarily prompt a meaningful discussion between the educator and student. Another weakness of this model is that the second step, which includes the suggestion for improvement, may not be fully received by the learner due to it being sandwiched by two areas of praise. This can be confusing to the learner. Several models of how to structure the feedback process within Level II fieldwork will be discussed next. See Box 8-6 for important tips on how feedback should be provided.

> **Box 8-7**
>
> **FWed:** *"Ok, you just finished working with Mr. Dwyer—what do you feel went well about the session?"*
>
> **Level II fieldwork student responds:** *"........"*
>
> **FWed:** *"I agree with you. You were successful in using neurodevelopmental treatment facilitation as a way to normalize his muscle tone prior to the ADL task. An area that you were not quite as successful was your use of handling skills to facilitate functional upper extremity movement within the occupation of dressing."*
>
> **FWed:** *"Tell me about what you noticed about your handling skills and key points of control used during the ADL part of the session?"*
>
> **Level II fieldwork student responds:** *"........"*

Ask Respond Tell

While the Sandwich Model may be a tactic to initiate feedback early during a Level II fieldwork as the experience progresses, the FWed should transition to feedback approaches that engage the student in a more active role, such as the Ask Respond Tell (ART) approach. ART, or also referred to as the Ask-Tell-Ask, is a useful method to promote bidirectional feedback. The steps include:

1. Ask the student what they think they did well

2. Reinforce and produce a new compliment

3. Tell the student an area to grow

4. Ask the student where they think they can grow (French et al., 2015)

The fourth and final step is important as it allows the student to exhibit self-directness and initiate and develop an improvement plan. See Box 8-7 for an example of ART.

Pendleton Approach

Moving along the feedback continuum, the Pendleton Approach stresses an even higher level of active involvement of the student within the feedback process. The Pendleton method of giving feedback is designed to make the learning experience constructive and the person receiving the feedback (i.e., the student) to be an active participant. It is an interactive approach that is intended to establish a conversation about performance (Pendleton et al., 1984). The FWed uses open-ended questions to prompt the learner to think and reflect on their performance (Hardavella et al., 2017). By both the student and the instructor highlighting positives, it can prevent defensiveness and lead to more of a constructive dialogue and plan to improve performance. Before initiating a conversation, the first and critical rule in Pendleton's method is to ensure that the student is ready for feedback. See Table 8-9 for an example of the Pendleton Approach.

Pendleton's rules are intended to promote a safe and supportive environment, to encourage and incorporate self-assessment, and to generate recommendations rather than criticisms. Creating a culture where feedback is expected is an important factor that contributes to success on fieldwork (Nicola-Richmond et al., 2017). See Box 8-8 for advice on giving feedback.

TABLE 8-9
EXAMPLE OF PENDLETON APPROACH

STEP	FIELDWORK EDUCATOR	STUDENT
Ensure that the student is ready for feedback.	*"Is now a good time to discuss your evaluation session you led with Ms. Volker?"*	
The student identifies what went well.	*"What went well?"* or *"What were you successful with during this patient session?"* Ensure that the student identifies strengths of the performance.	*"I think I was accurate in how I administered and interpreted the manual muscle test."*
The instructor reinforces what went well.	*"I thought you were successful in using appropriate hand placement during your testing of the upper extremity in against-gravity planes."* This can also introduce another area of good practice not related to what the student brought up.	
The student identifies what could have been improved.	*"What did not go so well?"* or *"Where was your performance less successful?"*	*"Yes, I agree with you that I need to review the appropriate techniques for manual muscle test during anti-gravity and gravity-eliminated planes."*
The instructor reinforces what could have been improved.	*"What I would have done differently during the gravity-eliminated test of the deltoid was to position the patient in supine instead of side-lying."*	
The instructor and student agree on an action plan for improvement.	*"What will you do differently next time?* *"How can this be achieved?"*	*"I am going to review my occupational therapy textbook over the weekend, and would love to set up a time to practice again on Monday if you are available."*

> **Box 8-8**
>
> To summarize, Adkoli (2017) provides some excellent advice in giving feedback as a clinical educator:
>
> - Be truthful and honest.
> - Keep it short and sweet.
> - Be nonthreatening and nonjudgmental.
> - Give feedback in real-time.
> - Show passion and a genuine concern for the learner's growth.

RECOGNITION OF LEARNING AND DIAGNOSING PERFORMANCE ISSUES

Clinical observation is an important skill throughout practice as an occupational therapy practitioner. Developing awareness of observation abilities is typically a precursor to didactic curricula on the evaluation process and subsequent intervention planning and implementation (Mackenzie & Westwood, 2012). The depth and breadth of observation skills is something that develops with time and experience, both within the role of practitioner and FWed. As a FWed, it is critical to hone observation skills geared toward recognizing signs that demonstrate the student is learning ("getting it") vs. at risk for learning challenges and problematic performance (i.e., red flag behaviors; Burns et al., 2006; Gutman et al., 1998). These may be observations that are made by the FWed during the implementation of some of the clinical teaching strategies discussed in this chapter. See Table 8-10 for observations and red flag indicators.

Consistent observations that the student is "getting it" should trigger the FWed to intentionally grade up certain expectations of the fieldwork experience to provide the just-right-challenge for the fieldwork student. Consistent or frequent red flag observations should not be overlooked. The FWed should keep documentation on these specific problematic behaviors, discuss with the student directly during regular feedback sessions, and communicate proactively with the AFWC. This may also lead to more formal remediation activities, such as a learning contract or performance improvement plan, which are discussed in Chapter 10.

TABLE 8-10

RECOGNITION OF LEARNING AND POTENTIAL PERFORMANCE ISSUES

OBSERVATIONS THAT THE STUDENT IS "GETTING IT"	"RED FLAG" INDICATORS OF PROBLEMATIC PERFORMANCE	CONNECTION TO OCCUPATIONAL THERAPY LITERATURE
Is self-confident but knows limits, ask for help appropriately	Lacks confidence, excessive reliance on supervision	Grenier (2015) determined that self-confidence enabled occupational therapy fieldwork student learning on fieldwork, whereas, whereas a lack of confidence was a barrier to learning.
Consistently articulates sound decision making	Is hesitant, presents less-focused plan or excessively misses information	Although models to predict students at-risk for failing fieldwork have been controversial in occupational therapy education, certain aspects of academic performance (e.g., anatomy grade, admission science GPA) have been proven to be predictors of future fieldwork performance (Whisner et al., 2019).
Seeks out and embraces constructive feedback	Is defensive, makes excuses, or places blame	Inability to accept, hear or respond to constructive feedback is a known attribute of a student that struggles with achieving success on fieldwork (Deluliis, 2017; Nicola-Richmond et al., 2016).
Collegial, team player, demonstrates respect for interprofessional collaboration	Not collegial	Emotional intelligence and professional communication skills have been correlated with higher fieldwork performance scores (Andonian, 2013; Andonian, 2017a; Brown et al., 2016; Tan et al., 2004; Tickle-Degnen, 1998). The importance of networking during the fieldwork experience is also noted as a facilitator of a successful fieldwork performance (James & Mussleman, 2005).
Organized, time-efficient	Inconsistent	Various aspects of intrinsic and extrinsic qualities of professionalism are known traits of a successful fieldwork student (Deluliis, 2017).
Generalizes knowledge and learning	The inability of the student to transfer knowledge or skill from one situation to another	A struggle to "get the big picture" during fieldwork is a noted common characteristic among failed fieldwork experiences, along with a lack of carryover from one patient encounter to another (James & Mussleman, 2005).

Adapted from Burns, C., Beauchesne, M., Ryan-Krause, P., & Sawin, K. (2006). Mastering the preceptor role: Challenges of clinical teaching. *Journal of Pediatric Health Care, 20*(3), 172-183. https://doi.org/10.1016/j.pedhc.2005.10.012

SUMMARY

Increasing awareness about the various styles and prompts that can be used during specific teaching encounters is valuable to the development of service competency within the FWed role. Understanding different ways to package and deliver feedback (whether focused on a student's strengths or growth areas) is also critical. Although many of the specific teaching tools discussed in this chapter originated in the training of medical students and other allied health professionals, they do provide a useful model for FWeds to add these strategies to their "FWed toolbox."

LEARNING ACTIVITIES

1. Your Level II fieldwork student completes the initial evaluation on a new client. You ask the student to provide an oral case presentation of the session:

   Maria is 55-year-old widow with major depressive disorder with complaints of difficulty sleeping, loss of appetite, and frequent aches and pains. She feels hopeless, and the nurses have found her yelling at people in her room when no one is actually there. She says she has trouble keeping track of all of her medications and things to do around her house. She recently has been ignoring her friends, family, and neighbors.

   Identify two clarifying and two probing questions that could be used to further examine the extent of the fieldwork student's knowledge.

2. Using Table 8-2 as a guide, create direct questioning prompts that can be used with Level II fieldwork students novice through proficient levels of skill acquisition (Dreyfus) and scaffold to higher levels of learning on Bloom's Taxonomy.

3. Using Tables 8-3 and 8-4, explain how each step in the OMP and 5MP models fosters effective and efficient teaching within Level II fieldwork.

4. It is week 3 for your Level II fieldwork student. You, the FWed, want to give feedback regarding their documentation skills, since your student is unable to finish assigned documentation by the end of the day. The notes are very detailed; however, many specifics are not necessary. You want to give guidance to improve your student's time management skills and go over the pertinent information to be included.

   Which feedback exchange model discussed in the chapter would you select to use (Sandwich Model, ART, Pendleton Approach), and why?

5. Table 8-10 outlines several examples of observable behaviors or attitudes that demonstrate that a student is "getting it" and indicative of learning. Within your practice setting, what are specific behaviors or attitudes that would indicate that the student is "getting it"?

REFERENCES

Adkoli, B. V. (2018). The role of feedback and reflection in medical education. *Journal of Basic, Clinical and Applied Health Science, 2*(1), 34-40. https://pdfs.semanticscholar.org/0aaa/0c442c85da07804a934751f4e95d1adc599b.pdf

American Occupational Therapy Association. (2020). Occupational therapy practice framework: Domain and process (4th ed.). *American Journal of Occupational Therapy, 74*(Suppl. 2). Advance online publication.

Anderson, L. W., & Krathwohl, D. R. (Eds.). (2001). *A taxonomy for learning, teaching and assessing: A revision of Bloom's Taxonomy of educational objectives: Complete edition.* Longman.

Andonian, L. (2013). Emotional intelligence, self-efficacy, and occupational therapy students' fieldwork performance. *Occupational Therapy in Health Care, 27,* 1-15. https://doi.org/10.3109/07380577.2012.763199

Andonian, L. (2017a). Emotional intelligence: An opportunity for occupational therapy. *Occupational Therapy in Mental Health, 33*(4), 1-9. https://doi.org/10.1080/0164212X.2017.1328649.

Andonian, L. (2017b). Occupational therapy students' self-efficacy, experience of supervision, and perception of meaningfulness of level II fieldwork. *The Open Journal of Occupational Therapy, 5*(2), 1-12. https://doi.org/10.15453/2168-6408.1220

Armson, H., Lockyer, J. M., Zetkulic, M., Könings, K. D., & Sargeant, J. (2019). Identifying coaching skills to improve feedback use in postgraduate medical education. *Medical Education, 53*(5), 477-493. https://doi.org/10.1111/medu.13818

Barnum, G. M., Guyer, M. S., Levy, L. S., & Graham, C. (2009). The supervision, questioning, and feedback model of clinical teaching: A practical approach. In T. G. Wiedner (Ed.), *The athletic trainer's pocket guide to clinical teaching* (pp. 85–99). SLACK Incorporated.

Bott, G., Mohide, E. A., & Lawlor, Y. (2011). A clinical teaching technique for nurse preceptors: The five-minute preceptor. *Journal of Professional Nursing, 27*(1), 35-42. https://doi.org/10.1016/j.profnurs.2010.09.009

Brown, T., Williams, B., & Etherington, J. (2016). Emotional intelligence and personality traits as predictors of occupational therapy students' practice education performance: A cross-sectional study. *Occupational Therapy International, 23*, 1-13. https://doi.org/10.1002/oti.1443

Burns, C., Beauchesne, M., Ryan-Krause, P., & Sawin, K. (2006). Mastering the preceptor role: Challenges of clinical teaching. *Journal of Pediatric Health Care, 20*(3), 172-183. https://doi.org/10.1016/j.pedhc.2005.10.012

Cantillon, P., & Sargeant, J. (2008). Giving feedback in clinical settings. *BMJ, 337*, 1292- 1294. https://doi.10.1136/bmj.a1961

Chinai, S. A., Guth, T., Lovell, E., & Epter, M. (2018). Taking advantage of the teachable moment: A review of learner-centered clinical teaching models. *Western Journal of Emergency Medicine, 19*(1), 28. https://doi.org/10.5811/westjem.2017.8.35277

Costa, D. M. (2006). The importance of feedback. [Electronic Version]. *OT Practice, 11*(16), 7–8. http://motfieldwork.pbworks.com/w/file/fetch/44901978/ImportanceFeedback.pdf

DeIuliis, E. (2017). Professionalism and fieldwork education. In E. DeIuliis (Ed.), *Professionalism across occupational therapy practice* (pp. 201-221). SLACK Incorporated.

DeIuliis, E. D., & Saylor, E. (2021). Bridging the gap: Three strategies to optimize professional relationships with generation Y and Z. *The Open Journal of Occupational Therapy, 9*(1), 1-13. https://doi.org/10.15453/2168-6408.1748

Dreyfus, S. E., & Dreyfus, H. L. (1980). *A five-stage model of the mental activities involved in directed skill acquisition.* California Univ Berkeley Operations Research Center.

Fletcher, K. A., & Meyer, M. (2016). Coaching model+ clinical playbook= transformative learning. *Journal of Professional Nursing, 32*(2), 121-129. https://doi.org/10.1016/j.profnurs.2015.09.001

French, J. C., Colbert, C. Y., Pien, L. C., Dannefer, E. F., & Taylor, C. A. (2015). Targeted feedback in the milestones era: Utilization of the ask-tell-ask feedback model to promote reflection and self-assessment. *Journal of Surgical Education, 72*(6), e274-e279. https://doi.org/10.1016/j.jsurg.2015.05.016

Furness, L., Tynan, A., & Ostini, J. (2020). What students and new graduates perceive supports them to think, feel and act as a health professional in a rural setting. *Australian Journal of Rural Health, 28*(3), 263-270. https://doi.10.1111/ajr.12607

Gazelle, G., Liebschutz, J. M., & Riess, H. (2015). Physician burnout: Coaching a way out. *Journal of General Internal Medicine, 30*(4), 508-513. https://doi.org/10.1007/s11606-014-3144-y

Giles, T. M., Gilbert, S., & McNeill, L. (2013). Nursing students' perceptions regarding the amount and type of written feedback required to enhance their learning. *Journal of Nursing Education, 53*(1), 23-30. https://doi:10.3928/01484834-20131209-02

Graziano, S. C. (2011). Randomized surgical training for medical students: Resident versus peer-led teaching. American *Journal of Obstetrics and Gynecology, 204*(6), 542-e1. https://doi.org/10.1016/j.ajog.2011.01.038

Grenier, M.L. (2015). Facilitators and barriers to learning in occupational therapy fieldwork education: Student perspectives. *American Journal of Occupational Therapy, 69*(2), 6912185070p1-6912185070p9. https://doi.org/10.5014/ajot.2015.015180

Gribble, N., Ladyshewsky, R. K., & Parsons, R. (2017a). Fluctuations in the emotional intelligence of therapy students during clinical placements: Implication for educators, supervisors, and students. *Journal of Interprofessional Care, 31*(1), 8-17. https://doi.org/10.1080/13561820.2016.1244175

Gribble, N., Ladyshewsky, R. K., & Parsons, R. (2017b). Strategies for interprofessional facilitators and clinical supervisors that may enhance the emotional intelligence of therapy students. *Journal of Interprofessional Care, 31*(5), 593-603. https://doi.10.1080/13561820.2017.1341867

Gutman, S. A., McCreedy, P., & Heisler, P. (1998). Student level II fieldwork failure: Strategies for intervention. *American Journal of Occupational Therapy, 52*(2), 143-149. https://doi.org/10.5014/ajot.52.2.143

Hardavella, G., Aamli-Gaagnat, A., Saad, N., Rousalova, I., & Sreter, K. B. (2017). How to give and receive feedback effectively. *Breathe, 13*(4), 327-333. https://doi.10.1183/20734735.009917

Houchens, N., Harrod, M., Fowler, K. E., Moody, S., & Saint, S. (2017). How exemplary inpatient teaching physicians foster clinical reasoning. *The American Journal of Medicine, 130*(9), 1113-e1. http://dx.doi.org/10.1016/j.amjmed.2017.03.050

Kolb, D. A. (1984). *Experiential learning: Experience as the source of learning and development.* Prentice-Hall.

Koski, K.J., Simon, R.L., & Dooley, N.R. (2013). Valuable occupational therapy fieldwork educator behaviors. *Work, 44,* 307-315. https://doi.org/10.3233/WOR-121507

Kotsis, S., & Chung, K. (2013). Application of the "see one, do one, teach one" concept in surgical training. *Plastic and Reconstructive Surgery, 131*(5), 1194-1201. https://doi.org/10.1097/PRS.0b013e318287a0b3

Kritek, P. A. (2015). Strategies for effective feedback. *Annals of the American Thoracic Society, 12*(4), 557-560.https://doi.org/10.1513/AnnalsATS.201411-524FR

Lazarus, J. (2016). Precepting 101: Teaching strategies and tips for successful preceptors. *Journal of Midwifery & Women's Health, 61*(1), S11 – S21. https://doi.org/10.1111/jmwh.12520

LeBaron, S. W., & Jernick, J. (2000). Evaluation as a dynamic process. *Family Medicine, 32*(1), 13-14.

Lefroy, J., Watling, C., Teunissen, P. W., & Brand, P. (2015). Guidelines: the do's, don'ts and don't knows of feedback for clinical education. *Perspectives on Medical Education, 4*(6), 284-299. https://doi.org/10.1007/s40037-015-0231-7.

Long, M., Blankenburg, R., & Butani, L. (2015). Questioning as a teaching tool. *Pediatrics, 135*(3), 406-408. https://doi.org/10.1542/peds.2014-3285

Lundgrén-Laine, H., & Salanterä, S. (2010). Think-aloud technique and protocol analysis in clinical decision-making research. *Qualitative Health Research, 20*(4), 565-575. https://doi.org/10.1177/1049732309354278

MacKenzie, D. E., & Westwood, D. A. (2012). Occupational therapists and observation: What are you looking at?. *OTJR: Occupation, Participation and Health, 33*(1), 4-11. https://doi.org/10.3928/15394492-20120928-01

Melvin, L., & Cavalcanti, R. B. (2016). The oral case presentation: A key tool for assessment and teaching in competency-based medical education. *JAMA, 316*(21), 2187-2188. https://doi.org/10.1001/jama.2016.16415

Naidoo, D., & van Wyk, J. (2016). Fieldwork practice for learning: Lessons from occupational therapy students and their supervisors. *African Journal of Health Professions Education, 8*(1), 37-40. https://doi. 10.7196/AJHPE.2016.v8i1.536

Neher, J. O., Gordon, K. C., Meyer, B., & Stevens, N. (1992). A five-step "microskills" model of clinical teaching. *Journal of the American Board of Family Practice, 5*, 419-424. https://doi.org/10.3122/jabfm.5.4.41

Nicola-Richmond, K., Butterworth, B., & Hitch, D. (2017). What factors contribute to failure of fieldwork placement? Perspectives of supervisors and university fieldwork educators. *World Federation of Occupational Therapists Bulletin, 73*(2), 117-124. https://doi.org/10.1080/14473828.2016.1149981

Nottingham, S., & Henning, J. (2014). Feedback in clinical education, part I: Characteristics of feedback provided by approved clinical instructors. *Journal of Athletic Training, 49*(1), 49-57. https://doi.org/10.4085/1062-6050-48.6.14

Onishi, H. (2008). The role of case presentations for teaching and learning activities. *Journal of Medical Science, 24*(7), 356-360. https://doi.org/10.1016/S1607-551X(08)70132-3

Orr, C. J., & Sonnadara, R. R. (2019). Coaching by design: Exploring a new approach to faculty development in a competency-based medical education curriculum. *Advances in Medical Education and Practice, 10*, 229. https://doi.org/10.2147/AMEP.S191470

Palamara, K., Kauffman, C., Stone, V. E., Bazari, H., & Donelan, K. (2015). Promoting success: A professional development coaching program for interns in medicine. *Journal of Graduate Medical Education, 7*(4), 630-637. https://doi.org/10.4300/JGME-D-14-00791.1

Pascoe, J. M., Nixon, J., & Lang, V. J. (2015). Maximizing teaching on the wards: review and application of the One-Minute Preceptor and SNAPPS models. *Journal of Hospital Medicine, 10*(2), 125-130. https://doi.org/10.1002/jhm.2302

Patterson, B., & D'Amico, M. (2020). What does the evidence say about student, fieldwork educator, and new occupational therapy practitioner perceptions of successful level II fieldwork and transition to practice? A scoping review. *Journal of Occupational Therapy Education, 4*(2). https://doi.org/10.26681/jote.2020.040210

Pendleton, D. (1984). *The consultation: An approach to learning and teaching* (No. 6). Oxford University Press.

Pintrich, P. R. (2000). The role of goal orientation in self-regulated learning. In M. Boeskaerts, R. Pintrich & M. Zeidner (Eds.), *Handbook of self-regulation* (pp. 451-502). Academic Press. https://doi.org/10.1016/B978-012109890-2/50043-3

Rodger, S., Fitzgerald, C., Davila, W., Millar, F., & Allison, H. (2011). What makes a quality occupational therapy practice placement? Students' and practice educators' perspectives. *Australian Occupational Therapy Journal, 58*(3), 195-202. https://doi.org/10.1111/j.1440-1630.2010.00903.x

Scheerer, C. R. (2003). Perceptions of effective professional behavior feedback: Occupational therapy student voices. *American Journal of Occupational Therapy, 57*(2), 205-214. https://doi.org/10.5014/ajot.57.2.205

Smith, J. R., & Lane, I. F. (2015). Making the most of five minutes: The clinical teaching moment. *Journal of Veterinary Medical Education, 42*(3), 271-280. https://doi.org/10.3138/jvme.0115-004R

Snyder, K. (2018). Exploring students' use of feedback during occupational therapy Level II fieldwork experiences. *Journal of Occupational Therapy Education, 2*(2), 1. https://doi.org/10.26681/jote.2018.020204

Stickrath, C., Aagaard, E., & Anderson, M. (2013). MiPLAN: A learner-centered model for bedside teaching in today's academic medical centers. *Academic Medicine, 88*(3), 322-327. https://doi.org/10.1097/ACM.0b013e318280d8f7

Tan, K., Meredith, P., & McKenna, K. (2004). Predictors of occupational therapy student's clinical performance: An exploratory study. *Australian Occupational Therapy Journal, 51*(1), 1-9. https://doi.org/10.1046/j.1440-1630.2003.00383.x

Tickle-Degnen, L. (1998). Working well with others: The prediction of students' clinical performance. *American Journal of Occupational Therapy, 52*(2), 1-10. https://doi.org/10.5014/ajot.52.2.133

Van De Ridder, J. M., Stokking, K. M., McGaghie, W. C., & Ten Cate, O. T. J. (2008). What is feedback in clinical education?. *Medical Education, 42*(2), 189-197. https://doi.org/10.1111/j.1365-2923.2007.02973.x

Weinholtz, D. (1983). Directing medical student clinical case presentations. *Medical Education, 17*(6), 364-368. https://doi.org/10.1111/j.1365-2923.1983.tb01121.x

Westcott, L. (2016). How coaching can play a key role in the development of nurse managers. *Journal of Clinical Nursing, 25*(17-18), 2669-2677. https://doi.org/10.1111/jocn.13315

Whiner, S. M., Geddie, M., Sechrist, D., & Wang, E. (2019). Examination of potential factors to predict fieldwork performance: A program evaluation project. *Journal of Occupational Therapy Education, 3*(1), 6. https://doi.org/10.26681/jote.2019.030106

Wolpaw, T., Papp, K. K., & Bordage, G. (2009). Using SNAPPS to facilitate the expression of clinical reasoning and uncertainties: A randomized comparison group trial. *Academic Medicine, 84*(4), 517-524. https://doi.org/10.1097/ACM.0b013e31819a8cbf

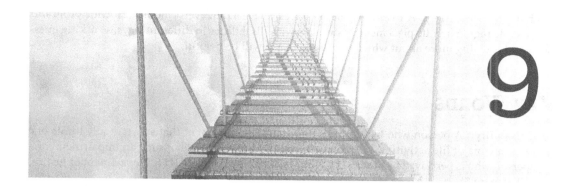

Reasonable Accommodations
Supporting Students With Disabilities in Level II Fieldwork

Rebecca L. Simon, EdD, OTR/L, FAOTA; Anna Domina, OTD, OTR/L; and Angela Lampe, OTD, OTR/L

In recent years the number of students with a disability entering post-secondary educational programs has increased, with statistics showing 12% of students at the post-baccalaureate level reporting a disability (National Center for Education Statistics [NCES], 2019; Ozelie et al., 2019). This represents a tremendous growth that directly impacts occupational therapy programs. The American College Health Association (2021) National College Health Assessment III found that 40.9% of respondents reported that anxiety negatively impacted their academic performance, 47.7% indicated that depression impacted academic performance, and 41.3% stated that stress had a negative impact. With this rise of post-secondary students with disabilities on college campuses, and the more common negative impact on academic performance, it is evident a disability can keep a student from completing their program(s) successfully. It is important that fieldwork educators (FWeds) are knowledgeable about how to navigate and successfully support a Level II fieldwork student that may disclose a disability.

This chapter will provide an overview of inclusion, how students with disabilities may be able to fully participate in Level II fieldwork experiences, the challenges and roles of each member of the fieldwork team, and best practice methods to design a Level II fieldwork experience for occupational therapy and occupational therapy assistant students that meets Americans with Disability Act (ADA) requirements. It is important to note there will be individual differences and challenges based on program policies and procedures, but this chapter is meant to provide a general guide for FWeds to help them better understand the requirements and needs of the students they supervise/

DeIuliis, E. D., & Hanson, D. (Eds.).
Fieldwork Educator's Guide to Level II Fieldwork (pp. 255-275).
© 2023 Taylor & Francis Group.

teach in practice settings. A FWed may be surprised to learn that even schools/academic programs in the same region handle placement of students with disabilities in different ways, so asking questions and learning more about which questions to ask will be helpful.

KEY WORDS

- **Disability:** "A person who has a physical or mental impairment that substantially limits one or more major life activities, a person who has a history or record of such an impairment, or a person who is perceived by others as having such an impairment" (U.S. Department of Justice, 2020, para 2).

- **Essential functions:** Those fundamental job duties that the person must be capable of performing with reasonable accommodations (U.S. Department of Education, 2021).

- **Family Educational Rights and Privacy Act (FERPA; 20 U.S.C. § 1232g; 34 CFR Part 99):** A federal law enacted in 1974 that protects the privacy of student education records

- **Invisible, or hidden, disability:** A disability that is not immediately apparent to others, for example, renal failure, diabetes, anxiety, depression, and chronic pain (Disabled World, 2020).

- **Technical standards:** The nonacademic criteria essential for the student to participate in the program; they include the attitudes, experiences, and physical requirements the student must possess to learn and perform the essential requirements of the program (Blackrock & Montgomery, 2016).

- **504 coordinator (i.e., disability services/accessibility officer):** The Section 504 regulations, at 34 C.F.R. § 104.7(a), require recipients that employ 15 or more persons to designate at least one person to coordinate its efforts to comply with Section 504 (Pub. L. No. 110–325). This individual or group of individuals supports students with identified disabilities within a college/university.

LEARNING OBJECTIVES

By the end of reading this chapter and completing the learning activities, the reader should be able to:

1. Understand the distinct nature of the needs of Level II fieldwork students with disabilities.

2. Recognize the roles of each party involved with placement of Level II fieldwork students with disabilities.

3. Utilize resources that can help with unexpected issues and understand the limitations of each party involved in the process.

19.4% of undergraduate   11.9% of postbaccalaureate

Percentage of students reporting one or more of the following disabilities: blindness or a visual impairment not corrected by wearing glasses; hearing impairment; orthopedic or mobility impairment; speech or language impairment; learning, mental, emotional, or psychiatric condition (e.g., serious learning disability, depression, attention deficit disorder); or other health impairment or problem (NCES, 2019).

13.3% of postbaccalaureate women compared to 9.9% of postbaccalaureate men reporting disabilites (NCES, 2019).

Postbaccalaureate students over the age of 24 were more likely to report a disability compared to their younger classmates as well as postbaccalaureate students who had served in the military (NCES, 2019).

Figure 9-1. Statistics pertaining to students with disabilities.

Major life activities for college students may range from seeing and hearing a didactic lecture, studying, taking tests and exams, cooking, hanging out with friends, and sleeping. Students with disabilities also experience social isolation and limited access to the necessary accommodations to complete classroom tasks (Lyman et al., 2016; Wilgosh et al., 2008). This impacts students exponentially since it is known that 23% of adult Gen Z-ers, the generation of people born in the late 1990s and early 2000s (Merriam Webster, n.d.), report they have been diagnosed with depression and 18% report a diagnosis of an anxiety disorder (American Psychological Association [APA] 2018). Mental health issues, including anxiety and depression, are real concerns for Gen Z-ers who may feel sad and nervous and show lack of interest, motivation, or energy in an academic or clinical setting (APA, 2018), which adds to the layers of issues a student with any disability may face. The stress and challenges of participating in a high stakes activity like Level II fieldwork can add to these issues, while forcing students to take a hard look at what they may need in an unfamiliar setting. See Figure 9-1 from more information from the National Center for Educational Statistics (2019) related to students with disabilities.

Under the Rehabilitation Act of 1973 (P.L. 93-112) and the Americans with Disabilities Act of 1990 (P.L. 101-476), public and private post-secondary institutions may not discriminate against and are required to provide accommodations to students who have a documented disability. See Table 9-1 for more information related to federal laws pertaining to postsecondary education and students with disabilities. Postsecondary institutions **must ensure** the academic and extracurricular activities, including fieldwork, are accessible to students with disabilities. Specific to Level II fieldwork, accommodations may include a variety of changes to the work and/ or environment to support students with visible physical disabilities as well as invisible disabilities, such as communication and information exchange, psychosocial issues, fatigue, or ergonomic needs. Accommodations and aids **must be provided** unless it is determined these requests would fundamentally alter the program or result in undue financial or administrative burdens (U.S. Equal Opportunity Employment Commission, 2008). To be considered "fundamentally altered" is a change that is so significant that it alters the essential nature of the goods, services, facilities, privileges, advantages, or accommodations offered (ADA.gov). For example, if an accommodation would cause a direct safety threat to a client that would mean the site would have the right to refuse it. For example, some sites may not allow an individual who is on crutches into a facility where a

TABLE 9-1

FEDERAL LAWS PERTAINING TO POSTSECONDARY EDUCATION AND STUDENTS WITH DISABILITIES

FEDERAL LAW	SPECIFICS AS APPLIES TO POST-SECONDARY EDUCATION INSTITUTIONS
Americans with Disabilities Act (ADA) "The ADA prohibits discrimination on the basis of disability in employment, State and local government, public accommodations, commercial facilities, transportation, and telecommunications. It also applies to the United States Congress." https://www.ada.gov/cguide. htm#anchor62335	**ADA Title II: State and Local Government Activities** Covers all activities of state and local governments; including public education **ADA Title III: Public Accommodations** including private education https://www.ada.gov/cguide. htm#anchor62335
Amendments Act of 2008 An act that amended the ADA of 1990.	"... reasonable modifications in policies, practices, or procedures shall be required, unless an entity can demonstrate that making such modifications in policies, practices, or procedures, including academic requirements in postsecondary education, would fundamentally alter the nature of the goods, services, facilities, privileges, advantages, or accommodations involved." (U.S. Equal Opportunities Employment Commission, 2008, Sec. 6[a][1][f].)
Rehabilitation Act of 1973, Section 504 "No qualified individual with a disability in the United States shall be excluded from, denied the benefits of, or be subjected to discrimination under any program or activity that either receives Federal financial assistance or is conducted by any Executive agency or the United States Postal Service." https://www.ada.gov/cguide. htm#anchor65610	A "program or activity" is among many things "a college, university, or other post-secondary institution, or a public system of higher education." https://www.govinfo.gov/content/pkg/ USCODE-2010-title29/pdf/USCODE-2010- title29-chap16-subchapV-sec794.pdf

child may elope (since they would hinder the safety if a child were to run away) or in a forensic mental health facility (where the crutch may be used as a weapon). As long as the accommodation does not fundamentally alter the nature of the program, modifying policies and procedures, such as allowing a service animal on-site or allowing a student to use technology to communicate, are other ways that postsecondary institutions may accommodate students with disabilities both within their programs and on fieldwork.

DISCLOSURE

It is ultimately the responsibility of the student in postsecondary institutions to request accommodations (Aquino & Bittinger, 2019; U.S. Department of Education, 2011). In postsecondary education settings the responsibility of disclosing a disability shifts from the team to the student, and this shift is significant for the Level II fieldwork experience. Therefore, an occupational therapy student with a disability should advocate for their needs in both the classroom and fieldwork environment. In addition to requiring the student to disclose a disability to faculty, the academic program is not allowed to disclose a disability to any fieldwork personnel without direct consent from the student themselves. This can be a challenge in many ways. Students who are new to disability services must self-navigate and essentially predict what might happen on a fieldwork site that is new to them, and perhaps even new to the academic fieldwork coordinator (AFWC). The AFWC must balance the needs of the student with their potential success on site, while not treating the student any differently so as to participate in ableism (Hutcheon & Wolbring, 2012), which would mean the coordinator, who may be able-bodied, is marginalizing someone with a disability.

In addition, a student may elect to request accommodations for the academic component of a program, but not disclose their disability for the fieldwork experience(s). AFWCs and faculty should positively support, and even empower, a student with a disability to disclose and request needed accommodations (Mamboleo et al., 2015). As students progress to Level II fieldwork, it is important that they have had a positive experience in their didactic and Level I fieldwork experiences. Students who have a positive experience disclosing and requesting accommodations as well as positive perceptions of instructors are more willing to disclose a disability (Mamboleo et al., 2015).

When a student opts to request an accommodation for either of their Level II fieldwork experiences, the student must follow the same procedures that they would to request accommodations in the classroom. However, there are several factors that may complicate this process. Under the Family Educational Rights and Privacy Act (FERPA), institutions must have written consent from the student before disclosing any information about the student's educational records (U.S. Department of Education, 2018), and colleges and universities often have specific rules and regulations about what an AFWC can disclose to sites about a student. The AFWC cannot disclose a student's disability to a site, nor can they place the student at a site based on their disability unless a specific accommodation is in place in advance of the placement process. Since it is the student's responsibility to initiate the request of accommodations, not knowing the site in advance can make it a logistical challenge. Both the student and the AFWC must work with the disability coordinator at the academic institution to try to predict what might be needed during the placement process, but then, once assigned to a fieldwork site, the student must work directly with the site and the school to further refine their accommodation needs. There are many ways this can be done, dependent upon the school's requirements, state and local laws, and the wishes of the student. A FWed should be prepared to ask questions prior to placement and know that sometimes those questions can be answered, and sometimes they cannot. This can be especially complicated for a full-time placement, which may have unexpected challenges arise.

Kennedy, an occupational therapy student, is placed in a hospital setting. Kennedy has disclosed that she has irritable bowel syndrome (IBS) to her AFWC, but not to the site. She has not requested any accommodations since she feels she will be able to use the bathroom in the hospital when needed. When Kennedy arrives on site, she learns that she will be following a practitioner who also does home health care 3 days a week. She immediately calls her AFWC because she is now afraid that she will not be able to complete the placement since she will not be able to have regular access to a bathroom. In this case, Kennedy must disclose her disability AFTER her placement, and work together with site, AFWC, and disability services to decide the next course of action. This now may cause her to delay graduation if no accommodations can be made and she must be placed elsewhere.

Box 9-1

CASE EXAMPLE

Louis is an occupational therapy assistant student who has a visual impairment that prevents him from driving independently. He has planned to utilize public transportation to attend fieldwork, which was initially 9 a.m. to 5 p.m. Monday through Friday.

Upon arriving to the site, he learns that his FWed has switched her schedule and now works 10 a.m. to 8 p.m. Tuesday through Saturday. This does not work with the transportation schedule, and he becomes nervous that he will not be able to independently arrive and depart. Louis is afraid to tell his site this information for fear they will dismiss him from the placement. He contacts his AFWC who advises him to be honest with the site. Louis continues to struggle and decides to withdraw from the placement vs. share his disability with the site since he is afraid the admission will limit his ability to obtain employment in the future.

Students who have had successful accommodations for a shorter, more flexible Level I placement may not realize the complexity of their Level II needs and overall expectations of entry-level practice. Conversely, if the student felt any form of stigma from faculty, therapists, and/or peers (Cole & Cawthon, 2015) during their Level I or academic experience, they may wish not to disclose or utilize accommodations for a site where they will be placed full time, and may feel their disclosure could impact employment. Flink (2017) identifies students who express feelings of "self-stigma," which is an "internalized negative reaction" resulting from a membership in a stigmatized group (p. 5). This feeling of self-stigma can make it difficult to cope with transitions and can be debilitating (Flink, 2017). See Box 9-1 for an example of how this self-stigma may be limiting.

Collins and Mowbray (2005) identify several barriers for disclosure of disability. Of the 12 barriers identified, the top 5 barriers were:

1. Fear of disclosing (39%)

2. Lack of knowledge (19%)

3. Fear of being stigmatized (19%)

4. Lack of specific supported education program, lack of staff or community referral sources (16%)

5. Not seeing themselves as having a disability or not wanting help (12%)

Collins and Mowbrary (2005) also report the most frequent issues for students with psychiatric disabilities are obtaining accommodations, coping with school, and attendance issues. These factors all may interfere with successful completion of fieldwork experiences and are certainly issues AFWCs have to address. For example, Ozelie et al. (2019) reported students who chose not to disclose their disability said that more breaks during the day and an altered daily schedule would have been helpful fieldwork accommodations. They also found that more than half of those surveyed (n=22, 51.16%) "felt their disability presented challenges during their fieldwork" (Ozelie et al., 2019, p.11). Creating a culture of openness to disabilities and understanding individual student needs would have been beneficial to their growth and development and potentially decrease some of the challenges experienced.

Jose is returning to a school system where he completed his 30-hour Level I placement. He has the same therapist as a FWed and is looking forward to returning to a placement where he would like to work in the future. Jose has an anxiety disorder and has not disclosed it to anyone since he has managed it quite well independently through his educational experience. When Jose arrives on site, he finds the full-time placement includes going to multiple schools and meeting with multiple teams. He also learns he has to report on an assessment during an Individual Education Plan (IEP) meeting as a part of his experience. Jose becomes more and more anxious as each day passes and is having a hard time getting out of his car to go into the schools. He returns home and begins to call in sick regularly. The FWed calls the AFWC who then calls Jose who discloses what is happening. This creates a conundrum because Jose does not wish to disclose his condition since he feels it will hurt his ability to get a recommendation from the site. However, he is fearful that he will not be able to continue and asks for another placement with one therapist in one school. The AFWC reminds him this may delay his graduation and cause confusion with the first school. Leaving the site also counts as a failure per the school's policy without a documented accommodation or medical note. This also creates a conflict for the AFWC in that they cannot tell the former site what happened nor can they let the future site know why he might need to stay in one school. The AFWC attempts to work with Jose to encourage disclosure, which may allow him to continue the current fieldwork experience successfully.

Educators, including FWeds, who have direct access to students with a disability, must recognize the need for support within this population and determine how to best serve students who can be equally as successful as their peers if given proper support (Simon, 2019). This is especially true for students with less visible disabilities, including mental health issues, who typically are the last to report (O'Shea & Meyer, 2016). Choosing to disclose a disability is a complicated decision for a postsecondary education student and poses specific challenges as they enter the unknown facets of a Level II fieldwork. Fieldwork sites will benefit from understanding their role in the process of disclosure and placement and what the limitations from the school may be, based on student choice. Sites must also be aware of the laws and resources available to support them. This can be a challenge, so working together with the school is essential. While a student must feel supported by AFWCs, faculty, and FWed when/if they choose to disclose a disability; it is important that the FWed feel supported as well. Sometimes knowledge of barriers to support is also important and should open honest discussion with the school prior to placement. These barriers can include resistance from management, lack of funds, productivity demands, and other unexpected issues that can arise.

In addition to the barriers cited above, students also sense there are invisible barriers, which may include judgment, social isolation, and self-doubt, which give them reason to not disclose their disability. AFWCs and faculty must be mindful of the student's perception of disclosing a disability and offer support as appropriate.

PROCESS FOR LEVEL II FIELDWORK ACCOMMODATIONS

The process for seeking fieldwork accommodations must be understood from a variety of contexts including the student, AFWC, and Level II fieldwork site to conceptualize best practices in providing appropriate support (see Boxes 9-2, 9-3, and 9-4). For students, this process of disclosing a disability starts very early in their academic career as described earlier. The student

BOX 9-2

KEY STEPS FOR STUDENTS REQUESTING ACCOMMODATIONS FOR LEVEL II FIELDWORK

1. Ensure paperwork is filed with the Office of Disability Services at the academic institution
2. Disclose the need for accommodations to the AFWC at the academic institution in preparation for fieldwork
3. Work with the AFWC and Office of Disability Services to develop/approve the accommodation request letter
4. Review feedback provided from Level II fieldwork site about accommodations requested
5. In some instances, may need to meet with AFWC and Level II fieldwork site in advance to discuss accommodation requests
6. Once Level II fieldwork site agrees to an accommodation request, keep a copy of the signed letter along with your other necessary paperwork for Level II fieldwork provided by the academic institution in your files.

should become familiar with the office of disability services at the school and begin to explore accommodations that are effective in their didactic learning. This early stage of accommodations in professional programs is ultimately important in informing the fieldwork accommodation process, as accommodations apply to both these aspects of a curriculum (Ozelie et al., 2019). Accommodations are based on the needs of each student to enable the student access to their education. Accommodations frequently requested by students for a Level II fieldwork may include extended time for documentation, documenting in a private or distraction-free space, need for breaks during the day, accommodations for lighting or vision, or an altered schedule (Ozelie et al., 2019).

Students seeking accommodations for fieldwork will need to work closely with the AFWC at the academic institution to implement the steps detailed in Box 9-2. The AFWC serves as the primary communicator with the Level II fieldwork site and will assist the student in the accommodation letter request process. The AFWC should have intimate knowledge of the occupational therapy program's technical standards, the Level II fieldwork standard objectives, as well as an understanding of essential functions for a therapist in the setting they are placing a fieldwork student. *Technical standards* are meant to describe the requirements students must meet to be able to participate in an educational program; these could include lifting and carrying a certain weight, reaching overhead, certain skills that need to be demonstrated, etc. *Level II site-specific objectives* are created on site and provided to school and student to clarify goals and relationship to curriculum as well as standard fieldwork evaluations, and *essential functions* are often found on site, which indicate requirements of employees for the job. An understanding of these documents should assist in making determinations of reasonable accommodations. Kezar and colleagues (2019) remind us that while technical standards do exist for academic programs, such as occupational therapy, **they are not standardized across academic institutions**. Therefore, not all technical standards are inherently compliant with ADA but can provide guidance in conjunction with the Level II fieldwork standard objectives for a specific fieldwork setting in selecting accommodations (Kezar et al., 2019).

As a rule of thumb, technical standards should include **what** needs to be accomplished, not **how** it needs to be accomplished. So, instead of saying a student must be able to see an obstacle to avoid it, they must detect the obstacle (which means a cane can be used or another tool to identify barriers is acceptable). While this is a task that can be done in a controlled environment, it is often difficult to predict the unexpected and allow for standards that will provide student success in any situation, including fieldwork, even though it is part of the student's learning experience.

Box 9-3

KEY STEPS FOR THE AFWC IN REQUESTING STUDENT ACCOMMODATIONS FOR LEVEL II FIELDWORK

1. Upon student disclosure of need for formal accommodations for Level II fieldwork experience, set up a meeting with student.

    a. Review with the student successful accommodations previously utilized in academic program and previous Level I fieldwork.

    b. Review with student the standard fieldwork objectives for practice settings of selected or potential placement.

    c. May use the fieldwork performance evaluation (FWPE) as a tool to review performance standards to ensure full review of possible reasonable accommodations for consideration.

2. Place student according to regular placement processes at the school for the Level II fieldwork experience if not already done.

3. Draft or review accommodation request letter for student review, taking into consideration standard fieldwork objectives and technical standards (letter may come from AFWC or Office of Disability Services, this will depend on the institution).

4. Work with student and Office of Disability Services to develop final version of accommodation request letter well in advance of Level II fieldwork experience dates.

5. Send request for accommodation letter **approximately 3 months prior** to the start of the Level II fieldwork experience.

6. Follow up with Level II fieldwork experience site regularly until response received.

7. Assist student in reviewing any feedback from Level II fieldwork site in regard to concerns or questions about accommodations.

8. Facilitate meeting with Level II fieldwork site and student if further discussion is warranted on accommodations request (representative from department of disability services at institution may also need to be present at meeting with fieldwork site).

9. If accommodations request is signed and approved by student and Level II fieldwork site, keep this on file for reference during the fieldwork experience.

10. If the accommodations request is not approved by one or both parties, start placement and accommodation process over with the student (return to steps 1 and 2).

11. In the event there are concerns regarding a cancellation or denial of accommodations for a Level II fieldwork placement in regard to accommodation-specific requests, seek legal counsel or advisement at the academic institution.

Utilizing this knowledge of behavioral fieldwork objectives and technical standards, the AFWC should work together with the office of disability services to set expectations with students seeking accommodations that will allow for a realistic understanding of the fieldwork setting, reasonable accommodations, and timetable to ensure agreement to an accommodation request(s) in a timely manner. To keep the process efficient and effective, the AFWC should facilitate open communication with the student, office of disability services, and the FWed or fieldwork site throughout the accommodations process. The fieldwork site is considered an extension of the academic institution through the affiliation agreement process. This reemphasizes that students are eligible for accommodation at the fieldwork site as they are in the postsecondary education setting. Through thoughtful collaboration and following the detailed steps in Box 9-3, the AFWC can provide a supportive environment to enhance the accommodation request process.

> ## Box 9-4
> ## KEY STEPS FOR THE LEVEL II FIELDWORK SITE IN SETTING UP STUDENT ACCOMMODATIONS FOR FIELDWORK
>
> 1. Develop a review process for fieldwork-related accommodation requests if it does not already exist at the fieldwork site.
> 2. Consider technical standards from the school or essential functions available from the employer (these should be available through your HR or department manager).
> 3. Ensure standard learning objectives for Level II fieldwork are available or request a copy from the academic institution.
> 4. Connect with legal department, HR, or rehab director if needed to determine if accommodations are considered reasonable in the fieldwork setting.
> 5. Review the accommodations request letter sent from the academic institution and ensure accommodations can be met as outlined.
> 6. If in agreement with accommodations request letter, sign, and return to the AFWC at the academic institution to indicate ability to accept and provide the accommodations.
> 7. If there are concerns in ability to meet the accommodations requested reach out to the AFWC with details of what can and cannot be met and what alternatives may be available.
> 8. Participate in meeting with AFWC and student to discuss accommodation requests and what is reasonable and appropriate as determined by the clinical setting. It is appropriate to ask the student to describe how they envision the accommodation being implemented in the clinical setting. **It is not reasonable** to request additional information about the student disability that was not already disclosed, or other information protected under FERPA. In situations where the site may be unsure of how to proceed it may be appropriate to seek assistance from HR or legal counsel at the fieldwork site. See Table 9-2 for tips for interviewing students with disabilities.
> 9. Request necessary and agreed upon adjustments from the AFWC and new letter to be sent for review based on the outcomes of the meeting.
> 10. If in agreement with accommodations request letter at this stage, sign and return the letter to the AFWC.
> 11. Prepare as needed for accommodations to be in place when student arrives on day one to the Level II Fieldwork site.
> 12. In the event where the accommodations request is seen as unreasonable and a meeting with the student and AFWC does not resolve the concern it is recommended to seek legal counsel or advisement at the Level II fieldwork site to determine next steps or if a cancellation of placement is appropriate in the situation.

Let's revisit the case of Kennedy, a Level II fieldwork student discussed earlier in the chapter. In the original example Kennedy did not disclose her disability prior to the start of fieldwork. Let's now review what it would look like if Kennedy had followed the steps for accommodation in preparation for fieldwork to set her up for success.

Kennedy, an occupational therapy student, has received her notification that her Level II will be in a hospital setting with possible home care visits. Kennedy has IBS, which she has on file with the office of disability services at her academic institution and has decided to notify her AFWC of her need for accommodations. The AFWC requests that Kennedy set up a meeting and in preparation

TABLE 9-2

TIPS FOR INTERVIEWING A STUDENT WHO HAS DISCLOSED A DISABILITY AND REQUESTS ACCOMMODATION

ASK THESE QUESTIONS AND/OR DO THESE THINGS

- When setting up the interview, ask about special accommodations the student might need, such as a quiet room for the interview, written material provided in an accessible format, or how to access the interview location using a wheelchair (National Center on Disability and Journalism, n.d.; U.S. Equal Employment Opportunity Commission, n.d.).

- Allow for extra time to complete the interview.

- During the interview, use person-centered etiquette and focus on the **person**, not the disability.

- Ask questions to discern whether or not the student is qualified to complete the fieldwork experience. These questions should focus on if the student can perform the essential functions of the fieldwork position (Butler, 2008).

- If a student discloses a disability and/or has a visible disability (e.g., is in a cast or uses a wheelchair), you can ask the student to describe or demonstrate how they would perform a fieldwork-related function with or without accommodation (Butler, 2008; U.S. Equal Employment Opportunity Commission, n.d.).

- Questions about the student's nonmedical qualifications and skills, such as their course work, work history, or leadership roles (Butler, 2008).

- You can ask if the student is able to meet time and attendance requirements (Butler, 2008).

- Ensure your questions are focused on the student's technical and professional knowledge, skills, and experiences instead of their disability (Butler, 2008).

(continued)

has her review the fieldwork objectives for her site and the FWPE. When they meet, Kennedy expresses her main concern is access to a bathroom and opportunities for breaks during the day, especially during home care visits. The AFWC verifies with Kennedy she has her disability on file with the university and then following the meeting contacts the office of disability services to collaborate on an accommodation letter that can be sent to the Level II fieldwork site. They discuss bathroom access, possible ideas for breaks, and potential shortened days to assist Kennedy during her fieldwork, which are outlined clearly in the accommodation letter. The AFWC then provides a copy of the draft letter for Kennedy to review and approve. With the student approval, the AFWC is ready to send the letter to Kennedy's Level II fieldwork site who reviews the accommodation letter. The fieldwork site contacts the AFWC with questions regarding the accommodations within 1 week and offers a possible solution in changing the FWed for the rotation to make it easier for Kennedy to access the restroom when needed. Kennedy is agreeable to this change in FWed, and the AFWC notifies the site. The AFWC and office of disability services, Kennedy, and the fieldwork site all maintain a copy of the fully signed accommodation letter, and Kennedy is now set up for a successful start to her Level II fieldwork with accommodations available to her as needed.

TABLE 9-2 (CONTINUED)

TIPS FOR INTERVIEWING A STUDENT WHO HAS DISCLOSED A DISABILITY AND REQUESTS ACCOMMODATION

DO NOT ASK THESE QUESTIONS

- Questions related to the nature or severity of the disability, prognosis, or treatment regime are prohibited (Butler, 2008).

- Do not ask questions about possible time away from the clinical rotation for management and treatment of the disability.

- Do not ask medically related questions (U.S. Equal Employment Opportunity Commission, n.d.).

- The following questions are examples of questions that cannot be asked during an interview process under the Equal Employment Opportunities Commission regulations from the ADA (Butler, 2008; U.S. Equal Employment Opportunity Commission, n.d.):

  - During the past year, how many days has your disability prevented you from engaging in your classroom or clinical learnings?

  - What medications do you currently take and how do they interfere with your daily routines and activities?

  - How did your disability happen?

  - What have doctors told you about your prognosis for your disability?

  - Have you ever received treatment for mental health problems?

  - How long can you stand?

  - How far can you walk?

Note: Due to limited information available specific to interview questions for fieldwork experiences, some of the information in this table was borrowed from literature related to job interview questions for persons with disabilities.

The example of Kennedy primarily demonstrates the role of the AFWC in facilitating the accommodations process for Level II fieldwork. However, another key contributor to this process is the fieldwork site. There are many considerations that the FWed and the fieldwork site also need to review prior to signing an accommodation request letter. The steps for the Level II fieldwork site in setting up student accommodations are detailed in Box 9-4.

Once accommodations are agreed upon by all parties, there are preparations that may need to be made at the fieldwork site for the student's arrival. These preparations may in part require consideration of changes in practice routines by the FWed or thoughtful consideration of space and equipment availability. Table 9-3 provides examples of environmental and practice routine changes in relation to common Level II fieldwork student accommodations.

While the accommodation process appears simple to follow from each of the key contributor's perspectives, there are many areas that can create confusion or difficulty in the accommodation process specific to Level II fieldwork accommodation requests. One common area of concern that may arise is when the Level II fieldwork site does not agree to one or more of the requested accommodations for the student placement. When this occurs, it is essential that the AFWC seek additional information from the Level II fieldwork site on the reasons the accommodations could

TABLE 9-3

EXAMPLES OF ENVIRONMENTAL OR PRACTICE ROUTINE CHANGES AT A FIELDWORK SITE TO SUPPORT STUDENT ACCOMMODATIONS

FIELDWORK SITE ROUTINE OR ENVIRONMENT	EXAMPLE OF CHANGE TO PRACTICE OR ENVIRONMENT
FWed would normally have student arrive at 8 a.m. and leave at 3 p.m., allowing the fieldwork student to take on the morning caseload.	The student has an accommodation to arrive late to fieldwork or adjust hours according to availability of public transportation due to a visual impairment that prevents driving. The FWed may have to start the day at 8 a.m. covering the initial patients and then allow the student to pick up mid-morning.
FWed checks all notes from students and COTAs at 3 p.m. each day.	The student has an accommodation in place for extended time on documentation. The student will not be able to have afternoon notes available at 3 p.m. as normally expected. The student should be allowed to remain at site (when site policy allows) to finish documentation and can submit for review at another agreed upon time such as 5 p.m. same day or 8 a.m. next day that allows for the full use of accommodations agreed upon.
FWed expects student to take on full caseload by end of the fieldwork experience which allows them time to focus on a special project at their place of employment.	The student has an accommodation for decreased caseload in place due to fatigue levels from a documented disability. The FWed may have to maintain 20% of caseload or more throughout the time of the Level II fieldwork to decrease student caseload and therefore will have less special project time for this one experience.
Occupational therapists in clinic like to use a vacant treatment space for private conversations or lunch meetings in the clinic.	The student has an accommodation in place for a quiet space with low lights due to a visual impairment that requires occasional breaks from the lighting in the other clinic spaces. The fieldwork site agreed to provide a separate room during the experience the student could access as needed. The occupational therapists in the clinic may be asked to find a different space for conversation or eating during this fieldwork experience to allow the space to be set up for the student needs.
No designated desk spaces at the fieldwork site, all therapists share space as needed during the day.	The student has an accommodation to keep extra food, drink, and medication at a designated space with locked cabinet or drawer for safety. The fieldwork site may need to designate a desk with a sign for fieldwork student during the experience and provide a key to lock one desk drawer to keep student items in a designated and secure space, which would change the general environment and routine in the office space for the fieldwork experience timeline.

not be met and what alternatives the site may be able to accommodate for the student. Level II fieldwork placements are long-term learning experiences, and it is necessary the agreement on accommodations is clear on all counts before the student begins the placement. It may be necessary for the AFWC to facilitate a meeting with the student and the Level II fieldwork site in instances of disagreement or uncertainty around accommodations. If this is not successful it may also be necessary to seek legal counsel at the academic institution if the student feels the site has refused reasonable accommodations. This is just one example of complications that can occur in the process for Level II fieldwork accommodations.

PROCESS FOR EVALUATION

Questions also often arise in relation to the assessment of students with a disability on fieldwork. If a student has accommodations in place for the Level II fieldwork experience, then these accommodations are considered reasonable in meeting the expectations and performance measures that are a part of the evaluation process. Level II fieldwork experiences are often evaluated by the FWed by using the Fieldwork Performance Evaluation (AOTA, 2020a). This evaluation covers six areas of student performance that indicate a student is prepared for entry-level practice at the completion of their Level II fieldwork experience; these can be found in Table 9-4. Within each area of student performance there are multiple skills that are evaluated. When a FWed evaluates a student with accommodations, it would be important to understand the accommodation in place so that the student can be fairly assessed. A student that requires double time for documentation should not be rated lower for the item on productivity standards if they are completing tasks within a reasonable time based on their accommodation. Table 9-4 provides common accommodation requests that may be approved for students and the sections within the FWPE where there are related performance measures.

THE VALUE OF INCLUSION

It is important to begin to look at students with disabilities as just another diverse population on campus, not through the lens of ableism (Hutcheon & Wolbring, 2012), which allows marginalization of those with disabilities by able-bodied individuals. As occupational therapy practitioners, we are taught to maximize independence and empower those with disabilities, yet do not always consider a disability as an asset to a practitioner. Many members of the occupational therapy community from underrepresented groups may face or be affected by the same discrimination as the clients they serve (AOTA, 2020b, p. 3). An understanding of the disability perspective may enhance a student's role as an active participant in fieldwork and may ultimately allow them to be a much better therapist once they learn to navigate the system. The AOTA (2020b, p. 1) affirms the inalienable right of every individual to feel welcomed, valued, a sense of belonging, and respected while accessing and participating in society.

As early as 1995, the literature was demonstrating a need to support occupational therapy students with disabilities (Kornblau, 1995). As stated by Chris Daughtry, "My unique position has proven to be an asset in working with patients I have treated in my career" (AOTA.org, Practitioners with Disabilities). In 1995, the Network of Occupational Therapy Practitioners with Disabilities was formed with the goal to have the occupational therapy profession world leaders in respecting and promoting equal access and inclusion for all people (NOTPD.org).

Heffron and Harrison (2017) recommend fieldwork sites assist in the process of creating a culture of acceptance by identifying core requirements and identifying how these can be met, including flexible practice options, providing training for FWeds on working with students with disabilities, and ensuring guidelines for practice in the setting are nondiscriminatory and somewhat

TABLE 9-4

EXAMPLES OF COMMON LEVEL II FIELDWORK ACCOMMODATION REQUESTS BASED ON LEVEL II FIELDWORK PERFORMANCE EVALUATION

SECTION FROM COMPETENCY EVALUATION	COMMON ACCOMMODATION REQUESTS APPROVED AT FIELDWORK SITES	ACCOMMODATION IN CLINICAL CONTEXT
Fundamentals for practice	Patient lifting restrictions. Additional individual with student to read monitors for student with visual impairment. Availability of student assistant to scan room for items the student requests.	Student may receive support from tech, FWed, or other individual at site to complete a transfer. Student can instruct another individual at the site how to complete a transfer with a client. Student may guide another designated individual to review certain aspects of the room or patient monitors during a session.
Basic tenets	Additional time for tasks that require gathering of materials such as research articles or client/family resources.	Student may be allowed to come early or stay late at the clinical location to gather materials for the day.
Screening and evaluation	Double time or time-and-a-half for chart review. Double time or time-and-a-half for documentation. Additional time for gathering of materials required to complete evaluation. Access to assessments that may be required of student in setting ahead of time. Ability to practice assessment that is new to student in setting prior to working with client. Provide printed template of evaluation if completed in EMR.	Student may come in early or stay late to complete chart review and documentation for clinical site without impact to their grade on the FWPE for time management. Student may be able to check out assessments or be provided additional notice on assessments to review. FWed may need to print or have printed materials available of various forms and flow sheets that the student may need to access.

(continued)

negotiable for students with disabilities. Through these processes, sites can be more accepting and sensitive to the culture of disability they may encounter and therefore continue to promote a more diverse workforce with approaches not always provided by nondisabled practitioners.

Creating fieldwork sites and fieldwork expectations that are inclusive of all students provides a much easier path for all students to succeed. Like the concept of universal design for learning,

	Table 9-4 (continued)	
	Examples of Common Level II Fieldwork Accommodation Requests Based on Level II Fieldwork Performance Evaluation	
SECTION FROM COMPETENCY EVALUATION	**COMMON ACCOMMODATION REQUESTS APPROVED AT FIELDWORK SITES**	**ACCOMMODATION IN CLINICAL CONTEXT**
Intervention	Additional time for tasks that require gathering of materials or set up. Patient lifting restrictions. Additional time for tasks that require gathering of materials such as research articles for intervention planning. Additional time for assignments such as intervention planning. Double time or time-and-a-half for chart review. Double time or time-and-a-half for documentation.	Student may have altered schedule to allow for set up time with clients if additional time is required. Student may have additional time outside of treatment times to complete treatment planning, may need to provide assignments earlier.
Management of occupational therapy services	Double time or time-and-a-half for documentation and billing. Additional time for tasks that require use of computer. Decreased number of clients on daily caseload.	An altered schedule may be necessary for some students with accommodations for extended time to allow for appropriate access to information that may be available only on a computer.

(continued)

which provides a framework to improve and optimize teaching and learning for all people based on how humans learn (CAST, 2018), the authors propose a similar structure for fieldwork. Utilizing concepts that will be needed to some may serve to be beneficial for all. For example, provision of a structured document that outlines objectives and expectations may help those students who need more organization and clear expectations, but may also assist all students in achieving clarity of expectations. Demonstrating tasks visually and allowing observation prior to interaction may encourage visual learners to be successful, but may also benefit students who wish to jump right in, but may not be ready to do so. Direct verbal and written feedback may benefit those who need to experience concrete examples to enhance learning, but may also benefit all students so that they may have a record of improvement over time. These are but a few examples of how cognitive strategies can assist all students, including those with mental health issues who may need more structure and repeated feedback. While much of this will be site-specific, it may be beneficial to begin to create a culture of acceptance and disability confidence. Lindsay et al. (2019) found that this culture of acceptance and desire to enhance the special skills employees with disabilities may have enhanced

TABLE 9-4 (CONTINUED)
EXAMPLES OF COMMON LEVEL II FIELDWORK ACCOMMODATION REQUESTS BASED ON LEVEL II FIELDWORK PERFORMANCE EVALUATION

SECTION FROM COMPETENCY EVALUATION	COMMON ACCOMMODATION REQUESTS APPROVED AT FIELDWORK SITES	ACCOMMODATION IN CLINICAL CONTEXT
Communication and professional behaviors	Double time or time-and-a-half for assignment completion. Double time or time-and-a-half for documentation. Permission to use notepad or clipboard to assist with organization and memory aids. Short breaks allowed during the day due to a student condition. Ability to eat and drink throughout the day due to student condition. Access to a private space for removal from sensory stimulation for short periods of time during day. Access to area and breaks for pumping for student who is nursing. Late arrival or early departure allowed with notice due to medical condition and need for medical care. Provided printed materials for frequently used medical terminology or materials student is expected to reference frequently.	Student may need to document in a separate space from other therapists. Students may need to wear noise canceling headphones during chart review or documentation in order to be in a busy therapist space. Be sure to communicate with the student prior to these times so they are not seen to be ignoring feedback. Student may have permission with accommodations to leave early or arrive late when necessary. Student may need to ask for breaks during the day even when the FWed may still be working with a client. Student may need to stay late or arrive early to be allowed extended time for documentation. Student may need to bring a clipboard with cues, checklists, or note sheets with them into patient rooms. One way to protect information on the clipboard is to have them place a solid-colored blank sheet of paper on top.

Adapted from American Occupational Therapy Association. (2020a). *Fieldwork performance evaluation for the occupational therapy student.* American Occupational Therapy Association.

social inclusion for those with disabilities in the workplace and broadened perspectives as a model for social change. If we can bring this attitude into the fieldwork environment, students with disabilities may experience more success, less stigma, and better outcomes as therapists; see Box 9-5.

BOX 9-5

SUMMARY OF RECOMMENDATIONS FOR FIELDWORK EDUCATORS OF STUDENTS WITH DISABILITIES

- Consider disability as an element of diversity. Help trainees understand and respond to client and family reactions to disability in a way that is both clinically appropriate and comfortable for the trainee.

- Interviewers may appropriately inquire how the trainee would explain their disability to a client and what accommodations the intern would need to perform the essential functions of the position.

- Routinely inquire to all trainees whether or not any accommodations are required, regardless of whether or not a disability is apparent.

- Learn about various options and types of accommodations that could potentially benefit trainees, staff, and clients. May consider attending the AOTA Fieldwork Educators Certificate Workshop for additional training.

- Assist as an advocate for securing appropriate reasonable accommodations.

- Be aware of the boundary between supervision and psychotherapy.

- Make supervision an opportunity to discuss all trainees' diversity variables, including disability.

- Resist the medicalization of a trainee with a disability; it is not appropriate to ask trainees specific questions about their disability for the sake of curiosity.

- Be able to process and problem solve reactions to disability with the trainee in supervision.

- Facilitate opportunities for trainees to make contact with psychologists with disabilities for mentorship.

- Assist trainees with disabilities to develop their own style of coping with systemic and attitudinal barriers.

- Include several resources on the social experience of disability, in the body of readings for the rehabilitation training experience and discuss it in supervision.

Adapted from Pilarski, C. R., Dunn, M., & Lund, E. M. (2013). Providing culturally competent supervision to trainees with disabilities in rehabilitation settings. *Rehabilitation Psychology, 58*(3), 233–244. https://doi.org/10.1037/a0033338

SUMMARY

The fieldwork placement process for students with disabilities is complex and requires multiple layers of communication, understanding, and can entail significant specific policy and procedural issues. It can be different for each student and each school, so FWeds need to be aware of the resources available to them and ask questions to ensure success. Empowering students to disclose their disability is important, but it is equally as important to respect their decisions not to disclose and to work with them in whatever way possible. FWeds and AFWCs must work in partnership with college and university disability service programs to ensure compliance with all regulations while maintaining an attitude of positivity and respect at all times. As students with disabilities increase in number, the environments they will need to thrive in must be flexible and adaptable to their needs and begin to consider how the culture of disability will grow and change the future of occupational therapy. Effectively supporting students with disabilities to engage in diverse fieldwork experiences not only benefits the fieldwork student but the occupational therapy profession as whole by promoting a more diverse workforce.

LEARNING ACTIVITIES

One of the most challenging aspects of fieldwork for students with disabilities is navigating the request for accommodations. The following activities introduce the learner to technical standards from multiple perspectives. FWeds can partner with fieldwork students and AFWCs to complete the following activities together as a learning experience.

1. **For the Fieldwork Student**

   Referring back to Box 9-2: Key Steps for Students Requesting Accommodations for Level II Fieldwork, write a script that may demonstrate best practices as a student in discussing accommodations with your AFWC at your educational institution for the first time. Consider things such as what to disclose, what assistance may you need in determining clinical accommodations, and what expectations do you have of your AFWC or your Level II fieldwork site in helping meet your accommodations.

2. **For the AFWC**

   Find your technical standards for your academic institution and compare them to the essential functions for a Level II fieldwork student placement. Consider how you would explain the importance of and the difference between these to fieldwork students. To FWeds.

3. **For the FWed**

   Contact AFWCs from occupational therapy programs that your site partners with. Request the technical standards from the academic institution. Compare the technical standards to the essential functions of the job of an occupational therapist at your facility. Describe in what ways they are similar and in what ways are they different. Why would this be important for you to know as a FWed of a Level II student with accommodations?

4. Another challenge that may occur when working with a fieldwork student who has a disability is understanding their desire not to disclose. Consider the following scenario:

   A fieldwork student has started at your site and discloses their disability on week 6 of the full-time placement.

   What is your next step? Why? What if, in the scenario above, the student is failing at the point where they disclose? What is your next step? Why? If your response is different from the scenario above, why?

5. Sometimes it is a challenge to determine what is covered under the Americans with Disabilities Act and what is not. It is also important to know both your rights and the student's rights. How might you react to the following situations?

   a. During week 2 of the placement, the student discloses that they are pregnant. What is your next step? Why? Is this a different response than a student who discloses a mental health issue? Why?

   b. While on a Level II placement, a student is exhibiting tics, swearing, and other inappropriate comments to clients who are adolescents in a school placement. Are you allowed to ask them if they have an identified disability? What are the next steps? What are you able to do immediately to address the situation?

   c. The student has been emailing you regularly prior to placement; you have a nice rapport and are excited for them to begin the placement. The week prior to starting, the student requests an American Sign Language interpreter as an accommodation. What is your next step? Why? Who is responsible for providing the interpreter? How do you determine if this is reasonable?

REFERENCES

American College Health Association. (2021). American College Health Association-National College Health Assessment III: Graduate/Professional Student Reference Group Executive Summary Fall 2020. https://www.acha.org/documents/ncha/NCHA-III_Fall_2020_Graduate_Reference_Group_Executive_Summary.pdf

American Psychological Association. (2018). Stress in America: Generation Z. https://www.apa.org/news/press/releases/stress/2018/stress-gen-z.pdf

American Occupational Therapy Association. (2020a). *Fieldwork performance evaluation for the occupational therapy student*. American Occupational Therapy Association.

American Occupational Therapy Association. (2020b). Occupational therapy's commitment to diversity, equity, and inclusion. *American Journal of Occupational Therapy, 74*(Suppl. 3), 7413410030. https://doi.org/10.5014/ajot.2020.74S3002

Americans with Disabilities Act Amendments Act, Pub. L. No. 110–325 § 3406 (2008).

Aquino, K., & Bittinger, J. (2019). The self-(un)identification of disability in higher education. *Journal of Postsecondary Education and Disability, 32*(1), 5-19. https://eric.ed.gov/?id=EJ1217454

Blacklock, B. and Montgomery, T. (2016). Understand technical standards in health science and medical education. *Disability Compliance for Higher Education, 21*, 7-7. https://doi.org/10.1002/dhe.30188

Butler, M. (2008). Interviewing applicants with disabilities for doctoral and postdoctoral internship positions. https://www.apa.org/pi/disability/resources/interviewing

CAST (2018). About Universal Design for Learning. https://udlguidelines.cast.org/ (retrieved November 18, 2020).

Cole, E.V. & Cawthon, S.W., (2015). Self-disclosure decisions of university students with learning disabilities. *Journal of Postsecondary Education and Disability, 28*(2), 163-179. https://eric.ed.gov/?id=EJ1074663

Collins, M., & Mowbray, C. (2005). Higher education and psychiatric disabilities: National survey of campus disability services. *American Journal of Orthopsychiatry, 75*(2), 304. https://doi.org/10.1037/0002-9432.75.2.304

Disabled World. (2020). Invisible disabilities: List and general information. https://www.disabled-world.com/disability/types/invisible/

Flink, P.J. (2017). Invisible disabilities, stigma, and student veterans: Contextualizing the transition to higher education. *Journal of Veterans Studies, 2*(2), 110–120. http://doi.org/10.21061/jvs.20

Heffron, J., & Harrison, E. (2017, March 30- April 2). Promoting a more diverse workforce through the inclusion of OT practitioners with disabilities [Conference session]. American Occupational Therapy Association, Philadelphia, PA, United States. https://www.aota.org/-/media/Corporate/Files/ConferenceDocs/onsite-guides/2017-annual-conference-centennial-onsite-guide.pdf

Hutcheon, E.J., & Wolbring, G. (2012). Voices of "disabled" post-secondary students examining higher education "disability" policy using an ableism lens. *Journal of Diversity in Higher Education, 5*(1), 39-49. http://dx.doi.org.jwupvdz.idm.oclc.org/10.1037/a0027002

Kezar, L. B., Kirschner, K. L., Clinchot, D. M., Laird-Metke, E., Zazove, P., & Curry, R. H. (2019). Leading practices and future directions for technical standards in medical education. *Academic Medicine, 94*(2), 520-527. https://doi/10.1097/ACM.0000000000002517

Kornblau, B. (1995). Fieldwork educational and students with disabilities: Enter the Americans with Disabilities Act. *The American Journal of Occupational Therapy, 49*(2), 139-145. https://doi.org/10.5014/ajot.49.2.139

Lindsay, S., Leck, J., Shen, W., Cagliostro, E. and Stinson, J. (2019). A framework for developing employer's disability confidence. *Equality, Diversity and Inclusion, 38*(1), 40-55. https://doi.org/10.1108/EDI-05-2018-0085

Lyman, M., Beecher, M.E., Griner, D., Brooks, M., Call, J., & Jackson, A. (2016). What keeps students with disabilities from using accommodations in postsecondary education? A qualitative review. *Journal of Postsecondary Education and Disability, 29*(2), 123-140. https://eric.ed.gov/?id=EJ1112978

Mamboleo, G., Meyer, L., Georgieva, Z., Curtis, R., Dong, S., & Stender, L. M. (2015). Students with disabilities' self-report on perceptions toward disclosing disability and faculty's willingness to provide accommodations. *Rehabilitation Counselors and Educators Journal, 8*(2), 8–19. https://www.ncbi.nlm.nih.gov/pmc/articles/PMC6474675/

Merriam Webster. (n.d.). Generation Z. In Merriam-Webster.com dictionary. Retrieved March, 15, 2021,from https://www.merriam-webster.com/dictionary/Generation%20Z

National Center for Educational Statistics. (2019). Fast facts: Students with disabilities. https://nces.ed.gov/fastfacts/display.asp?id=60

National Center on Disability and Journalism. (n.d.). Tips for interviewing people with disabilities. https://ncdj.org/resources/interviewing-tips/

O'Shea, A., & Meyer, R. H. (2016). A qualitative investigation of the motivation of college students with nonvisible disabilities to utilize disability services. *Journal of Postsecondary Education and Disability, 29*(1), 5-23. https://eric.ed.gov/?id=EJ1107472

Ozelie, R., Delehoy, M., Jones, S., Sykstus, E., & Weil, V. (2019). Accommodation use by individuals with disabilities in occupational therapy fieldwork. *Journal of Occupational Therapy Education, 3*(4). 1-18. https://doi.org/10.26681/jote.2019.030407

Pilarski, C. R., Dunn, M., & Lund, E. M. (2013). Providing culturally competent supervision to trainees with disabilities in rehabilitation settings. *Rehabilitation Psychology, 58*(3), 233-244. https://doi.org/10.1037/a0033338

Simon, Rebecca L. (2019). Using a faculty community of practice to support college students with mental health needs. (Publication No. 13884593) [Doctoral dissertation, Northeastern University]. ProQuest Dissertations and Theses Global.

U.S. Department of Education. (2011). Students with disabilities preparing for postsecondary education: Know your rights and responsibilities. https://www2.ed.gov/about/offices/list/ocr/transition.html#note

U.S. Department of Education. (2018). Family educational rights and privacy act (FERPA). https://www2.ed.gov/policy/gen/guid/fpco/ferpa/index.html

U.S. Department of Education. (2021). Disability Employment 101: Appendix IV. https://www2.ed.gov/about/offices/list/osers/products/employmentguide/appendix-4.html

U.S. Department of Justice. (2020). A guide to disability rights laws. https://www.ada.gov/cguide.htm

U.S. Equal Opportunities Employment Commission. (2008). ADA Amendment Act of 2008. https://www.eeoc.gov/statutes/ada-amendments-act-2008

U.S. Equal Employment Opportunity Commission. (n.d.). Job applicants and the ADA. https://www.eeoc.gov/laws/guidance/job-applicants-and-ada#

Wilgosh, L., Sobsey, D., Cey, R., & Scorgie, K. (2008). Life management of post-secondary students with disabilities. *Developmental Disabilities Bulletin, 36*(1&2), 199-224. https://eric.ed.gov/?id=EJ828957

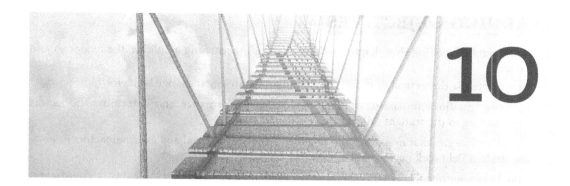

Supporting the At-Risk Fieldwork Student

Bridget Trivinia, OTD, MS, OTR/L
and Caryn Reichlin Johnson, MS, OTR/L, FAOTA

Poor performance during Level II fieldwork creates challenges for everyone involved, as there are many stakeholders in the fieldwork education paradigm: the academic program and faculty, the student, the service recipient, and the fieldwork site and educator (Recker-Hughes et al., 2014; Trivinia & Johnson, 2019). The reasons for poor performance, which may lead to failure of the fieldwork experience, can be multidimensional and complex. Although these situations are rare, they can be very time consuming and highly stressful for the student and fieldwork educator (FWed; Nicola-Richmond et al., 2017). Furthermore, failure of a fieldwork experience can have a significant impact on the student's progression in their academic program, finances, and self-image (Nicola-Richmond et al., 2017). Utilizing a systematic approach to analyze and remediate fieldwork challenges is critical, as it can provide a standardized method to assess situations and promote changes needed to prevent repeat issues, facilitate communication and collaboration among stakeholders, and provide opportunities for change, ultimately reducing the time and effort involved in problem mitigation and student remediation (Myers & Covington, 2019).

Learning contracts are typically used to address student underperformance. A learning contract is "… a written agreement between teacher and student which makes explicit what a learner will do to achieve specific learning outcomes" (Gallant et al., 2006, p. 223). This chapter will address how to recognize when a learning contract is needed during Level II fieldwork. Furthermore, the authors will provide a model of how to navigate the learning contract process using a systematic and evidence-based approach to identify problems, set measurable goals, and develop strategies to facilitate goal attainment.

DeIuliis, E. D., & Hanson, D. (Eds.).
Fieldwork Educator's Guide to Level II Fieldwork (pp. 277-320).
© 2023 Taylor & Francis Group.

LEARNING OBJECTIVES

By the end of reading this chapter and completing the learning activities, the reader should be able to:

1. Appreciate the theoretical foundations of student readiness to change behavior.

2. Evaluate situations impacting student's fieldwork performance and determine the factors contributing to the student's difficulty.

3. Identify strategies that might be used to address specific internal and external factors impacting student fieldwork performance.

4. Collaborate with stakeholders including the student, FWed, academic fieldwork coordinator (AFWC), and/or site clinical coordinator of fieldwork (CCFW) to systematically assess student performance and develop learning contracts to promote successful completion of the Level II fieldwork experience.

5. Develop measurable goals and timeframes for performance improvement that can be objectively evaluated.

6. Apply principles that protect and respect students' rights.

7. Conclude an unsuccessful fieldwork experience in a fair, sensitive, and dignified manner.

THEORETICAL FOUNDATION

"Learning is the process whereby knowledge is created through the transformation of experience" (Kolb, 1984, p. 38). Fieldwork experiences serve as the platform for this learning to occur. Just as theory is foundational to occupational therapy practice, theory is essential for student learning and facilitation of behavior change when challenges arise. Both the Transformative Learning Theory and the Transtheoretical Model of Behavior Change (Merriam & Baumgarnter, 2020; Prochaska, 2008) play key roles in addressing student challenges and facilitating their success through the utilization of learning contracts.

For positive behavior change to occur, a student must develop an awareness of the challenge, an "aha" moment when the "lightbulb goes on" and they suddenly experience an issue with more insight, recognition, or comprehension. Transformative Learning Theory focuses on the process by which an adult examines, questions, and modifies their perceptions and assumptions about their experiences (Cranton, 2016; Wang & Torrisi-Steele, 2019). This can lead to a change in their understanding, thereby influencing behavior needed to successfully implement a learning contract. A student must develop an awareness of the identified challenging behavior, then reflect, in order to identify possible causes of poor performance and begin the process of change. Box 10-1 provides an example of a student continuing to demonstrate unsafe performance despite the FWed verbally addressing the behavior. Once the student experiences the "aha" moment, behavior change occurs, and improved performance is the result.

While the Transtheoretical Model of Behavior Change (Stages of Change Model) is often utilized in health promotion practice, it can also be useful in understanding student behavior and the development learning contracts. This model identifies five stages in which an individual progress through in order to change a behavior: precontemplation, contemplation, preparation, action, and maintenance (Figure 10-1). The model suggests that readiness to benefit from a learning contract requires that the student be in the preparation stage, intending to take action in the immediate future and/or may have taken steps to improve behavior. This is followed by matching an optimal intervention to the current stage of readiness. (Reitz & Graham, 2019). It is imperative

BOX 10-1

Joe is currently in week 5 of his Level II fieldwork placement at Friendship Subacute Rehabilitation Center. The FWed has instructed him on proper patient guarding/handling techniques during dynamic standing balance tasks. On two occasions, the FWed has had to speak with Joe about being either too far away from the patient or too busy talking with the patient to notice the safety concerns. Today, Joe was properly guarding a patient during a similar activity when the patient lost their balance and Joe needed to take action to prevent a fall. Although the patient did not fall, Joe reported feeling "shook up" after the session. The FWed and Joe had a serious discussion following the incident in which Joe reported understanding the importance of proper guarding of patients during any functional standing activities. New changes in his verbal and nonverbal communication suggested that he had experienced that "a-ha" moment.

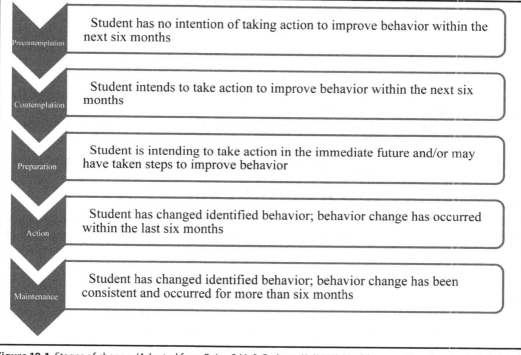

Figure 10-1. Stages of change. (Adapted from Reitz, S.M. & Graham, K. (2019). Health promotion theories. In B.A.Schell & G. Gillen (Eds.), *Willard & Spackman's occupational therapy* (13th ed., pp. 675-692). Wolters Kluwer.)

that the AFWC works closely and continually with the FWed and students to help identify their level of readiness for accepting the need for change, their ability to prepare for change, and finally implementing the changes included in the learning contract.

Box 10-2 offers an example of how the Stages of Change Model can be applied to student performance in Level II fieldwork. Applying the stages of this model creates a framework to understand student performance and facilitate behavior change through a structured approach, including the use of learning contracts when appropriate.

> **BOX 10-2**
>
> Macy is a Level II occupational therapy assistant student at a general outpatient facility. According to the 8-week schedule, she has fallen short in a few areas. For one, Macy should be able to complete a SOAP note independently by week 3. It is the end of week 3 and the FWed has expressed concern several times about the need for Macy to improve her documentation skills. Macy has been in the precontemplation stage. Although the FWed has provided extensive feedback on SOAP notes completed during the first 3 weeks, there has been little to no integration of feedback or change, and it appears she is unaware of her poor performance.
>
> Following the next supervision meeting, Macy verbalizes awareness of the need to improve and a desire to do so, but offers no clear plan for how this will occur. She is in the contemplation stage.
>
> The FWed encourages Macy to develop a specific plan to improve her skills. At Macy's midterm review (week 4), they discuss her underperformance and decide to initiate a learning contract. Macy clearly understands the degree of concern and expresses the desire to improve her performance by the end of the 8-week experience. She purchases a documentation text as a resource. Macy and the FWed develop a plan for her to gain additional practice writing SOAP notes by writing notes for all treatment sessions, not just for those for which she is responsible, along with established timelines and goals for improvement. This suggests Macy has advanced to the Preparation Stage. She is now more likely to carry over the action steps of a learning contract.

A BLUEPRINT FOR SUCCESS: STEPS IN CREATING A LEARNING CONTRACT

The first steps in creating a learning contract are to establish a positive context and a time for all parties to meet to finalize and implement the learning contract. A learning contract should be viewed as a "blueprint for success" (Trivinia & Johnson, 2019, p. 24), and not as a threat or punishment. If a student perceives the learning contract as a penalty for their performance, they may have more difficulty embracing it as something that will benefit them. It is essential that everyone involved views it as a tool that will assist both the student and the FWed, uniquely designed for that student to target priority issues and implement strategies to achieve successful completion of fieldwork. "A well-developed learning contract will be objective, transparent, methodical, measurable, collaborative, student-centered, individualized, and respectful of each student's right to due process" (Trivinia & Johnson, 2019, p. 25).

Both the student and FWed typically view the stakes to be very high, and both have usually invested a great deal of time and effort into the fieldwork experience by the time the need for a learning contract is determined. The student and FWed/CCFW have often had multiple conversations with the AFWC prior to the learning contract meeting. Having collected data from all parties involved, the AFWC, who usually has more experience with learning contracts than students or FWeds, should draft a learning contract and share it with all involved parties before the meeting, requesting and incorporating feedback, and revising as needed. The meeting is then likely to proceed more smoothly and take less time out of everyone's busy schedule. This initial meeting usually takes 1 to 2 hours. It is important to plan time for the AFWC and student to meet together afterward to process what has occurred and address the student's questions and concerns.

A learning contract should be structured and comprehensive, leaving as little room for guesswork as possible. Considerations for each section of the learning contract are reflected in Appendix A (Learning Contract Template) and described as follows:

1. Document date of meeting and attendees
2. Define student's strengths and needs:

   a. Areas in which student is doing well.

   b. Areas in which problems have been identified with specific examples to illustrate challenges.

The experience of receiving a learning contract is often a traumatic one that may undermine self-confidence and heighten emotions. In fact, many FWeds are reluctant to broach the need for a learning contract because they are afraid of how the student will react. The learning contract begins with the student's strengths, as students benefit from hearing that they are not doing poorly in everything, and that they are doing well in some, perhaps the majority, of areas.

Use objective terminology and examples that describe the student's performance. Relate your description to the expectations of the fieldwork schedule, Fieldwork Performance Evaluation (FWPE), and the site-specific learning objectives (SSLOs) where possible, so the student can understand where they stand in relation to expectations (e.g., not performing at expected level of independence, in a timely manner, safely, effectively, or accurately). During the learning contract meeting, it is often useful to have the student acknowledge or ask for clarification about the FWed's observations.

3. Identify significance of the problem:

   a. Explain why the behavior is a problem.

   b. Explain its impact on patients/clients, FWed, facility, student learning.

Students often react defensively when being presented with the possibility of failure. Objectively presenting the ways their behavior impacts their FWed, the facility, their patients/clients, and themselves facilitates recognition of the behaviors identified as problematic. For example, it could impact patients in terms of safety, outcomes, or their trust in their occupational therapist or belief that occupational therapy will benefit them. It could impact the FWed's productivity, personal time, or relationship with patients/clients. The facility may be concerned with the impact on revenue, reputation, or compliance with regulations. Students may experience concern about their ability to develop skills required to pass the fieldwork experience, or feel an impact on their sleep, mood, or ability to learn.

4. Establish measurable goals:

   a. Provide measurable baseline and target performance levels.

   b. Describe how the new behavior should look.

   c. Establish goals and timelines that are realistic and achievable.

The goals for the student must be measurable just as they are for our patients/clients. It is not unusual for the student to believe their performance level is better than the FWed reports, so providing a baseline level of their current performance level, with examples, is essential. Identify measurable target performance levels the student needs to achieve within a designated period of time. Most learning contracts give the students 2 weeks to achieve the goals. Consider the timeliness, quality, quantity, and level of consistency required for the expected performance.

- *How far below expectation is the student at this point in their placement?*

- *How far along is the student in their placement, and how much time is available to work on the goals?*

- *Can the student have 1 or 2 weeks to gradually improve to the target level (e.g., from a current level of 40% of the time up to 60% after 1 week and up to 80% after 2 weeks?) or does the student need to demonstrate an immediate change in performance to a higher level, such as with safety issues?*

TABLE 10-1
EXAMPLES OF MEASURABLE GOALS

PROBLEM AREA	MEASURABLE GOAL	PERFORMANCE EXPECTATION
Professional behavior (time management): Does not provide treatment plans prior to beginning of treatment session as required.	Student will complete daily treatment plan on 6 of 8 patients prior to the beginning of treatment session 8 out of 10 days over the next 2 weeks.	Begins immediately, but does not expect perfection Expects consistent performance over the next 2 weeks at improved level Aligns with FWPE/SSLOs Sets students on path to catch up to 12-week schedule expectations
Safety: Unsafe line management during bed mobility and patient transfers (student forgets to position lines, or positions them incorrectly prior to transfers, gives confusing cues to patients).	For the remainder of the fieldwork experience, student will position all lines so that patient can come to sitting position in bed and transfer to wheelchair safely 100% of the time.	Expects 100% compliance Expects consistent performance Begins immediately Aligns with FWPE/SSLOs
Communication: Student is overly wordy in verbal communication, using too many words when giving instructions and confusing her clients with intellectual and developmental disabilities resulting in decreased client engagement and increased frustration.	By 2 weeks from now, student will simplify instructions to clients, using no more than 5 to 6 words per sentence, 90% of the time.	Gradual improvement over a period of time is acceptable Aligns with FWPE/SSLOs Sets students on path to catch up to 12-week schedule expectations

- *Is there room for occasional error? For example, when is it acceptable for performance to be 80% to 90% instead of 100%? Most novice therapists are not perfect, and it is not always necessary for a student to achieve a 100% performance rate. Percentages may be upgraded as the fieldwork experience progresses.*

As a rule of thumb, 2 weeks is usually a reasonable amount of time to achieve goals in a learning contract. However, a common exception to this time frame is in the area of safety, where risky performance is often not acceptable. When setting measurable goals, think about what is realistic to achieve within a 2-week period, what absolutely must change immediately and what can be given some time to develop. Table 10-1 provides examples of a variety of considerations for developing strong measurable goals.

5. Determine how goals will be measured:

   a. Determine how data will be collected.

   b. Determine who will contribute to the data.

   c. Establish how the student's performance over the period of the learning contract will be measured and documented.

Address mechanism(s) for how student performance will be assessed. You need more than the FWed's guesstimate at the end of 2 weeks. Students may be reluctant to trust that the FWed will evaluate them fairly and objectively when the stakes are so high. They may think they are doing well when the FWed is not observing them, and that the FWed does not see their "good" performance. Therefore, it is important to agree upon a method of evaluation that is objective and can be trusted by all involved.

6. Identify strategies to achieve goals:

   a. Identify strategies the student will be responsible for implementing (e.g., research, studying, behavior change, habit development).

   b. Identify strategies the FWed will be responsible for implementing (e.g., mechanisms and timing of feedback, availability, direct observation, agreed-upon level of cueing).

This is typically the most collaborative part of the learning contract process. Each student experience is unique, and the variety of strategies that can be developed to promote success is limitless. Over time, the experienced AFWC and CCFW will develop a repertoire of strategies that can be commonly called upon in a variety of situations, helping to manage the very time-consuming nature of learning contract development.

It is essential that students understand when poor performance might result in failure of the fieldwork experience. It is not uncommon for FWeds and AFWCs to prevaricate, fearing an emotional response on the part of the student or damage to the supervisory relationship. They may even have concerns about students becoming depressed or harming themselves. However, **students are entitled to know if there is a possibility they could fail the experience**, and the final meeting to address failure of the experience and termination of the placement should never be the first time the possibility of failing the experience is mentioned. All academic programs should have strategies for addressing concerns about a student's mental health, whether the student is on fieldwork or in the classroom.

7. Establish time frame and consequences for failure to achieve goals

Timeframe and consequences must be clearly stated in the learning contract, making it evident to all involved, right from the beginning, what the consequences are for meeting or failing to meet the goals of the learning contract. Possible outcomes include the following:

- In most cases, achieving the goals sets the student on the right path and they continue to a successful conclusion of the fieldwork experience.

- Occasionally, the student achieves the goals but remains at risk, necessitating a second, or even a third, learning contract (time permitting).

- In some cases, failure to achieve the goals, while concerning, is not egregious enough to necessitate failure of the fieldwork experience. The FWPE allows for a degree of limited competence (items scored as "Emerging Performance" on FWPE), except in the areas of safety and ethics, as long as the passing score is achieved.

- Unfortunately, in some cases the student's failure to achieve the goals does result in termination of the fieldwork placement.

8. Include signatures of all attendees

Although a learning contract is not a legal document, signatures imply an understanding of and agreement to the arrangements. This may need to occur electronically.

COMMON CAUSES OF STUDENT DIFFICULTY IN FIELDWORK

Why is one student successful and yet another student experiences challenges in the fieldwork setting? Identifying the causes of student difficulty in the fieldwork setting can be quite challenging for all stakeholders. Literature suggests confidence, professionalism, and setting or environment are important factors to a successful fieldwork experience (Patterson & D'Amico, 2020). Poor performance typically shows up in one or more areas. There is often an overlap of challenges increasing the complexity of the situation.

Factors impacting student performance may be seen as internal or external. Internal factors with which students most typically struggle include professional behavior, performance, clinical reasoning, and safety (Potter, 2018). Professional behavior areas that students most frequently struggle with include time management, interpersonal communication, and organization (Potter, 2018). Students may also have difficulty administering performing evaluations and interventions in a timely, organized, appropriate, and effective manner. Still, other students struggle with the clinical reasoning process or verbalizing their clinical reasoning. Many of these challenges can ultimately lead to poor safety adherence.

Student performance may also be affected by outside influences, or external factors, such as the FWed and the environment. A FWed may have communication or organizational challenges resulting in difficulty providing feedback to the student and/or unclear student expectations. Additionally, the FWed may have a supervisory style that conflicts with a student's learning style (Costa, 2015; Trivinia & Johnson, 2019). The learning environment may also impact the student's performance. Settings that are particularly fast paced, serve patients with higher levels of acuity, are over- or understimulating, or are not supportive of the student can contribute to underperformance (Trivinia & Johnson, 2019).

Internal Factors Affecting Student Performance

This next section will provide an in-depth overview of common internal factors that might influence a student's performance on Level II fieldwork, which includes communication, clinical reasoning, professional behavior, and safety. Strategies for addressing each factor's issues will be identified and learning contract examples will be provided to illustrate their use in addressing performance issues.

Communication

Effective communication is a complex process requiring a well-developed set of skills and is foundational to all successful relationships (Davis & Rosee, 2015). In Level II fieldwork, this holds true for not only the student-client relationship, but the student-interprofessional team and student-FWed relationships as well. The student's ability to communicate and engage with a client often predicts their effectiveness in understanding the client's needs as well as motivating and teaching the client, thereby impacting outcomes (Davis & Rosee, 2015; Plourde, 2019). Communication is also important within interprofessional teams, and a student's ability to communicate effectively can impact their standing as a member of such a team (Davis & Rosee, 2015). The stakes are high in Level II fieldwork, and a student must be able to ask questions of their FWed to clarify concepts, seek guidance and support when needed, and address challenges they are encountering.

BOX 10-3

Tips for the FWed/CCFW

Prior to the start of the fieldwork experience

- Develop SSLOs and a comprehensive weekly schedule that outlines student expectations week by week (As described in Chapters 4 and 5 of this book).
- Set clear expectations prior to the start of the fieldwork experience. This can be done through both verbal and written formats.
- Identify preferred methods of communication and feedback. As the FWed, inform the student if you prefer questions during a session or after. Ask the student how they feel about being questioned during a session or if they prefer, when feasible, to have you ask questions in the absence of the client after the session is over.
- Identify a time for regularly scheduled feedback meetings.

During the fieldwork experience:

- Utilize the SSLOs and weekly schedule to communicate expectations.
- Follow through with the preferred methods of communication and feedback as determined prior to the start of the experience.
- Utilize multiple sources of feedback (e.g., verbal, written, video).
- Balance feedback with both positive and constructive statements and have the student paraphrase/reflect on the feedback to ensure mutual understanding (as discussed in Chapter 8 of this book).
- Be mindful of your verbal and nonverbal communication to ensure a clear message is conveyed to your student.
- Determine how performance is being impacted by skills rather than personality and focus on skill development because it is not helpful to try to change a personality.

(continued)

Conversely, the FWed must be able to provide the student with clear expectations as well as positive and constructive feedback during the experience. The communication process is complex, as it involves overlapping relationships between multiple parties consisting not only of verbalization of thoughts and feelings, but also nonverbal aspects including eye contact, body posture, gestures, facial expressions, and volume and tone of voice (Davis & Rosee, 2015; Plourde, 2019). This may stem from generational communication preferences and lack of engagement in traditional face-to-face and verbal communication. For example, Gen Y or Millennials prefer the use of text and social media over telephone calls, and approximately 57% of Gen Z or Centennials use messaging apps to communicate (Plourde, 2019). Differences in the manner in which students and FWeds articulate thoughts, feelings, wants, and/or incongruence between the verbal and nonverbal aspects of communication may result in obstacles to behavior change. Box 10-3 offers suggestions for both students and FWeds to assist them in establishing good communication strategies prior to fieldwork as well as implementing good communication habits during the fieldwork experience. The learning contract example that follows provides an example of how you might develop a learning contract for a student demonstrating significant shortcomings in the area of communication.

Box 10-3 (CONTINUED)

Tips for the Student

Prior to the start of the fieldwork experience:

- Review the SSLOs and comprehensive weekly schedule that outlines student expectations week by week. Develop a list of questions you may have and ask the FWed in one communication, either via email or in person. By asking the questions in one communication, you are demonstrating your level of organization and respect of the FWed's time.
- Discuss preferred methods of communication and feedback. *Do you learn best when you receive written, verbal, and/or video feedback? Do you prefer a combination of feedback? How do you respond to feedback provided "in the moment" (i.e., in front of a client)?* Keep in mind safety is priority so it is not always feasible for a FWed to provide feedback in your preferred method when client safety is at risk as the FWed will have to address an issue immediately.
- Ask the FWed if they prefer questions during or after a session.
- Identify a time for regularly scheduled feedback meetings.

During fieldwork experience:

- Utilize the SSLOs and weekly schedule to determine if you are meeting expectations.
- Follow through with the preferred methods of communication as determined prior to the start of the experience.
- If you are having challenges, respectfully request a time to meet with the FWed. Be prepared to clearly identify the challenge and a possible solution to address the challenge.
  - Be sure to use "I" statements. Instead of "You haven't given me any feedback," try "*I am unsure if I am meeting expectations and believe I could benefit from more specific feedback.*"
  - Be solution oriented. Instead of "What can I do to improve?" try "*I would like to propose a weekly meeting, at your convenience, at the end of the week, either before our first client, during lunch, or after our last client. For each meeting, I will develop a list of areas I feel that I am meeting expectations and areas in need of improvement. For those areas in need of improvement, I will develop a list of strategies to improve my performance.*"
- Be mindful of your verbal and nonverbal communication to ensure a clear message is conveyed to your FWed and client.
- Make sure your words match your audience. Utilize professional terminology when engaging with other professionals. Modify your language to layman's terms when working with clients.

Example of a Learning Contract to Address Communication

SCENARIO: Cameron is an occupational therapy assistant student completing an 8-week Level II placement in a school for children with learning differences. This site exclusively uses the collaborative model of fieldwork education (two students to one FWed, refer back to Chapter 2 as necessary to better understand this fieldwork supervision model). Currently in week 5 of an 8-week placement, Cameron demonstrates strengths in collaboration with FWed, COTA, SLP, SLP student; consultation with transition team; daily documentation, annual review preparation; planning and implementing evaluation; planning intervention; and professional behaviors. She is struggling with articulating the value of occupation and the values and beliefs of occupational therapy to others (SSLO #s 4, 5), communicating clearly and effectively verbally and nonverbally to students and staff in this school setting (SSLO #32), using language appropriate to some students and groups at the school (SSLO #35), and during some intervention sessions (larger groups, older children). She also has difficulty modifying, upgrading, or terminating the task approach, environment, or intervention plan based on the child's response when necessary (SSLO #s 24, 25). The focus of this example has been narrowed to one area—the student's hesitation to engage verbally and nonverbally with children and team.

Student Name _____ Fieldwork Site _____

Date _____ In Attendance _____

Areas in which the student is doing well:

Areas in which problems have been identified (relate these to SSLOs):

DESCRIBE PROBLEMATIC STUDENT BEHAVIOR	WHY IS THIS BEHAVIOR A PROBLEM (IMPACT ON PATIENTS, FWED, FACILITY, STUDENT LEARNING?)	MEASURABLE GOALS: (BASELINE AND TARGET PERFORMANCE LEVELS; WHAT WE WANT THE NEW BEHAVIOR TO LOOK LIKE)	HOW WILL THE GOAL BE MEASURED?	IDENTIFY STRATEGIES TO ACHIEVE THE GOAL	
				What will student do?	What will FWed do?
Student hesitates to join in when groups are being led by her fellow speech language pathology student or another staff member, resulting in insufficient verbal and nonverbal communication.	Student's clients and colleagues have the impression that Cameron is an observer, rather than a participant. This may result in a child not receiving the assistance needed, and Cameron's FWed and peers not having confidence to rely on her. In addition, it affects rapport building with staff and students in that they may not develop trust in her abilities as an occupational therapy assistant. Then it also reflects poorly on occupational therapy in general.	Student will actively participate in groups, whether leading them or not, 60% of the time within 1 week, 75% of the time within 2 weeks, and 90% of the time within 3 weeks. Current level of participation is about 40%.	Direct observation by FWed, occupational therapist, or speech language pathologist	Student will move around the room when the group is working to monitor their responses. Student will respond to student or staff contributions with positive comments or verbal or nonverbal cues. Student will seek out opportunities to articulate the value of what the group is doing in the form of reiterating the instructions, focusing on progress being made, or repeating or demonstrating the process based on student need. Student will role play and inform FWed the night before how she will put forth the directions and determine how modifications will be made based on FWed's feedback. Student will discuss alternative group models with peer in order to maximize her opportunities for leadership, such as alternating leadership and backup roles, and alternating preparatory and main activity responsibilities. Student will reflect on strategies she has utilized to achieve these goals, what went well, what did not go well, what she would do differently next time and why, and email the reflections to FWed.	Attend sessions with student and be available to role play upon request. Obtain information from others when not in attendance personally. Provide feedback after the session and inform what went well and what could have been done differently. Provide measurable data on how much student has improved at the end of each week.

REFLECTION QUESTIONS FOR THE FWED

1. What might some causes be for the student's behavior? If the student's personality traits play a role, how can you address the issue without making it about personality?

2. How does integrating the SSLOs into a learning contract help the student and FWed?

3. Can you think of any other ways to make the goals measurable?

4. What might be an "aha" moment for this student? How could you assess readiness for change?

Clinical Reasoning

Students learn the basics of clinical reasoning in their academic program. During Level II fieldwork, they are expected to apply and develop a higher level of skill with these concepts. Studies show students believe that clinical reasoning skills are critical to success in fieldwork (Patterson & D'Amico, 2020) and that they place a high value on the FWed's ability to facilitate their clinical reasoning (Rodger et al., 2014). Literature also suggests students require strong clinical reasoning skills for successful fieldwork experiences (Potter, 2018; Silberman et al., 2018). Refer back to Chapter 7 for best practice strategies of how to facilitate clinical reasoning during Level II fieldwork.

Difficulty with clinical reasoning can be hard to tease out. It is easy to make assumptions about the reason someone behaves a certain way, and it is important to take a moment to question those assumptions. Take, for example, the student who demonstrates unsafe practice, such as a poorly executed functional transfer. *Why did the student perform an unsafe transfer? Was it inexperience with that specific transfer technique or could it have been that they could not problem solve how to set up the environment?* Likewise, think about the student who presents the FWed with a poorly designed treatment plan. *Was it because they did not give themselves enough time the night before to do a good job, or might it have been that they could not clinically reason the best way to up- or downgrade an activity for a particular client?* Many students are better at clinical reasoning than they or their FWeds realize, but do not know how, or are lacking the skill or confidence, to verbalize it.

When trying to determine if the student's problematic performance is related to clinical reasoning, ask yourself if the student is able to:

- Hypothesize the cause of the client's occupational performance deficits
- Provide an answer when you ask "why" or "what if"
- Suggest a variety of appropriate upgrades and downgrades for activities
- Reflect on a variety of possible outcomes
- Predict how the client should respond to the intervention
- Apply precautions when designing or implementing activities
- Provide a rationale/theoretical framework for their actions
- Connect outcomes of assessment to occupational performance
- Provide a hypothesis about the impact of the client's condition on their occupational performance
- Suggest hypotheses about why the intervention will improve performance, or why an intervention was not successful
- Describe the outcome of a treatment session and how they might adjust it to achieve better results in the future

---

BOX 10-4

Tips for the FWed/CCFW

- Describe the student's clinical reasoning in measurable terms—because you cannot see what the student is thinking, you need to reflect on their actions so that you can verbalize and/or document your observations.
- Provide specific examples to the student that illustrate your observations.
- Describe their performance quantitatively and qualitatively. Rather than writing "Student is unable to provide appropriate upgrades and downgrades," include measurable data such as *"Student provides a plan for appropriate upgrades/downgrades 50% of the time for less complex patients, and 25% of the time for more complex patients."*
- Assign the Clinical Reasoning Worksheet (Appendix B) for homework and review it prior to the next treatment session.

Tips for the Student

- Remind yourself that your FWed has a responsibility to understand your clinical reasoning. When they question you, it does not necessarily mean they think you have done something wrong—they may just be trying to clarify what they think you are thinking.
- If you are having trouble articulating your clinical reasoning, get into the habit of speaking out loud to the patient/client about what you are doing and why. This will force you to think about and verbalize your clinical reasoning while at the same time demonstrating your clinical reasoning to your FWed.
- If you are having trouble in the area of treatment planning and/or up- and downgrading, submit written treatment plans to your FWed ahead of time, including a plan A, plan B, and plan C for each activity you have planned, in the event the session does not go as planned.
- Use the Clinical Reasoning Worksheet (Appendix B) as a tool to examine, illustrate, develop, and share your clinical reasoning.

Strategies to promote clinical reasoning in a learning contract (Rodger et al., 2014) may include:

- Reflective writing (refer to Appendix B for a structured approach to elicit the student's clinical reasoning and reflections)
- Self-rating
- Questioning (refer to different types of questioning strategies in Chapter 8)
- Reflection in action
- Collaborative discussion
- Scheduled reflection time

Since we cannot see into the mind to determine the substance of a student's clinical reasoning, we depend on their actions to inform us. And because students require clear feedback in order to change, we must provide them with information they can use, in a form they can integrate, to make the needed changes. Box 10-4 offers some valuable tips for developing goals and strategies when a student needs to improve clinical reasoning skills. The following learning contract example incorporates some of those strategies and provides an example of how you might develop a learning contract for a student demonstrating significant shortcomings in the area of clinical reasoning.

Example of a Learning Contract to Address Clinical Reasoning

SCENARIO: Devin is an occupational therapy student completing week 8 of 12 in a day program for adults with intellectual disabilities. Clients receive occupational therapy services one to two times a week. The FWed is on-site 2 days per week. Devin demonstrates good communication skills and therapeutic use of self and interacts well with clients and team members. Although he demonstrates the ability to identify deficits, perform evaluations, plan treatment, and implement intervention, Devin struggles when it comes to explaining why he has selected the activities and what criteria he will use to determine how to progress the client toward their goals. The FWed questions whether Devin is using effective clinical reasoning to develop the treatment plans and make decisions.

Student Name _____ Fieldwork Site _____

Date _____ In Attendance _____

Areas in which the student is doing well:

Areas in which problems have been identified (relate these to SSLOs):

DESCRIBE PROBLEMATIC STUDENT BEHAVIOR	WHY IS THIS BEHAVIOR A PROBLEM (IMPACT ON PATIENTS, FWED, FACILITY, STUDENT LEARNING?)	MEASURABLE GOALS: (BASELINE AND TARGET PERFORMANCE LEVELS; WHAT WE WANT THE NEW BEHAVIOR TO LOOK LIKE)	HOW WILL THE GOAL BE MEASURED?	IDENTIFY STRATEGIES TO ACHIEVE THE GOAL	
				What will student do?	*What will FWed do?*
When probed by the FWed about rationale for intervention plan, student requires moderate prompting to state hypotheses for why deficits exist and why proposed interventions should be effective. For example, student has difficulty explaining why an environmental adaptation would be preferable to teaching a new skill.	In order to optimize treatment planning and intervention, accurate understanding of the basis for the client's performance deficit is necessary. Otherwise, the client may not benefit from the intervention. The FWed must be confident of the student's clinical reasoning in order to give them the autonomy needed to meet the requirements for successful completion of fieldwork.	By the end of 2 weeks, student will independently verbalize two to three appropriate possible hypotheses about cause of performance deficits prior to each treatment session (student currently offers only one hypothesis). Student will also independently propose at least one appropriate intervention for each of the possible hypotheses, with a sound rationale for each, as well as one acceptable up- and downgrade (currently requires assist to state rationale 50% of the time). Student will independently provide sound rationale for how intervention plan will be modified or maintained for the next client session.	FWed will assess student's clinical reasoning daily, based on observation or review of clinical reasoning worksheets. On days that FWed is not on-site, student will email information reflecting on session outcomes for the day and plans for the next day.	Use clinical reasoning worksheet

Verbalize clinical reasoning (rationale for actions, occupational performance and treatment hypotheses) while talking with/treating patients

Verbalize clinical reasoning to FWed during meetings research a variety of activities, up- and downgrades appropriate to client population.

Student will complete and submit clinical reasoning worksheets by 8 p.m. each day. | Be available to listen to/read student's clinical reasoning, and be careful not to jump in too soon, so that student has time to present clinical reasoning without cueing.

Read clinical reasoning worksheets and provide feedback within 24 hours.

Provide specific daily feedback to give student a barometer on progress (e.g. "all of your hypotheses about occupational performance limitations were accurate today; however, you needed cuing when describing rationales for proposed interventions for two of the five clients.") |

REFLECTION QUESTIONS FOR THE FWED

1. What might some causes be for the student's behavior?

2. How do you think the setting or supervision model may be impacting the student's performance?

3. Suggest additional ways to make the goals measurable.

4. Identify additional strategies for providing the student with feedback on how they are progressing.

Professional Behavior

Professional behavior is deemed as essential for success in fieldwork (Campbell & Corpus, 2015; Hackenberg & Toth-Cohen, 2018; Koenig et al., 2003; Robinson et al., 2012). Professional behaviors include demonstration of initiative, reliability, time management, organization, self-directed learning, professional reasoning or problem-solving ability, use of professional terminology, written and verbal communication, interpersonal skills including the ability to demonstrate empathy, ability to establish and maintain personal and professional boundaries, and engagement in the fieldwork and supervisory experience (Campbell & Corpus, 2015; Davis & Rosee, 2015; Philadelphia Region Fieldwork Consortium, 2003). Studies have indicated the most common reason students have been unsuccessful in fieldwork is not due to lack of preparation of the academic or knowledge but poor professional behaviors (Hackenberg & Toth-Cohen, 2018; James & Musselman, 2006). FWeds are often more inclined to support a student challenged with understanding a concept than one who demonstrates poor professional behavior, believing that if the student is not putting forth their full effort, why should the FWed work harder? Box 10-5 offers suggestions for how students and FWeds can proactively address professional behavior expectations based on Level I fieldwork experiences, as well as strategies that can promote strong professional behaviors in Level II fieldwork. This next learning contract example involves a student demonstrating unprofessional behaviors in the context of mental health concerns.

Box 10-5

Tips for the FWed/CCFW

- When developing relationships with the academic programs, inquire as to how they facilitate professional behavior development throughout the curriculum. Development of professional behavior is a process.
- When you have Level I students, make a point of providing them with feedback on professional behavior. Be sure to document on the Level I fieldwork evaluation form if a student is lacking in this area or needs to strengthen a professional behavior. This will facilitate behavior change prior to the start of Level II fieldwork. **Do not** take the approach that "this is only a Level I fieldwork experience." Level I is foundational to Level II fieldwork. Students uninformed of challenging behavior during Level I fieldwork often respond in disbelief and/or become defensive when challenges are addressed in Level II fieldwork, as they perceive it as the "first time" they are hearing this kind of feedback. The AFWC can address professional behavior issues more effectively when proper documentation is in place.
- Prior to the start of the experience, have the student complete a professional behavior self-assessment, developing objective and measurable goals with corresponding detailed plans on how they will improve in the self-identified areas.
- Address any "red flags" or unprofessional behavior immediately. Not addressing these behaviors when they occur may lead the student to believe they are acceptable and often result in a student feeling surprised and defensive when addressed later.
- During weekly meetings, review student performance regarding clinical/practice skills and professional behavior. Students need to be aware of the areas they need to improve upon, and they need to know what they are doing well so they perpetuate the positive behaviors.

Tips for the Student

- Prior to the start of your fieldwork experience, ask the FWed about their expectations. This includes clinical/practice skills and professional behavior.
- Review feedback you have received in your Level I fieldwork experiences to determine if you need to focus on improving any professional behaviors.
- In preparation for weekly supervision meetings, reflect and self-assess your performance. Be sure to consider clinical/practice skills and professional behavior. Develop objective and measurable goals with corresponding detailed plans to improve your performance.
- Actively participate in your weekly supervision meeting. Identify those areas you believe you are demonstrating solid performance in. Share those areas in which you have identified a need for improvement, including the goals and plans you have established. Monitor your progress through self-reflection and self-assessment. Communicate with your FWed for feedback as appropriate.
- Take initiative and be prepared for sessions by reviewing what you learned in school and practicing newly required skills ahead of time.

Example of a Learning Contract to Address Professional Behavior

SCENARIO: Brady is an occupational therapy student in week 7 of a 12-week Level II fieldwork experience at an acute rehab facility. The FWed contacts the school with concerns about her professional behavior. Brady is doing well with designing and implementing treatment plans, developing rapport with all types of patients, constructing functional programs to increase level of independence and return to occupational roles, and constructing/integrating creative devices to compensate for deficits and improve occupational performance. However, Brady struggles with the ability to regulate emotions and can be seen in tears several times every day. This constitutes unacceptable professional behavior, and impacts Brady's productivity; ability to communicate with patients, FWed, and staff; and implement intervention. The FWed confides concerns about the student's mental health to the AFWC, and states they are afraid to give Brady any constructive feedback, anticipating a negative reaction. The academic program is aware of Brady's history of anxiety and depression but has not (at the student's request) disclosed it to the fieldwork site.

Student Name _____ Fieldwork Site _____

Date _____ In Attendance _____

Areas in which the student is doing well:

Areas in which problems have been identified (relate these to SSLOs):

DESCRIBE PROBLEMATIC STUDENT BEHAVIOR	WHY IS THIS BEHAVIOR A PROBLEM (IMPACT ON PATIENTS, FWED, FACILITY, STUDENT LEARNING?)	MEASURABLE GOALS: (BASELINE AND TARGET PERFORMANCE LEVELS; WHAT WE WANT THE NEW BEHAVIOR TO LOOK LIKE)	HOW WILL THE GOAL BE MEASURED?	IDENTIFY STRATEGIES TO ACHIEVE THE GOAL	
				What will student do?	What will FWed do?
Student becomes emotionally overwhelmed at points during the day, resulting in inability to put sentences together in a coherent way, panic attacks, crying, disengagement, and inability to take in and respond to feedback.	Coherent speech, therapeutic use of self and emotional regulation are integral elements of the occupational therapy process. The occupational therapist must be able to engage with patients for the duration of the treatment session and throughout the day and respond in the moment during treatment sessions in a way that conveys commitment and interest in the patient. Failure to do so deprives the patient of the full benefit of therapy, results in decreased productivity, and may have a negative effect on the patient emotionally.	Student must be able to regulate emotions throughout the day to the degree that she can effectively communicate/ engage with patients and staff and complete fieldwork responsibilities. Student is currently demonstrating effective emotional regulation and therapeutic use of self skills 75% of the time to FWed, 80% for patient care, 75% to other staff members.	By week 8, student will maintain emotional regulation in order to interact/ communicate effectively with patients and staff 90% of the day. By week 9, student will engage in 100% of patient and supervisory meetings with no loss of emotional control.	Sleep prep for increased quality of rest

Weekly counseling

More exercise

Journaling after stressful treatment days

Intermittent supportive text messages from friends/family

Take a stress break for 20 minutes mid-day as needed

Express and reflect pros/cons of the day in journal

Utilize resources to maintain regulation. Communicate/meet with AFWC one or two times per week to ensure effective communication and emotional regulation. | Provide feedback using 1 to 10 scale at the end of each day about goal attainment

Allow time throughout the day for student to ask questions regarding her performance.

Adjust caseload as follows:

1. Four patients for the next week

2. Five patients for the following 2 weeks

3. Six patients (full caseload) after that until completion of fieldwork. |

REFLECTION QUESTIONS FOR THE FWED

1. What might some causes be for the student's behavior? Knowing that the student has a history of anxiety and depression, how can the AFWC address the FWed's concerns about the student's mental health? Should this be reflected in the learning contract?

2. Do you think the behavior is serious enough to put the student at risk for failing? Why?

3. How will the student's future performance be measured? Can you think of any other ways to make it measurable?

4. Do you think the strategies address the underlying problem? Can you think of any additional strategies for either the student or FWed?

Safety

As occupational therapy practitioners, we are committed to the safety and well-being of the recipients of our services (AOTA, 2015). The area of safety is considered so critical that two criteria on the AOTA FWPE tool address safety and require students to achieve a score of "Proficient Performance" to receive a passing score on the fieldwork experience (AOTA, 2020). However, safety is one of the areas often identified as a challenge in fieldwork (Cardell et al., 2017; Potter, 2018; Trivinia & Johnson, 2019). Challenges with the internal factors previously discussed (communication, clinical reasoning, and professional behavior) can all contribute to unsafe practice, along with deficient knowledge base, underpreparedness of the student, unclear expectations, poor interpersonal skills, and the level of acuity in the environment, and can play a role in unsafe decision making and actions (Cardell et al., 2017; Nicola-Richmond et al., 2017; Potter, 2018; Silberman et al., 2018).

It is critical to tease out the underlying cause of the unsafe behavior in order to develop a learning contract targeting the factor in need of attention. It is not unusual for a learning contract to require 100% goal attainment when it comes to safety, as the care and safety of the patient is the highest priority. You may want to consider the following questions when developing your plan:

- Are you familiar with the curriculum of the academic program? Does the student appear to have been adequately prepared by the academic program to meet the demands of your specific setting? For example, is this a fast-paced, high-acuity environment requiring students to arrive prepared with a specific skill set?

- Did the student prepare to complete the task at hand? If the student was expected to complete an assessment, did they practice administering it prior to the actual patient session? (Refer back to professional behavior strategies discussed earlier in this chapter.)

- As the FWed, were you clear on your expectations? Was there any room for misunderstanding between what you stated to the student and what the student understood was to be completed?

- Is the student able to clearly articulate expectations to the client? (Refer back to communication strategies in Box 10-3.)

- Does the student ask clarifying questions of the FWed if unclear of expectations?

- Is the student able to provide appropriate reasoning for their decision making and actions?

Box 10-6

Tips for the FWed/CCFW

- When a student demonstrates unsafe behaviors, **address it immediately**. This is critical for client safety. Additionally, failure to immediately address it may give the student the impression their behavior is acceptable resulting in reinforcement of bad habits and continuation of unsafe practices.
- Reflect and assess all possible contributing factors to determine potential causes of unsafe behavior.
- Have the student reflect on the incident. Ask them to identify factors impacting their ability to perform task(s) safely. Then have the student identify the steps they should have taken to ensure client safety. Collaborate with the student to develop a plan to facilitate their performance.
- Utilize video recording of behavior (Eeckhout et al., 2016; Fukkink et al., 2011), with client and student consent, to allow the student to view unsafe behavior firsthand, in an effort to more rapidly facilitate behavior change.

Tips for the Student

- If challenged with safe performance of a clinical/practice skill, speak with your FWed. Arrive at the meeting prepared to reflect on the situation and identify factors that contributed to unsafe performance, as well as how you could have completed the task safely. Identify how you will improve performance. Note, increased repetition does not increase safety. Insight and behavior change increase safety.
- When performing the task in the future, consider verbalizing the steps of the task to the FWed either before or during task completion. Follow up with FWed to ensure your performance met expectations.
- Role play/practice at home with family or friends to improve skills.
- Develop and memorize lists of sequences or environmental set-ups needed for safe practice.

- At what point of the placement is competence in the safety skill expected? Is this a higher-level skill that the student needs more time to practice?
- When determining the level of performance expected for the goal, consider the expectations for new, entry-level therapists as a guide. Can there be any flexibility or is a 100% safe performance level essential?

Box 10-6 offers tips for both the student and FWed when a student has difficulty demonstrating safe practice. This next learning contract example illustrates ways of handling situations involving safety, where 100% goal attainment is required.

Example of a Learning Contract to Address Safety

SCENARIO: Sandy is an occupational therapy assistant student in week 5 of an 8-week placement. Sandy demonstrates professional behaviors including appropriate dress, punctuality, and flexibility. She collaborates with her occupational therapy FWed and the interdisciplinary team to enhance the educational experience. Sandy is open to constructive feedback and responds in a professional manner, is pleasant to patients and staff, and is hard working and dedicated to this affiliation. However, she is demonstrating inadequate safety awareness specifically related to functional transfers and line management, and her anxiety about this skill area is increasing daily.

Student Name _____ Fieldwork Site _____

Date _____ In Attendance _____

Areas in which the student is doing well:

Areas in which problems have been identified (relate these to SSLOs):

DESCRIBE PROBLEMATIC STUDENT BEHAVIOR	WHY IS THIS BEHAVIOR A PROBLEM (IMPACT ON PATIENTS, FWED, FACILITY, STUDENT LEARNING?)	MEASURABLE GOALS: (BASELINE AND TARGET PERFORMANCE LEVELS; WHAT WE WANT THE NEW BEHAVIOR TO LOOK LIKE)	HOW WILL THE GOAL BE MEASURED?	IDENTIFY STRATEGIES TO ACHIEVE THE GOAL	
				What will student do?	*What will FWed do?*
Student has demonstrated inconsistent safety awareness including patient handling, functional transfer/ guarding techniques, and line management during transfers/ activity requiring frequent cueing and intervention from FWed.	These inconsistencies can result in injury to the patient and compromise patient comfort as well as overall confidence in the therapist.	Effective immediately, student will: • Demonstrate safe patient handling techniques 100% of the time (currently at 60% of time). Student will educate patients regarding appropriate safety techniques with minimal cueing from FWed. • Describe to FWed the plan to keep lines organized during handling prior to handling the patient 100% of the time (currently at 75% of the time) • Execute safe patient handling, incorporating plan for keeping lines organized throughout the entire session 100% of the time (currently at 75% of the time) • Verbally identify and demonstrate understanding of the environmental implications, prior to start of each session, 100% of the time (currently at 75% of the time) • Anticipate potentially hazardous situations with functional transfers and mobility 100% of the time (currently at 60% of the time). For example, consistently block patients' knees to prevent buckling, recognize when it is appropriate to use a lift vs. attempt a transfer, discuss with FWed proper hand placement prior to execution of transfers/mobility.	FWed will observe student at each session, either from inside or outside of the room.	Employ relaxation techniques when indicated Develop a script of how lines will be managed and discuss plan with FWed prior to instituting it Develop a plan for each treatment session addressing all points listed previously and share with FWed at the beginning of the day or each session Develop an outline of the transfer process to be used and share the outline with FWed to convey clinical reasoning and safety awareness Practice using correct body mechanics during transfers with friends and family. Video and self-critique.	Provide feedback for every area of improvement using a 1 to 10 scale at least three times every week Provide positive feedback by describing specific instances in which success was observed. In the areas identified for improvement, provide modeling

REFLECTION QUESTIONS FOR THE FWED

1. What are some possible causes for this problem?

2. What do you think is an appropriate timeline to require progress? How much progress would you require? Why? By when?

3. Can you think of any other ways to make the goals measurable?

4. Are there ways the FWed can assess how the student is progressing without being in the room, which is sometimes perceived as "hovering" and increases student anxiety.

External Factors Affecting Student Performance

Now, let's review external factors that might impact student performance on Level II fieldwork, which might include supervision, the preparation of the FWed, and the learning environment at the fieldwork site.

Supervisory Issues Impacting Student Success

Multiple studies have demonstrated that the student-supervisor relationship is key to a successful fieldwork experience (Andonian, 2017; Christie et al., 1985a; Christie et al., 1985b; Patterson & D'Amico, 2020; Rodger et al., 2014). While the FWed is typically the student's mentor, role model, and greatest support, there may be situations when supervisory behaviors negatively impact student success rather than promoting it. Costa (2015) identifies several such behaviors, including the FWed using an inflexible teaching style, absence of clear expectations, inadequate orientation at the beginning of the placement, insufficient time spent modeling for and observing the student in action, personality differences, and failure to provide balanced feedback. Grenier (2020) describes several supervisory behaviors that negatively impact student learning, including "disengagement, a high need for control, closed-mindedness, lack of communication, lack of experience, and intimidation" (p. 3). These behaviors may add to growing tensions resulting in both student and FWed becoming frustrated and student performance declining, ultimately impacting the patient/client outcomes (Bolding et al., 2020).

FWed Preparation and Training

Just as the student must be adequately prepared for the fieldwork experience, so must the FWed. While some occupational therapy practitioners have completed the AOTA Fieldwork Educator Certificate Program (approximately 10,000 as of this writing), not everyone can develop the skills needed to be an effective FWed without training. A FWed without the necessary training may not know how to individualize the fieldwork programs for students with different needs or learning styles. They may not realize the importance of setting clear expectations through a well-developed orientation, schedule, and SSLOs. They may need to develop methods for communicating with students and providing a balance of positive and constructive feedback that do not come naturally to them. They may not recognize that "effective supervisors adapt their supervision approach" to the student's learning style (Nicola-Richmond et al., 2017), rather than expecting the student to adapt to them. They may not know when to reach out to the AFWC for support. They may not know what they do not know. In addition, the unprepared FWed may experience difficulty managing their own responsibilities in addition to their student responsibilities (Ozelie et al., 2015). Box 10-7 suggests some questions FWeds might ask themselves to determine if the issues they are facing with supervising a student may be linked to their own professional development as an educator.

> ### Box 10-7
>
> Occupational therapy practitioners practice at different levels of experience, ranging from novice to expert. FWeds fall into the same continuum of experience. AOTA and state regulations provide guidance regarding minimum qualifications needed to accept Level II fieldwork students, but individuals' levels of readiness will vary, and practitioners with as little as 1 year of practice experience may be willing or required to train Level II students. The AOTA Self-Assessment Tool for Fieldwork Educator Competency (AOTA, 2009) is an excellent resource for practitioners who are interested in identifying their strengths and areas that could benefit from further development. And remember, the AFWCs are also excellent resources and very invested in helping you to improve your skills. You do not need to be an expert to work with fieldwork students! Here are some questions to help you reflect on your own level of development as a FWed.
>
> - Am I prepared? What have I done to prepare?
> - Does my supervisory style tend to be controlling or flexible?
> - What do I know about various teaching and learning styles?
> - What is my preferred way of communicating?
> - Do I have any biases (e.g., gender, race, age)?
> - Do I know how to recognize if my student is struggling and when it would be appropriate to reach out to the AFWC?
> - Does my fieldwork program offer an adequate level of structure?
> - Am I clearly stating my expectations, both performance and behavioral?
> - How would I get support if I find myself in a challenging situation?

Learning Environment

Managing the power differential inherent in the student-FWed relationship requires skill, flexibility, and sensitivity. It is often influenced by the culture of the fieldwork setting. While most settings are welcoming and student-friendly, students may occasionally find themselves in a setting that is socially challenging. Students have reported sites that "expected me to break down in tears at least once before midterm" or "had a culture of hazing." The term "incivility" has been used to describe a spectrum of behaviors that range from subtle verbal or nonverbal slurs (e.g., eye-rolling, exclusion, swearing) to overt bullying (e.g., intimidation, humiliation, physical abuse). Incivility in clinical education has been studied in a variety of health professions and found to "lead to stress, loss of confidence, mistakes, disengagement, and decreased patient outcomes" (Bolding et al., 2020, p. 1). Fieldwork students exposed to incivility report "anxiety, loss of confidence, struggling with critical thinking, dreading reporting to work, and doubting their ability to continue in the profession" (Bolding et al., 2020, p. 1).

Bullying is considered one of the more severe acts of incivility. A recent study found that 16% of 247 respondents, all recent occupational therapy graduates, reported severe experiences of bullying by their FWeds or other staff or students (Bolding et al., 2020). Bolding and her colleagues surveyed occupational therapy (master's and doctoral level) and occupational therapy assistant students in order to examine the issue of bullying and other types of incivility in occupational therapy fieldwork. Participants were provided with a definition of bullying ("a situation where individuals persistently and over a period of time perceive themselves to be on the receiving end of negative actions from one or several persons and where the target of bullying has difficulty in defending him or herself") and asked to complete a survey (Bolding et al., 2020, p. 5).

Box 10-8

Tips for the AFWC

- As the AFWC, you are responsible for both advocating for the student and supporting the FWed, even though this might, at times, feel at odds. Both may need to develop their respective skill sets. While the criticisms of the student's performance may be justified, the method for delivering feedback must be acceptable. FWeds will appreciate the effort you put into helping them work with a student who is not responding to them in the way they wish.
- Guide those involved to recognize the need to focus on the student's performance, not their personal traits.
- Extra time and energy may be required of you in order to prevent escalation and address the needs of all involved. You may even need to learn some new skills yourself, such as how to work with FWeds who have challenging personalities or who may demonstrate (but not recognize that they have) implicit bias. Follow up with both student and FWed at least weekly until the situation has been resolved.
- You may hear differing versions of "the truth." Rarely is one truth or the other the "real" one. Help those involved to question their assumptions and to look at things differently than they have in the past.
- You will most likely have more influence over the student's behavior than the FWed's behavior. Set realistic goals for what you hope to accomplish.
- Two heads are better than one. If the situation is not improving, obtain support from colleagues in your program and in the AFWC community so that you can learn as much about the student, the fieldwork site, and the FWed as possible.

(continued)

The most frequently reported negative actions, experienced on a weekly or daily basis by 13% to 22% of participants, included excessive monitoring of the student's work, persistent criticism of the student's work, repeated reminders of the student's mistakes, being ignored or excluded, FWed withholding information affecting the student's performance, exposing the student to an unmanageable workload, and ignoring the student's views. Additional negative actions, reported to occur "now and then or monthly," were experienced by 20% to 36% of participants and included being ordered to work below their level of competence, being given tasks with unreasonable targets or deadlines, experiencing humiliation or ridicule, and encountering a hostile reaction upon approaching the FWed.

Bullying cannot be tolerated, and when bullying and other types of incivility occur in occupational therapy fieldwork settings, academic programs may need to take actions that are beyond the scope of a learning contract and beyond the scope of this chapter. However, when it is determined that a learning contract is appropriate, it must be approached with great care. This type of learning contract must provide strategies for both the FWed and the student and be presented in such a way that it does not put the student at even greater risk. Box 10-8 provides key pointers to help the FWed, student, and AFWC navigate this sensitive issue and move everyone toward successful completion of the fieldwork experience.

Box 10-8 (CONTINUED)

Tips for the FWed/CCFW

- Question your assumptions.
  - Consider some ways the student's academic experience, life situation, personal attributes, and fit with the fieldwork setting, FWed, and clients may be impacting their behavior. Then, do the same for yourself.
  - Ask yourself how your teaching style, your experience as a student, your experience supervising past students, and personal feelings about the student or the academic program they came from affects the way you interact with the student.
- Ask the student for examples of behaviors that are impacting them negatively. Just as we hope students can accept feedback without becoming defensive, it is important for you to accept feedback without becoming defensive.

Tips for the Student

- If you believe you are being treated unfairly or being bullied and are not comfortable addressing it directly with your FWed, reach out to the CCFW at the fieldwork site, if there is one, and ask for a time to meet with them. Reach out to your AFWC immediately as well.
- If you have concerns that the FWed is not aware of the efforts you are making to improve your performance, try this three-step process for enhancing their awareness. After your sessions with service recipients:
  1. State what your goals were for the session and how you planned to implement the session, highlighting the strategies you used to improve your performance and differences between what you have done in the past and what you did in the current session.
  2. Provide an assessment of how it went. If it went well (met your expectations for the session), reflect on the successful outcome and why you think it went well. If it did not go as well as you hoped, reflect on possible reasons it did not go as well.
  3. Offer a plan and rationale for how you will modify your approach for the next session.

Example of a Learning Contract to Address Supervisory Issues

SCENARIO: It is week 4 in a 12-week placement and the occupational therapy student, Anton, is not meeting expectations for timeliness and initiative. The FWed contacts the AFWC to express concerns. During this conversation, the AFWC picks up on remarks that indicate a bias toward the student, who is in a racial minority. While a number of approaches are indicated, this section is limited to the development of a learning contract designed to direct the focus toward the student's performance (rather than the student's personal characteristics) and collection of measurable data on which his performance will be judged. In collaboration with the student and FWed, mutually agreeable strategies are developed. The AFWC will maintain weekly contact with the Anton and FWed to monitor the situation and provide support as needed.

Student Name _____ Fieldwork Site _____

Date _____ In Attendance _____

Areas in which the student is doing well:

Areas in which problems have been identified (relate these to SSLOs):

DESCRIBE PROBLEMATIC STUDENT BEHAVIOR	WHY IS THIS BEHAVIOR A PROBLEM (IMPACT ON PATIENTS, FWED, FACILITY, STUDENT LEARNING?)	MEASURABLE GOALS: (BASELINE AND TARGET PERFORMANCE LEVELS; WHAT WE WANT THE NEW BEHAVIOR TO LOOK LIKE)	HOW WILL THE GOAL BE MEASURED?	IDENTIFY STRATEGIES TO ACHIEVE THE GOAL	
				What will student do?	*What will FWed do?*
Student arrives late to fieldwork at least one time per week	Late arrival on a repeated basis demonstrates disrespect for other staff and the institution. It inconveniences the staff who need to follow a schedule, disrupts patient treatment schedules, and affects therapist productivity.	Effective immediately, lateness will not be tolerated. Over the next week, student will target arrival for 7:45, but arrive no later than 8 a.m. daily. Over the remaining 6 weeks of the placement, student will have no late arrivals.	Arrival time will be documented by staff daily	Student will set alarm 30 to 45 minutes earlier. Student will take an earlier bus to the fieldwork site each day. In the event the FWed is not in the office at the time of arrival, student will have arrival time confirmed by receptionist. Student will take photo of clock on office wall upon arrival if no one is available to confirm his arrival time.	FWed will be available to the extent possible to confirm student arrival time. FWed will provide verbal and/or written feedback on student's progress/ compliance in this area. FWed will positively reinforce student's success at arriving on time.

REFLECTION QUESTIONS FOR THE FWED

1. How would you address the issue of bias?
2. Are there other ways to ensure the student is being evaluated fairly, on their performance and not their personal characteristics?
3. Identify some additional strategies either the student or the FWed can employ.
4. How should the academic program handle assigning fieldwork students to this site in the future?

ASSESSING PERFORMANCE IN THE UNDERPERFORMING STUDENT

Assessment of skills should be objective and systematic. Several resources will facilitate the methodical assessment of performance: SSLOs, the fieldwork site's 12-week schedule (8-week for OTA programs), and AOTA's FWPE (AOTA, 2020). Each tool may be used itself or with another resource based on the specific needs of the assessment and specific student challenges. Fieldwork sites should develop SSLOs specific to their site and for each different practice setting within the site. Weekly schedules should also be developed, 8-week (occupational therapy assistant) and 12-week (occupational therapist). These tools assist in communicating student expectations for the fieldwork placement. Refer back to Chapters 4 and 5 for a more in-depth overview of how to create/utilize SLLOs, weekly schedules, and orientation plans. Difficulties may arise at any point during a fieldwork experience.

> Once the fieldwork educator has determined that a student is experiencing difficulty, they need to assess the student's performance and identify areas of concern. Assessment of performance should be objective, systematic and based on multiple sources of evidence [e.g., documentation, weekly feedback forms, comments from team members and clients]. (Trivinia & Johnson, 2019, p. 24)

Most well-designed fieldwork programs already have several methods for assessing student performance at their disposal, including their weekly schedule, weekly feedback forms, SSLOs, and the AOTA FWPE.

The AOTA FWPE may be used as a formative assessment at any point in the student's placement to provide objective measures of performance, yielding information on both strengths and areas of need. When concerned that a student is falling behind, comparing their performance to the site's weekly schedule expectations provides additional data about how far behind the struggling student may be. Sites that have well-developed SSLOs will be able to apply them to help identify areas of need and narrow the focus on areas for remediation. Most importantly, weekly feedback forms that provide specific feedback on strengths and weaknesses, progress, or lack thereof, will help the student and AFWC better understand the problems at hand. Chapter 12 will provide a more detailed view of the important role that a FWed has with evaluation during Level II fieldwork.

COLLABORATIVE DEVELOPMENT OF LEARNING CONTRACTS

A student who has experienced challenges during fieldwork generally encounters a sequence of steps that will lead to improved performance, dismissal, or failure of the experience. This usually begins with the FWed recognizing concerns regarding the student's performance based on the AOTA FWPE criteria, progression with the fieldwork schedule, or achievement of SSLOs. At this time, the AFWC frequently becomes involved to discuss and help remediate those concerns. Remediation often involves implementing a learning contract. Occasionally, an extension of the fieldwork experience is needed to allow additional learning and/or time to reach established goals. Ultimately, if those goals are not achieved, the placement is terminated and the student is removed from the experience, either by decision of the academic program or at the request of the site. The academic program is responsible for determining a grade for the student, if any, at this time (Silberman et al., 2018). Of course, the ultimate goal is for the student to improve their performance and successfully complete the fieldwork experience. A learning contract can facilitate this positive outcome.

Fieldwork is challenging, and deliberately so. The FWed must progress the student from beginner to entry-level, with many potential learning challenges along the way. Some students struggle more than others, and when the likelihood of successful completion of fieldwork becomes questionable, intervention is required. Learning contracts are the preferred intervention, as they provide a framework to support the student toward successful completion of fieldwork. Only by understanding the perspectives of both the FWed and the student, which often differ significantly, can the AFWC successfully guide the process. "When unsatisfactory performance by a Level II student has been identified, the fieldwork educator should contact the AFWC, request a site visit or phone conversation, and collaborate with the AFWC to determine the need for and parameters of a learning contract" (Trivinia & Johnson, 2019, p. 25). Students, FWeds and AFWCs are all stakeholders who should collaborate in developing learning contracts. AFWCs are responsible for guiding the process, advocating for the students, and supporting both the student and the FWed. This requires ongoing communication, often over a protracted period of time. The "ability [of the AFWC] to manage conflict as well as to analyze student, fieldwork educator and contextual elements of the learning environment," along with ready access by phone, email, and face-to-face meetings are important to establishing the necessary support, respect, and trust to progress the at-risk student toward successful completion of fieldwork (Evenson et al., 2015, p. 4). Table 10-2 summarizes the steps used to create a learning contract.

RIGHTS AND RESPONSIBILITIES

All stakeholders, including the academic program, the student, the fieldwork site, and fieldwork coordinator, have rights and responsibilities throughout the process of developing a learning contract (Trivinia & Johnson, 2019). Awareness of student rights is of great importance. The Family Educational Rights and Privacy Act (FERPA) protects students by regulating how and what information may be shared, including but not limited to academic history, previous fieldwork performance, and medical and learning conditions (U.S. Department of Education, 2018). When a FWed has reason for concern, feedback regarding performance must be provided, as the student has a right to due process (Schenarts & Langenfeld, 2017; Trivinia & Johnson, 2019). Students also have the right to receive timely feedback. This includes the receipt and review of supporting evidence such as copies of feedback forms from weekly supervision meetings, written feedback previously provided on daily/progress notes, assessments, evaluations and treatment plans as well as timely notification of decisions (Trivinia & Johnson, 2019).

TABLE 10-2
STEPS FOR CREATING A LEARNING CONTRACT

STEPS	DESCRIPTION
Step 1: Identify the problem	FWed/CCFW recognizes there is a problem and that previous measures put in place to support student success are not working.
Step 2: Initiate communication between stakeholders	FWed/CCFW contacts the AFWC for support. When it becomes clear the student is at risk for failing, the collaborative team begins developing a learning contract.
Step 3: Collect data	FWed collects and evaluates evidence that illustrates the issues. Tools that can help to provide objective baseline data include the FWPE, SSLOs, weekly feedback forms, the 8- or 12-week schedule, and email communications.
Step 4: Draft learning contract	AFWC collects additional information from the student and FWed/CCFW and drafts a learning contract to be reviewed and revised by FWED/CCFW and student prior to a formal meeting.
Step 5: Finalize learning contract	Student, FWed/CCFW, and AFWC meet to review, rework, finalize and sign learning contract.
Step 6: Implement learning contract	Implement learning contract and re-evaluate, usually 2 weeks later.
Step 7: Evaluate outcome	Determine further action (continue fieldwork with or without additional learning contract or terminate fieldwork experience at that time)

Adapted from Trivinia, B.A. & Johnson, C.R. (2019). Blueprint for success: Measurable learning contracts for level II fieldwork students at risk for failing. *OT Practice, 24*(7), 24-27. .

By the time the decision is made to develop a learning contract, it is likely that there has already been a good deal of communication between the AFWC and FWed/CCFW and between the AFWC and the student. The importance of thorough documentation by the FWed and AFWC cannot be emphasized enough. At the conclusion of the learning contract, some students will receive a failing grade and typically have the right to contest the grade. Documentation of communications with the student and fieldwork site, and between the FWed and the student, over the course of the placement is integral to justifying the academic program's decision. The right to challenge any negative data or witnesses, to be supported by a person of their choosing, and inclusion of objections to allegations in permanent record is within the student's prerogative (Scanlan, 2001). Once a student has been informed that they are at risk for failing, a learning contract should be promptly implemented with measurable goals and a specific time for re-evaluation established. It is imperative that an appropriate amount of time be provided to allow student progress. Learning contracts should use a systematic methodology to help guide this process (Trivinia & Johnson, 2019).

In most cases, the learning contract provides the guidance, while the student and FWed implement the strategies needed to improve performance and reach the goals of the learning contract, leading to a successful completion of the fieldwork experience. Occasionally, it becomes clear that the student is making steady or significant progress even though the goals of the learning contract have not quite been achieved within the designated time period, or the need for new or different goals has arisen. When justified, the AFWC and fieldwork site have the prerogative to extend and/or revise the learning contract as they see fit.

TERMINATING A FIELDWORK EXPERIENCE

Learning contracts set the stage for remediation and usually result in successful completion of the fieldwork experience. FWeds have a responsibility to evaluate student performance, assess professional suitability, and ensure that students meet entry-level competencies. Failing a student is rarely an easy decision, and some FWeds may encounter barriers when the time comes to make that determination. "Fieldwork educators have often said that failing a student is the most difficult task encountered" (Costa, 2015, p. 514). Barriers to failing a student may result in lack of action, often referred to as failure to fail. Some examples of obstacles to failing a student include:

- The desire to avoid confrontation or student distress
- Wanting to pass students who were trying their best
- Feeling pressure from the academic institution to pass a student
- Lack of certainty and evidence required to fail a student
- Reluctance to fail a student they like or have grown close to
- Concern about the psychological and financial impact on the student
- Not having the time required to document performance that would support a failing grade
- Fear of legal consequences

Some FWeds may feel that failing a student reflects negatively on them. Others may not trust their own judgment or may question whether they have enough experience as a FWed to make this decision. Still others are unwilling to take responsibility for such a major decision (Luhanga et al., 2014; Nicola-Richmond et al., 2017). Regardless, academic and FWeds are bound by the AOTA *Code of Ethics* to confer the grade that was earned. Imagine a situation where an academic program gives a student a passing grade, even though the FWed gave that student a failing score for unsafe practice. Upon graduation, that student enters the workforce and injures a client. Have the educators involved violated the principle of nonmaleficence (do no harm) by knowingly passing a student who was unqualified? Have they violated the principle of veracity (truthfulness, candor, and honesty) by giving a passing score to a student who merited a failing score? Despite the challenges we face when failing a student, we have an ethical and professional responsibility to the public and the profession to ensure the students we graduate are adequately prepared to practice.

Termination of the fieldwork experience is usually an emotionally challenging experience for all involved. There is often concern about the mental health of the student following a fieldwork failure, and the need for counseling or other forms of support should be explored with the student. The FWed often sees the experience as a personal failure as well and may require support to view it as a learning experience and build on it so that the anticipation of future students does not provoke anxiety. (Note: Most FWeds have commented that they learned so much more about being a good FWed from fieldwork experiences that were challenging and warranted extensive communication, time, commitment, and creativity than the ones that ran smoothly).

It is the responsibility of the AFWC/academic program to determine grades for the academic course in which the student is enrolled in for fieldwork and ultimately remove the student from the fieldwork experience, once the decision is made (Trivinia & Johnson, 2019). There may be a variety of options for moving forward, and they will depend on the policies of the individual academic program. Some programs provide options for student withdrawal from the placement if the decision is made early on. Most academic programs allow students to repeat one time after failing a placement and dismiss the student if there is a second failure (Costa, 2015). The AFWC must be prepared with the knowledge of all options ahead of time, since the student will probably ask these questions at or prior to a termination meeting. For example:

BOX 10-9

Tips for the AFWC

Before the termination meeting:

- Communicate with the student and FWed/CCFW regularly over the term of the learning contract so that you can provide ongoing and honest feedback on a regular basis, ensuring the student has a realistic idea of how their performance is (or isn't) progressing.
- Throughout the course of the learning contract, reinforce the criteria for successfully completing fieldwork to the student and ensure they understand the consequences of failing.
- **Document all** phone calls, emails, and meetings with the student, FWeds, and CCFWs.
- Consult with the fieldwork site regarding the outcome of the learning contract ahead of time. If the student is likely to fail, they should be prepared. A student should never be taken completely by surprise.
- Confer with the fieldwork site to determine if there is a need to have security present.
- Discuss with the fieldwork site who will lead the meeting. This may be a function of the level of experience of those involved.
- Answer questions the student has about the consequences of failing a fieldwork experience in terms of progression through the program, financial implications, GPA, etc.
- Schedule time at the end of the meeting to meet with the student individually.

During the termination meeting:

- Have a box of tissues handy.
- Emphasize how much the student has learned despite the outcome of the learning contract.
- Present the outcomes of the learning contract in a clear, objective, and empathetic way.
- Allow the student to appropriately express their emotions and ask questions.
- Preserve the student's dignity.

After the termination meeting:

- At the end of the meeting, confirm that the student has a plan to speak with someone who can provide support (e.g., friend, family member, therapist); assess their mood/frame of mind; determine that they can get home safely.
- Follow up with the FWed/CCFW.
- Document the meeting.

(continued)

- *How does the academic program determine if failure to achieve the goals of a learning contract results in failure of the fieldwork experience?*
- *Will the student receive a grade of "withdrawal," "fail," or are there other options?*
- *If the student fails, are they dismissed from the program?*
- *What are the policies regarding repeating a fieldwork experience? Readmittance to the program? Wait until the fieldwork course is offered again in the curriculum?*
- *What are the financial implications?*
- *Is there a grievance process available to the student?*
- *What documentation should go into the student's academic record?*

When a student does not meet the criteria of the learning contract and a decision is made to terminate the experience, a meeting is scheduled to bring closure to the experience. Box 10-9 provides some tips for successfully preparing for and navigating these difficult situations.

Box 10-9 (CONTINUED)

Tips for the FWed/CCFW

- Consider the best time for the meeting. The end of the day is usually best. Usually, 1.5 to 2 hours is sufficient.
- Be prepared to justify your conclusions with objective and measurable data and examples.
- Be empathetic and supportive of the student. As hard as this is for you, it is even harder for them.
- Arrive at the meeting with a list of everything that the student will need to do at the conclusion of the meeting (e.g., turn in ID, return any borrowed books, complete any unfinished notes, say good-bye where appropriate).
- Remind yourself that not all fieldwork experiences are the right fit for all students.
- Reflect on how so much more can be learned about being a FWed when you have experienced a challenging situation.

Tips for the Student

- Know that you are not alone in this experience, and that the vast majority of students go on to be successful in their next placement.
- Understand that not all fieldwork placements are the right fit for every student, and work with your AFWC to identify a placement that will be a better fit for you next time.
- Accept that you need to work on areas of need, even if you don't agree with everything that occurred.
- Prepare to have support available after the meeting has ended.
- Obtain information about your rights and responsibilities from the academic program.
- Determine the impact that failing a placement will have on your academic progress. Most programs have policies and procedures in place that address remediation.
- Embrace the remediation process. It is critical to preparing you for success in the next placement.

Plan carefully for the actual termination meeting. When the student fails to achieve the goals of the learning contract and the decision is made to terminate the placement, it is best to give the student an indication of this likelihood ahead of time, as the meeting will go better if the student is not surprised. In the fieldwork resource *The Essential Guide to Occupational Therapy Fieldwork Education*, Costa (2015) provides the following recommendations:

- Open the meeting by stating that everyone will have the opportunity to speak.
- Begin by reviewing the student's strengths and accomplishments.
- Then review the limitations in the student's ability to achieve entry-level competence.
- State the consequences of terminating the placement, as specific to each academic program.
- The person with the best relationship with the student should be the person to actually tell the student they have failed the placement.
- "Allow the student to leave in a way that preserves his or her dignity. The student may or may not want to say goodbye to staff, other students, or patients …. If the student wants to make a quick exit, you may want to ask how he or she wants his or her departure explained to others" (Costa, 2015, p. 514).

For obvious reasons, it is best to have the meeting in person whenever possible. Consider whether there is a need to alert the security personnel on site about the meeting. Think about how the student can maintain their dignity at the conclusion of the meeting, and how follow-up with the academic program will occur. The student will typically need to complete some unfinished business, turn in their ID badge and fieldwork manual, and remove all their belongings from the premises immediately following the meeting. They may have questions for the AFWC, and they may be overwrought and need some time to collect themselves with support from the AFWC. At the conclusion of the fieldwork experience, the FWed should provide a completed FWPE along with a written report summarizing the student's fieldwork experience to the AFWC.

The academic program should follow up with the student and consider the possibility of a remediation plan to prepare the student for another fieldwork experience. The AFWC should also follow up with the FWed/CCFW to analyze what went right/wrong, and to provide support and resources to address any skills or areas needing development. The follow-up process with the student can play a critical role in helping the student to maintain hope and dignity, regardless of whether another fieldwork experience is possible. Follow-up with the site is often critical to maintenance of the relationship with the site/FWeds for future student learning opportunities.

SUMMARY

Well-designed learning contracts offer a systematic process to help students who are experiencing obstacles to completing fieldwork successfully. They minimize speculation and bias, while providing timely support and clear expectations to promote student success. Although time consuming, this collaborative process will ensure recognition of students' rights and result in higher levels of satisfaction for all stakeholders. When properly executed, the learning contract supports the learning process for everyone involved. Academic programs and AFWCs learn from each experience how to develop better policies and procedures, prepare their students for fieldwork experiences more effectively, and meet the continuing education needs of their fieldwork community. FWeds and CCFWs learn more about the strengths and limitations of their fieldwork programs, how to better develop and clarify expectations of students, and how to enhance their supervisory skill sets. Finally, students develop insight regarding their strengths and weaknesses and strategies to enhance their skills. Through addressing their challenges in the learning contract process, students become intimately acquainted with the persistence and discipline that is required to foster change. Although it might not be the journey they intended to take, those who go on to work in the profession become better therapists through the experience.

LEARNING ACTIVITIES

1. **Clinical Vignette re: Substandard Documentation and Caseload Management**

   It is week 6 of a 12-week placement. Sam is a Level II student in a school-based setting and is consistently late with submitting treatment plans to the FWed for review prior to child's treatment time (on time 20% of the time). Sam is also consistently late with submitting documentation following treatment (on time 40% of the time). In addition, important information is missing from daily documentation. The FWed has observed that Sam interacts well with the children, who enjoy and are engaged in the well-thought-out and creative activities provided, and they respond to him in a positive way. A midterm review has been completed using the FWPE, and Sam's performance is deemed unsatisfactory. He reacts with surprise to these concerns and becomes defensive when the FWed suggests contacting the AFWC for support. Sam has not reached out previously to the AFWC. During a conversation with the AFWC about implementing a learning contract, Sam expresses concerns about the way the FWed is supervising and becomes upset at the possibility of failing the placement, which would result in feelings of shame, additional expenses, and not graduating with the class.

a. Activity for the FWed: Develop a learning contract for Sam using the Learning Contract Template provided (Appendix A), following the steps previously described in the section entitled "A Blueprint for Success: Steps in Creating a Learning Contract."

2. **Clinical Vignette re: Failure to Fail**

Halfway through an occupational therapy assistant student's 8-week placement, Dave, a registered occupational therapist, recognizes he has concerns about his student Sara's performance. Dave has worked with two occupational therapy students in the past, but Sara is his first occupational therapy assistant student, and when she begins to fall behind the 8-week schedule, Dave becomes concerned about her performance and questions his expectations. Although Sara develops excellent relationships with patients, at midterm she is behind performance expectations in both caseload and documentation. In weekly feedback meetings Dave emphasizes Sara's strengths, and he keeps his constructive feedback "gentle" since Sara tends to be quiet and lacks confidence. He and Sara agreed early on to verbal feedback meetings weekly, and they have not been using the written feedback forms provided by the school. Not wanting to discourage his student, and questioning his own judgment, Dave provides generous scores on the FWPE midterm that do not truly reflect Sara's level of performance. When reviewing the midterm report that Dave submitted, the AFWC sees no reason to be concerned. Dave does not want to bother the AFWC yet, and tries a few strategies on his own, with poor results. By then, it is week 6 of the 8-week placement, and it becomes clear that Sara is unlikely to be able to reach and sustain entry-level competence within 2 weeks.

a. Reflection questions for fieldwork students:

- If you could go back in time, what would you suggest that Dave do differently?

- Develop three to five questions Sara could ask to obtain more specific feedback from Dave.

- Identify two to three tools and/or resources that were at Sara's disposal that would have enabled her to assess her own performance level more accurately.

- How could Sara "give permission" to Dave to give her more appropriate and honest feedback?

- Consider a scenario where Sara scores below the passing score on her final FWPE. How would you support her? What advice would you give her?

b. Reflection questions for FWeds/CCFWs:

- List three to five resources Dave's student fieldwork program should have in place prior to accepting a Level II student. Focus on resources that help to assess student performance.

- At what point should Dave have contacted the AFWC? Explain your reasoning.

- List three forms of documentation that Dave should be using to justify passing or failing Sara.

- What actions should be taken at this point in order to avoid passing a student who is not meeting entry-level competencies, or to avoid failing a student who may have the potential to pass?

- List three strategies Dave can use to provide constructive feedback more effectively to Sara.

- If, at the end of 8 weeks, Sara does not demonstrate entry-level competencies, why might Dave feel reluctant to fail her?

- Consider a scenario where Sara's final score totals 1 or 2 points below the passing score on the final FWPE. Would you question whether she should fail the placement? Would you feel differently if she scored more significantly below the passing score?

   c. Reflection questions for AFWCs:

- List two to three goals you would include in a learning contract for Sara.

- Identify two to three strategies you would suggest to ensure more effective communication between Dave and Sara.

- Identify two to three options that would give Sara a chance to achieve entry-level competence.

- What measures can you put in place to ensure that Sara does not pass the fieldwork experience unless she has achieved entry-level competence?

- Consider a scenario where Sara's final score totals 1 or 2 points below the passing score on the final FWPE. You have been involved with a learning contract and believe the score to be an accurate reflection of the student's performance. What would you say to the FWed to help them understand the justification for and value of failing the student when she is "so close" to passing?

ADDITIONAL RESOURCES

Internet resources:

- American Occupational Therapy Association—resources for FWeds, students, and AFWCs (https://www.aota.org/Education-Careers/Fieldwork.aspx)

- National Board for Certification in Occupational Therapy—resources for FWeds, students, and AFWCs (https://www.nbcot.org/)

- Philadelphia Region Fieldwork Consortium (http://www.philaotfwconsortium.org/)

- New England Occupational Therapy Education Council (https://neotecouncil.org/)

Books:

- *The Essential Guide to Occupational Therapy Fieldwork Education: Resources for Educators and Practitioners*, Second Edition, by Donna M. Costa (AOTA, 2016)

Courses:

- Fieldwork Educator Certificate Program (https://www.aota.org/Education-Careers/Fieldwork/Workshop.aspx)

REFERENCES

American Occupational Therapy Association. (2009). The American Occupational Therapy Association Self-Assessment Tool for Fieldwork Educator Competency. https://www.aota.org/-/media/Corporate/Files/EducationCareers/Educators/Fieldwork/Supervisor/Forms/Self-Assessment%20Tool%20FW%20Ed%20Competency%20(2009).pdf

American Occupational Therapy Association. (2015). Occupational therapy code of ethics. *American Journal of Occupational Therapy, 69*. https://doi.org/10.5014/ajot.2015.696S03

American Occupational Therapy Association. (2020). Fieldwork performance evaluation (FWPE) rating scoring guide. Retrieved from https://www.aota.org/Education-Careers/Fieldwork/performance-evaluations.aspx

Andonian, L. (2017). Occupational therapy students' self-efficacy, experience of supervision, and perception of meaningfulness of Level II fieldwork. *The Open Journal of Occupational Therapy, 5*(2). https://doi.org/10.15453/2168-6408.1220

Bolding, D. J., Dudley, T., Dahlmeier, A., Bland, L., Castro, A., & Covarrubias, A. (2020). Prevalence and types of incivility in occupational therapy fieldwork. *Journal of Occupational Therapy Education, 4*(1). https://doi.org/10.26681/jote.2020.040111

Campbell, M.K., & Corpus, K. (2015). Fieldwork educators' perspectives: Professional behavior attributes of Level II fieldwork students. *Open Journal of Occupational Therapy, 3*(4), 1-13. https://doi.org/10.15453/2168-6408.1146

Cardell, B., Koski, J., Wahl, J., Rock, W., & Kirby, A. (2017). Underperforming students: Factors and decision-making in occupational therapy programs. *Journal of Occupational Therapy Education, 1*(3). https://doi.org/10.26681/jote.2017.010301

Costa, D. M. (Ed.). (2015). *The essential guide to occupational therapy fieldwork education: Resources for educators and practitioners* (2nd ed.). AOTA Press.

Christie, B. A., Joyce, P. C., & Moeller, P. L. (1985a). Fieldwork experience, part I: Impact on practice preference. *American Journal of Occupational Therapy, 39*, 671-674. https://doi.org/10.5014/ajot.39.10.671

Christie, B. A., Joyce, P. C., & Moeller, P. L. (1985b). Fieldwork experience, part II: The supervisor's dilemma. *American Journal of Occupational Therapy, 39*, 675-681. https://doi.org/10.5014/ajot.39.10.675

Cranton, P. (2016). *Understanding and promoting transformative learning: A guide to theory and practice* (3rd ed.). Stylus.

Davis, L. & Rosee, M. (2015). Tuning in to communication nuances: Connecting with clients and colleagues. In L. Davis & M. Rosee (Eds.), *Occupational Therapy Student to Clinician: Making the Transition* (pp. 47-63). SLACK Incorporated.

Eeckhout, T., Gerits, M., Bouquillon, D., & Schoenmakers, B. (2016). Video training with peer feedback in real-time consultation: Acceptability and feasibility in a general-practice setting. *Postgraduate Medical Journal, 92*(1090), 431–435. https://doi.org/10.1136/postgradmedj-2015-133633

Evenson, M. E., Roberts, M., Kaldenberg, J., Barnes, M.A., & Ozelie, R. (2015). Brief report- national survey of fieldwork educators: Implications for occupational therapy education. *American Journal of Occupational Therapy, 69*(2). http://dx.doi.org/10.5014/ajot.2015.019265

Fukkink, R. G., Trienekes, N. & Kramer, L. J. C. (2011). Video feedback in education and training: Putting learning in the picture. *Educational Psychology Review, 23*(1), 45-63. https://doi.org/10.1007/s10648-010-9144-5

Gallant, M., Mac Donald J., & Higuchi, K. A. (2006). A remediation process for nursing students at risk for clinical failure. *Nurse Educator, 31*(5), 223 - 227. https://doi.org/10.1097/00006223-200609000-00010

Grenier, M.-L. (2015). Facilitators and barriers to learning in occupational therapy fieldwork education: Student perspectives. *American Journal of Occupational Therapy, 69*(Suppl. 2), 6912185070. http://dx.doi.org/10.5014/ajot.2015.015180

Hackenberg, G., & Toth-Cohen, S. (2018). Professional behaviors and fieldwork: A curriculum based model in occupational therapy. *Journal of Occupational Therapy Education, 2*(2), 1-16.

James, K. L., & Musselman, L. (2006). Commonalities in level II fieldwork failure. *Occupational Therapy in Health Care, 19*(4), 67-81. https://doi-org.db.usciences.edu/10.1080/J003v19n04_05

Koenig, K., Johnson, C., Morano, C. K., & Ducette, J. P. (2003). Development and validation of a professional behavior assessment. *Journal of Allied Health, 32*(2), 86-91.

Kolb, D. A. (1984). *Experiential learning: Experience as the source of learning and development.* Prentice Hall.

Luhanga, F. L., Larocque, S., MacEwan, L., Gwekwerere, Y. N., & Danyluk, P. (2014). Exploring the issue of failure to fail in professional education programs: A multidisciplinary study. *Journal of University Teaching & Learning Practice, 11*(2). http://ro.uow.edu.au/jutlp/vol11/iss2/3

Merriam, S. B. & Baumgartner, L. M. (2020). *Learning in adulthood: A comprehensive guide.* (4th ed.). Josey-Bass.

Myers, K., & Covington, K. (2019). Analysis of clinical education situation (ACES) framework: Identifying the root cause of student failure in the United States. *Journal of Educational Evaluation for Health Professions, 16.* https://doi.org/10.3352/jeehp.2019.16.11

Nicola-Richmond, K., Butterworth, B., & Hitch, D. (2017). What factors contribute to failure of fieldwork placement? Perspectives of supervisors and university fieldwork educators. *Journal of World Federation of Occupational Therapists, 73*(2), 117-124. https://doi.org/10.1080/14473828.2016.1149981

Ozelie, R., Janow, J., Kreutz, C., Mulry, M. K., & Penkala, A. (2015). Supervision of occupational therapy level II fieldwork students: Impact on and predictors of clinician productivity. *American Journal of Occupational Therapy, 69*(1). https://doi.org/10.5014/ajot.2015.013532.

Patterson, B., & D'Amico, M. (2020). What does the evidence say about student, fieldwork educator, and new occupational therapy practitioner perceptions of successful level II fieldwork and transition to practice? A scoping review. *Journal of Occupational Therapy Education, 4*(2). https://doi.org/10.26681/ jote.2020.040210

Philadelphia Region Fieldwork Consortium. (2003). *Philadelphia Region Fieldwork Consortium Level I Fieldwork Student Evaluation* (2nd ed.).

Plourde, M. A. (2019). Communicating across generations and cultures. In K. Jacobs & G.L. McCormack (Eds.), *The Occupational Therapy Manager* (6th ed., pp. 409-418). AOTA Press.

Potter, K. (2018). Why are students failing clinical? Clinical instructors weigh in. *Teaching and Learning in Nursing, 13*(2), 75-77. https://doi.org/10.1016/j.teln.2017.12.006

Prochaska, J. O. (2008). Decision making in the transtheoretical model of behavior change. *Society for Medical Decision Making, 28*(6), 845-849. https://doi.org/10.1177%2F0272989X08327068

Recker-Hughes, C., Wetherbee, E., Buccieri, K., Fitzpatrick Timmerberg, J., & Stolfi, A. M., (2014). Essential characteristics of quality clinical education experiences: Standards to facilitate student learning. *Journal of Physical Therapy Education, 26*, 48-55.

Reitz, S. M., & Graham, K. (2019). Health promotion theories. In B. A. Schell & G. Gillen (Eds.), *Willard & Spackman's occupational therapy* (13th ed., pp. 675-692). Wolters Kluwer.

Robinson, A. J., Tanchuk, C. J., & Sullivan, T. M. (2012). Professionalism and occupational therapy: An exploration of faculty and students' perspectives. *Canadian Journal of Occupational Therapy, 79*(5), 275-284. https://doi.org/10.2182/cjot.2012.79.5.3

Rodger, S., Thomas, Y., Greber, C., Broadbridge, J., Edwards, A., Newton, A., & Lyons, M. (2014). Attributes of excellence in practice educators: The perspectives of Australian occupational therapy students. *Australian occupational therapy journal, 61*(3),159-167. https://doi-org.proxy1.lib.tju.edu/10.1111/1440-1630.12096

Scanlan, J. M., Care, W. D., & Gessler, S. (2001). Dealing with the unsafe student in clinical practice. *Nurse Educator, 26*(1), 23-27. https://doi.org/10.1097/00006223-200101000-00013

Schenarts, P. J., & Langenfeld, S. (2017). The fundamentals of resident dismissal. *The American Surgeon, 83*(2), 119-126. https://doi.org/10.1177%2F000313481708300210

Silberman, N., LaFay, V., Hansen, R. L., & Fay, P. (2018). Physical therapist student difficulty in clinical education settings: Incidence and outcomes. *Journal of Physical Therapy Education, 32*(2), 175-182. https://doi.org/10.1097/JTE.0000000000000046

Trivinia, B. A., & Johnson, C. R. (2019). Blueprint for success: Measurable learning contracts for level II fieldwork students at risk for failing. *OT Practice, 24*(7), 24-27.

U.S. Department of Education. (2018). Family educational rights and privacy act (FERPA). https://www2.ed.gov/policy/gen/guid/fpco/ferpa/index.html

Wang, V. X., & Torrisi-Steele, G. (2019). Critical theory and transformative learning: Some insights. *Journal of Adult and Continuing Education, 25*(2), 234-251. https://doi.org/10.1177%2F1477971419850837

APPENDIX A
Learning Contract Template

Student Name _____ Fieldwork Site _____

Date _____ In Attendance _____

Areas in which the student is doing well:

Areas in which problems have been identified (relate these to SSLOs):

Failure to achieve these goals by _____ (date) may result in failure of the fieldwork experience.

FWed Signature _____ Date _____

Student Signature _____ Date _____

STUDENT BEHAVIOR (INCLUDING BASELINE/ CURRENT PERFORMANCE LEVEL)	WHY IS THIS BEHAVIOR A PROBLEM (IMPACT ON PATIENTS, FWED, FACILITY, STUDENT LEARNING?)	GOAL (WHAT WE WANT THE NEW BEHAVIOR TO LOOK LIKE)	HOW WILL THE GOAL BE MEASURED?	IDENTIFY STRATEGIES TO ACHIEVE THE GOAL	
				What will student do?	*What will FWed do?*
1. Behavior					
2. Behavior					
3. Behavior					
4. Behavior					

APPENDIX B
Clinical Reasoning Worksheet

Name _____ Date _____

CLIENT DIAGNOSIS/ CONDITION	Typical impairments (how do individuals with this condition typically appear? Symptoms?)	Typical interventions and rationale/theory (what are some interventions commonly used with individuals with this condition?)	
ASSESSMENT OF INDIVIDUAL	Occupational performance challenges (based on *OTPF-4*)	What did you see/hear/feel that makes you say that? (Observations of occupational performance, occupational performance assessment results supporting your assessment)	Occupational performance goals (e.g., self-care, leisure)
	Impairments: Performance components, personal characteristics/factors, environmental factors contributing to challenges (based on *OTPF-4*)	What did you see that makes you say that? (Observations, assessment results, documentation to support this?)	Impairment related goals (e.g., improvement in ADLs, transfers, strength)
	Individual's strengths	What did you see that makes you say that? (Observations, assessment results, documentation to support this?)	How will you incorporate these strengths in treatment?
TREATMENT PLANNING	Focus of intervention (e.g., strength, range of motion, balance, ADLs)	Treatment plan (activity or environmental adaptation) to address this need	Planned possible upgrades and downgrades
RATIONALE	What is your hypothesis about this individual's challenges? (The individual has difficulty with ___ because ...)	What is your treatment hypothesis? (If I provide this intervention I expect ___ to happen)	What is the theory/ evidence/rationale behind your treatment hypothesis?
INTERVENTION/ PLAN	What occurred? (Individual's response to intervention)	Reflection on how it went (effective, not effective? according to plan or surprises?)	What will you do same/ differently next session to progress toward goal?

Unit III

Conclusion and Reflection of the Level II Fieldwork Experience

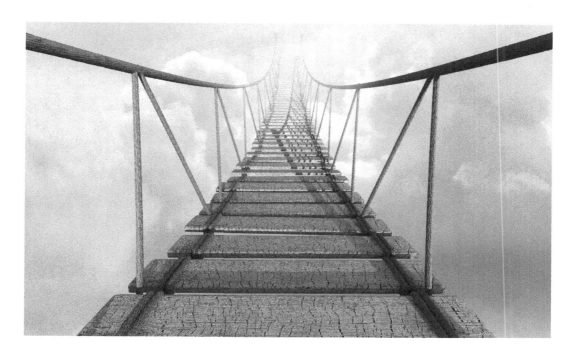

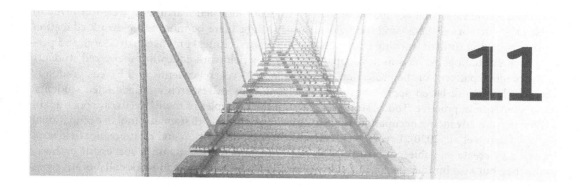

Value-Added Fieldwork
Building Practice Capacity

Patricia Laverdure, OTD, OTR/L, BCP, FAOTA

The value of Level II fieldwork education has long focused on the opportunity for occupational therapy students to develop "competence in applying the occupational therapy process and using evidence-based interventions to meet the occupational needs of a diverse client population" (American Occupational Therapy Association [AOTA], 2016, p. 7012410060p1). The Accreditation Council for Occupational Therapy Education (ACOTE) requires that Level II fieldwork be designed to "develop competent, entry-level, generalist" (2018, p. 41) occupational therapy practitioners who can effectively address client needs and articulate the value of the services provided to them. In addition, the fieldwork experience provides students the opportunity to expand their skills in knowledge translation, clinical reasoning, communication, leadership, advocacy, and management. The experience is intended to socialize students to a deep understanding of occupation and to the very ethos of the profession itself (Cohn, 2019) and serves as a critical "bridge" between academic education and occupational therapy practice (AOTA, 2016, p. 2).

Since its inception, fieldwork has offered students a pathway to practice; a means to expand critical thinking and clinical reasoning in the practice environment. To the profession it has provided a means to empower students to translate its body of knowledge in the care of clients, thereby advancing the practice of occupational therapy. To the clever academic and fieldwork teams working with them, it enables the identification and closure of gaps in practice. Yet, little attention has

DeIuliis, E. D., & Hanson, D. (Eds.).
Fieldwork Educator's Guide to Level II Fieldwork (pp. 323-344).
© 2023 Taylor & Francis Group.

been paid to the value that occupational therapy students and their learning experiences bring to fieldwork educators (FWeds) and the fieldwork site. Might there be more to fieldwork education than establishing student learning objectives, pacing guides, clinical practice instruction, and performance evaluation? At its outset, occupational therapy fieldwork education socialized students to the practice patterns of the profession. Over the next 25 years, academic and FWeds gradually adopted the science-based approaches of its emerging body of research and facilitated students' use of evidence in practice. Today, students, through the examples of their FWeds, are once again embracing and advancing occupation as both a core construct and therapeutic tool of occupational therapy (Canty et al., 2020). Leveraged creatively, through innovation and relationship, fieldwork experiences create valuable opportunities to not only launch students on a successful pathway to practice but also build capacity in fieldwork students and educators to work collaboratively as change agents in complex health care, social, and education systems.

In this chapter, I explore strategies for enhancing the value of the educational experience for the fieldwork student and the value of the fieldwork placement to the FWed and the placement site. I will explore the concept of "What's in it for me?" and shift the paradigm of fieldwork from volume to value; from a means to give back to the profession to a powerful mechanism to build capacity of practitioners, value of our profession, and efficacy of our service delivery systems. I will discuss and reflect a vision of a value-added fieldwork experience.

KEY WORDS

- **Altruism**: The demonstration on unselfish concern for the welfare of others.
- **Burnout**: A condition of overcommitment or overextension that is unmet by commensurate reward.
- **Value-added**: The difference between the value of a product and the costs associated with producing it.
- **Value-added education**: The quantitative progress made by students beyond that which might be typically expected of the student body.
- **Value-added fieldwork**: The sustaining value contributions made to the student, FWed, and the fieldwork placement by the fieldwork experience.
- **Value-based health care**: Health care services in which value outcomes are prioritized over the volume of services provided and ensure that outcomes of value to the client undergird all decision making.

LEARNING OBJECTIVES

By the end of reading this chapter and completing the learning activities, the reader should be able to:

1. Demonstrate the congruency of value-added fieldwork with trends in the delivery of health care services in a value-focused market and the development of the profession.
2. Identify the characteristics, key tools, and collaborative relationships required to envision and enact an innovative value-added learning experience in the Level II fieldwork across practice settings.
3. Articulate the benefits of a value-added learning experience to students, FWeds, and the academic institution.

BOX 11-1

Take a moment to examine your sense of altruism and your altruistic motivations to engage in fieldwork education. Jot down your reflections to the following questions:

1. What are the reasons that you are motivated to educate occupational therapy students?
2. What role does altruism play in your decision to education students (i.e., giving back to the profession)? What are the long-term costs and benefits of your altruism?
3. Describe a situation in which you were burdened by a fieldwork education experience. How did that experience make you feel? What did you do to resolve your feelings?
4. Describe a situation in which you felt like you, your patients, and/or your practice benefitted from a fieldwork education experience. What did you or the student do to facilitate that experience?
5. How might you maximize the opportunities to add value to your fieldwork placements?

IS ALTRUISM ENOUGH?
VALUE FOR THE FIELDWORK EDUCATOR

Across the professional literature, stewardship, altruism, and a solid sense of goodwill and satisfaction are identified as key considerations in the decision to train students in one's practice setting. Evenson et al. (2015) identifies personal satisfaction as one of the top five perceived benefits of occupational therapy practitioners who participate in fieldwork education. Altruism, one of the core values of the profession, is defined as "the demonstration on unselfish concern for the welfare of others" (AOTA, 2020a, p. 36) from which many of us obtain satisfaction in our work. Through our commitment to caring for and attending to the needs of others, occupational therapists demonstrate this professional prerequisite. Staying beyond contracted hours to ensure effective patient treatment plans and documentation, going the extra mile in professional service to patients and programs, and taking on the extra work to serve as FWed to support student education are altruistic behaviors that exemplify the cultural stereotype of an effective if not "good" occupational therapy practitioner. While altruism may provide a vantage from which to pitch and develop fieldwork placements and programs, it has proven a hard characteristic to leverage to sustain it. Consider for a moment the reasons you decided to accept your first student. Did your FWed from when you were an occupational therapy student inspire you and you wanted to give back to the profession? Was your merit raise, job promotion, or move up the clinical ladder tied to working with fieldwork students? Using the guided reflection in Box 11-1 to consider the reasons that you are interested in fieldwork education.

Altruist behaviors provide an important foundation perhaps for the development of ethical code and literacy; however, in fieldwork these behaviors may be anachronistic. "*Giving back*," "*I wouldn't be here if I did not have a dedicated FWed*," and "*It's my duty to the profession*," seem quite noble considerations in developing fieldwork experiences. Yet, Zeman and Harvison (2017) suggest that balancing professional duties with the emotional energy required for patient care in complex systems can lead to burnout. Rogers and Dodson (1988) describe burnout as a condition of overcommitment or overextension that is unmet by commensurate reward. An emerging body of literature suggests, in fact, that altruism in the face of complex work responsibilities and duties may threaten practitioner resilience and contribute to disengagement, stress, anxiety, and burnout (Maslach et al., 2001; Wilkinson et al., 2009). As a result, altruism has emerged as a contested attribute in health care professionalism and ethics (Harris, 2017).

Practitioner well-being has become an important priority for AOTA (n.d.), while at the same time developing and maintaining fieldwork experiences are critical to the advancement of the profession and its workforce. Care for one's self, reciprocal and meaningful engagement with others, and commensurate reward for one's efforts equip practitioners with the tools to support those who are served by the profession (AOTA, 2020a). Reciprocity and reward are not concepts commonly associated with fieldwork, yet studies suggest that they may sustain medical altruism, particularly in complex, fragmented, and episodic health care systems (Feldman, 2017; Jones, 2002). It appears that reciprocal benefit plays an important role in sustaining altruistic behaviors.

Though not explicitly examined in occupational therapy fieldwork education research, academic FWeds have been employing reciprocity and reward in their relationships with FWeds for some time. In my own practice, I have provided training and guidance, access to library resources, and continuing education credits as common reciprocal and rewarding advantages to support FWeds with whom I work. My occasional on-site visit, replete with university and occupational therapy swag and resources and, of course, the requisite tray of cookies, provides sought-after engagement and recognition needed to mitigate disenfranchisement and disengagement and promote ongoing commitment to student education. In return, academic FWeds receive a glimpse into current practice that is then shared with program faculty to support currency of the academic program.

Short of the exception of the student project designed with the dual purpose of enhancing student learning in the fieldwork setting and providing valuable knowledge or material resource to the FWed and practice, little has been invested in considering the opportunity for reciprocal reward received either directly or indirectly from the fieldwork student, despite the fact that it is often in this reciprocity that "benevolence to one individual increases the chances of receiving help directly in return or indirectly from others" (Jones, 2002, p. 624). Deriving value from students during the fieldwork experience, it stands to reason, may be an important tool to translate knowledge from academic education and occupational therapy practice for students and FWeds alike. In addition, it well may be a vehicle that reduces the burden of overextension, burnout, and fieldwork education disengagement.

Could it be that fieldwork can benefit you, the FWed, in ways beyond your desire to give back to the profession?

Benefits of Value-Added Fieldwork to Health Care Settings and Practitioners

Medical education systems have been exploring the development of partnerships for reciprocal capacity building for some time though a great deal of this research has focused on clinical research and knowledge translation and implementation (Monroe-Wise et al., 2014; Rabin et al., 2016). Though medical education internships, like occupational therapy fieldwork experiences, have been an instructional signature of the profession's educational approach since its inception, little focus has been placed on the use of this integral partnership as a tool to build capacity of health care practice settings and practitioners. A number of medical institutions have begun to explore the possibility of advancement of international health care systems through the development of partnerships in medical student training (Drobac & Morse, 2016; Rabin et al., 2016). The resulting concept of equity in partnership, in which the university, site, and student mutually benefit has shown promise in increasing student placement opportunities, developing the effective delivery of learning intervention that is relevant for the environment, enhancing opportunity for real-life application of acquired knowledge and skills of practitioners and staff, promoting development of sustainable career advancement trajectories, and moving health markets and practice forward (Crump & Sugarman, 2008; Drobac & Morse, 2016; Frenk et al., 2010; Rabin et al., 2016).

Imagine if you were to receive just as much, if not more, than the student or the educational institution as a result of the fieldwork experiences you provide! What might that look like?

Value-Added Fieldwork: Congruent With the Values-Based Health Care System

Value-added is a now familiar term derived from the field of economics to distinguish the difference between the value of a product and the costs associated with producing it. The construct represents not only the knowledge, materials, supplies, and labor required to bring the product to market, but the projected value the product will bring to the consumer. The economic value enhancements provide incentive to consumers to purchase the product at the price at which it is being sold. In the field of health care, the economic construct of value-added places a definitive value on the health outcomes clients achieved for every dollar spent (Porter, 2010). The construct of value-added in health care was initially met with skepticism. Fearful that the cost containment implied by the proposition of adding value to service delivery would decrease the quality and accessibility of health care, there was initial resistance to shifting service delivery measures from volume (number of services provided) to the value of the service for the consumer (health care outcomes).

Value, argues Porter in his 2010 *New England Journal of Medicine* commentary, is defined as "outcomes relative to costs [and] cost reduction without regard to the outcomes achieved is dangerous and self-defeating, leading to false 'savings' and potentially limiting effective care" (p. 2477). Collecting costs associated with client care across the entire care cycle and evaluating them against client outcomes supports health care accountability and structural cost reductions (e.g., reallocation of spending, elimination of non-value adding services, improving health care processes particularly those that are client-centered, and advancing health care innovation) improves long-term health care and quality of life outcomes for clients (Porter, 2010). Following in the footsteps of evidence-based practice, the construct of value is prominent in today's health care market. Some suggest that this signals a transition from evidence-based practice to value-based medicine in which the best available evidence and clinical expertise is made understandable by the client and the client's values, preference, and concerns are considered as clients enter into shared decision making with health care professionals (Brown et al., 2005; Greenhalgh et al., 2014).

A value-based health care system is one in which value outcomes are prioritized over the volume of services provided and ensure that outcomes of value to the client undergird all decision making (Porter & Teisberg, 2006, 2007) and are explicitly measured and analyzed across the entire care cycle (Porter, 2009). Marzorati and Pravettoni (2017) argue that health care is moving toward a model that prioritizes (1) client-centered and empowered approaches, (2) client engagement and participation, (3) client well-being and satisfaction (psycho-cognitive medicine), and (4) predictive and preventative care (Figure 11-1). Not only are these priorities in alignment with the AOTA's (2015) value proposition that occupational therapy is a valuable client-centered, evidence-based, and cost-effective service, but they characterize the key learning objectives for occupational therapy fieldwork experiences. While health care professions, service providers, and health care payers have been slowly advancing these priorities, occupational therapy fieldwork and academic educators have been building their and their students' capacities to approach client care in this critical way for some time.

The Centers for Medicare & Medicaid Services (CMS) have been a leading proponent in the structural transition from volume to value in health care reimbursement (2017). Driven by exponential increases in health care costs and little accountability, CMS has implemented a number of value-based programs over the last decade (e.g., End-Stage Renal Disease Quality Incentive Program, Hospital Value-Based Purchasing Program, Value Modifier Program [also called the Physician Value-Based Modifier], Hospital Acquired Conditions Reduction Program, and Hospital Readmission Reduction Program) culminating in Patient Driven Payment Model for skilled nursing facilities that went into effect on October 1, 2019 and the Patient Driven Grouping Model for home health that went into effect on January 1, 2020 (CMS, 2019a, 2019b, 2019c). The CMS shift from fee for service to value-based reimbursement is:

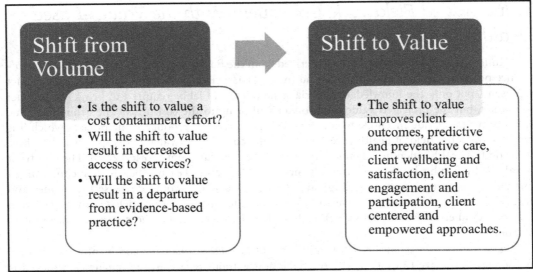

Figure 11-1. The shift from volume to value in health care.

- Based on the premise that high-quality care improves client health outcomes, increases satisfaction, and reduces health care costs
- Relies on a foundation of client-centered care
- Requires reliable quality measures to identify the outcomes of intervention and projects the need for future support
- Aligns with AOTA's stance that occupational therapy is a client-centered, evidenced-based, valuable, and cost-effective health care service (Tickle-Degnan, 2002; Lamb & McCarley, 2019; Miller, 2018; Scott & Eminger, 2016)

As occupational therapy practitioners and their teams transition to value-based reimbursement systems, what has become clear is that (1) occupational therapy is solidly grounded upon the founding principles of value-based care, (2) occupational therapy practitioners can play a significant role in identifying and assessing client-centered outcomes that empower engagement and participation and improve satisfaction and well-being, and (3) academic educators, FWeds, and students have capacity-building needs around value-driven health markets that can be addressed through collaboration (Laverdure et al., 2020a). Some service delivery systems have been impacted more significantly than others by value-based reimbursement.

How has yours been impacted?

Has that impact trickled down to your student program?

Have you leveraged your association with the academic institutions and students that you work with to advance the value of your service delivery?

Box 11-2 offers guided reflection questions to help you consider these impacts and what they might mean to your student program, practice, and site.

BOX 11-2

- In what ways has the volume to value trends impacted your practice and your practice setting?
- How have you leveraged your training in client-centered and occupation focused care in identifying client-centered outcomes that empower engagement and participation and improve satisfaction and well-being?
- What ways might you collaborate with academic institutions and students to maximize value?

Extending Value to Multiple Stakeholders Through Collaboration

In academia, value-added refers to the quantitative progress made by occupational therapy and occupational therapy assistant students beyond that which might be typically expected of the student body (Department of Health, 2015). Students, however, enter fieldwork prepared to (Laverdure et al., 2020b):

- Share research literacy skills and evidence-based practice
- Work within the parameters of value-based care
- Provide client-centered care (evaluation, client-centered and occupation-based assessment and intervention planning)
- Collect data for progress monitoring and outcomes measurement (e.g., activities of daily living, instrumental activities of daily living, quality of life, home safety, vision, ergonomics, driving, fall risk, swallowing, and mental health)
- Use collaborative team decision-making approaches

While fieldwork is designed to align with ACOTE (2018) standards and program curricula, fieldwork programs vary quite considerably. What is important for the purposes of capacity building is that (1) student learning objectives clearly align with the standards, the program's learning outcomes, and the site's expectations, (2) students demonstrate the distinct value of occupation in learning process and outcomes, and (3) students produce explicit positive occupational outcomes for service recipients. When fieldwork experiences are intentionally aligned with the program objectives, when occupation and its dimensions are explicitly linked to occupational therapy practice, and when experiences are anchored to the development of skills to meet the occupational needs of society, fieldwork experiences are primed to build capacity of academic faculty, FWeds, and students alike. Table 11-1 highlights the value-added capacity-building considerations for occupational therapy fieldwork.

Creating value-added innovative experiences in fieldwork requires that academic educators, FWeds, and students work together to examine the program, site, and student learning objectives, and consider the collective needs and interests of all involved. Students need fieldwork experiences to advance their knowledge of occupation and its dimensions; build the clinical reasoning skills to meet the present and future occupational needs of individuals, communities, and populations; and to strengthen their professionalism and competence in career responsibilities (Laverdure et al., 2020b). As students learn within the parameters of client-centered, occupation-based, theory-driven, and evidence-informed care and activate their reflection skills in occupational therapy practice, they enact AOTA's Vision 2025 (AOTA, 2017).

TABLE 11-1

BUILDING CAPACITY THROUGH COLLABORATION

ACOTE STANDARDS AND AOTA GUIDANCE FOR FIELDWORK CONSIDERATION 1

Through the collaboration between academic faculty and FWeds, students are given the opportunity to achieve the competencies necessary to meet the present and future occupational needs of individuals, communities, and populations.

Fieldwork Educators	Students	Academic Educators
Fieldwork experiences address the occupational needs of clients and may promote opportunities for FWeds to effect change in their practice settings in the following ways: • Clarifying the distinct value of occupational therapy and articulating its full scope of practice. • Expanding community/population health approaches (population-based/ occupation-based population health approaches). • Advancing education, advocacy, policy changes that improve client outcomes. • Create wellness and prevention programs (e.g., health disparities). • Address occupational justice issues that may affect patient care (e.g., access). • Reduce the impact of health disparities in the facility/region.	Fieldwork experiences facilitate the development of the attitudes and skills of an entry-level practitioner, including not simply the assumption of a full patient caseload, but also the responsibility for independent learning influencing lifelong career trajectories.	Program objectives are addressed, and student learning outcomes improve.

(continued)

THE VISION OF THE VALUE-ADDED FIELDWORK

Innovation becomes possible when focus is placed on collaborative learning objectives rather than simply maintaining traditional scheduling practices (e.g., two 8- [occupational therapy assistant] and 12- [occupational therapy] week fieldwork experiences, across two different sites) and traditional pacing guides. There are, in fact, no ACOTE (2018) standards that require students to maintain a full-time, one-on-one client caseload at the end of the fieldwork experience to demonstrate entry-level competence. Productivity expectations are not ACOTE requirements and may, in fact, inhibit the development of clinical reasoning and client-centered care. Instead, academic educators, FWeds, and students who align the fieldwork learning objectives to their collective interests and needs may positively influence the value outcomes of the learning experience as well as their own professional trajectories.

Adding value to the fieldwork experience by including innovative learning opportunities can occur at any point along the fieldwork placement. Critical examination of ACOTE (2018)

TABLE 11-1 (CONTINUED)
BUILDING CAPACITY THROUGH COLLABORATION

ACOTE STANDARDS AND AOTA GUIDANCE FOR FIELDWORK CONSIDERATION 2

The fieldwork experience is designed to link and actualize knowledge of occupation and its dimensions and the distinctiveness of occupational therapy in the unique learning context. Fieldwork is designed to transmit the philosophical core values and beliefs that enable ethical practice (client centered, occupation based, theory driven, and evidence informed).

Fieldwork Educators	Students	Academic Educators
In collaboration, students and FWeds produce explicit positive occupational outcomes for service recipients. FWeds build capacity in value and occupation-based practice.	Students demonstrate the imperative value of occupation in learning the occupational therapy process and outcomes and engage intentionally in learning activities that connect practice to occupation.	Academic faculty build a community of educators and collaborators to teach students the value of occupation in health and wellness.

ACOTE STANDARDS AND AOTA GUIDANCE FOR FIELDWORK CONSIDERATION 3

The fieldwork experience is designed to provide the student with the opportunity to carry out professional responsibilities under the graded supervision and ongoing evaluation of qualified personnel serving as a role model.

Fieldwork Educators	Students	Academic Educators
Fieldwork supervision focuses explicitly on occupation in the structure or application of learning and strengthens FWed's knowledge and application of the value of: • Occupation as a therapeutic tool • Theory in practice • Clinical reasoning	Students are responsible for active participation in the supervision process and build the skills of collaborative learning through: • Creation and completion of learning objectives • Completion of assigned learning activities and assignments • Proactive and ongoing communication with the FWed • Continual self-assessment and reflection • Participation in formal and informal assessments	Academic faculty build knowledge of occupational therapy theory, evaluation, and intervention in current practice, which influences research development, implementation and dissemination and education.

(continued)

standards, program objectives, academic and FWed capacity, motivation and collaboration (and sheer will), and student preparation provides the necessary foundation for successful value-added experiences in traditional, nontraditional (research, administration, educational), and role-emerging placements. Many FWeds wait for the last 3 to 4 weeks of a student's placement to consider the

TABLE 11-1 (CONTINUED)

BUILDING CAPACITY THROUGH COLLABORATION

ACOTE STANDARDS AND AOTA GUIDANCE FOR FIELDWORK CONSIDERATION 4

The fieldwork experience is designed to promote the transfer of knowledge, clinical reasoning, and reflective practice in the promotion of meaningful occupation and the dimension of occupation.

- Students demonstrate the imperative value of occupation in learning process and outcomes.

- Students produce explicit positive occupational outcomes for service recipients.

Fieldwork Educators	Students	Academic Educators
As students gain clinical and leadership skills and those skills are effectively leveraged to promote positive client outcomes, FWeds can articulate the value proposition of their services and the fieldwork education program. Shifting the narrative from volume (productivity) to value (client outcomes) can enable FWeds the opportunity to build skills in advocacy for change.	Fieldwork experiences provide students: • Opportunities to apply the occupational therapy process • Structured opportunities for reflection of the occupational therapy process in action • In-depth learning opportunities to deliver occupational therapy services to clients to include individuals, communities, and populations • Innovative opportunities to build skills in team collaboration, communication, and leadership	With the shift from volume and productivity metrics to high-quality client outcomes, the value to fieldwork education opportunities becomes more visible. Rather than relying on altruism for fieldwork placements, value-added outcomes drive interest in and availability of fieldwork placements.

(continued)

unique value-added opportunities, assuming that a student's level of productivity and patient care is approaching entry-level skill. However, the coronavirus global pandemic brought tremendous innovative collaboration among academic educators, FWeds, and students who modeled the way to enact value-added opportunities throughout fieldwork. What we learned is that these novel value-added activities not only provided effective formative learning activities that resulted in competent practice but that they enhance the capacity of the FWeds they work with and their client's outcomes. Fieldwork was upended by the coronavirus, but important and lasting outcomes were realized:

- Students and FWeds alike focused on competency outcomes that extended beyond the role of direct practice activities and include all our professional roles including educator, advocate, and researcher.

- Students, FWeds, and academic educators were energized by creative and collaborative opportunities that enabled all to develop their capacities beyond simple application of therapy procedures to analysis and evaluation of our therapeutic methods to advance practice approaches.

TABLE 11-1 (CONTINUED)
BUILDING CAPACITY THROUGH COLLABORATION

ACOTE STANDARDS AND AOTA GUIDANCE FOR FIELDWORK CONSIDERATION 5

The fieldwork experience is designed to promote effective administration and management of occupational therapy service provision.

Fieldwork Educators	Students	Academic Educators
Innovative fieldwork designs often include the development of administration and management skills and practices that link explicitly to access to occupational therapy services or promote optimal participation in occupations of meaning for individuals, communities, and/or populations. FWeds can leverage student skills to advance program evaluation and development.	Students engage intentionally in learning activities that support their ability to manage, organize, and promote occupational therapy services.	Innovation in fieldwork education influences research, collaborative partnership in emerging practice, and educational opportunities.

Adapted from ACOTE, 2018; AOTA, 2012, 2016, 2018a, 2018b; Laverdure et al., 2020b.

- Students, fieldwork and academic educators, and site administrators mobilized their collective and collaborative energies and passion to address and close gaps in service delivery and value-based outcomes.

In a recent meeting of the Virginia Occupational Therapy Education Council (2020), my colleagues and I considered our vision of a value-added fieldwork across a number of practice settings. Using the areas of performance on the AOTA (2020b) Fieldwork Performance Evaluation (FWPE), we considered the ways in which we might develop value-added fieldwork contributions across specific practice areas. Table 11-2 includes some of the exemplars that were developed in the areas of acute care, skilled nursing, and outpatient pediatric services. In all of the activities indicated, students demonstrated their knowledge and application of the occupational therapy process, FWeds and their practice sites built greater capacity and added value to their client outcomes, and academic programs expanded their understanding of current value-based occupational therapy practice.

Shortly after the start of the COVID-19 pandemic, I received a call regarding the impending fall 2020 fieldwork placements at a large school district for five students (two doctor of occupational therapy, two master of science occupational therapy, and one occupational therapy assistant) from institutions across the state of Virginia. Given the shift from in-class education to remote learning, the fieldwork coordinator was struggling to imagine a way to proceed with the placements. In the conversation that ensued, we considered the many challenges facing the school district and its occupational therapy staff (e.g., remote learning and the associated privacy considerations, hybrid learning environments and educational team collaboration, support, and

TABLE 11-2

VALUE-ADDED FIELDWORK CONTRIBUTIONS IN ACUTE CARE, SKILLED NURSING, AND OUTPATIENT PEDIATRIC SETTINGS

AREAS OF PERFORMANCE ON THE FIELDWORK PERFORMANCE EVALUATION (AOTA, 2020B)	ACUTE CARE	SKILLED NURSING	OUTPATIENT PEDIATRICS
Basic tenets	Develop a quick reference guide of diagnoses, their associated condition, and precautions commonly seen in the acute care setting	Develop a quick reference guide to strengthen understanding of the communicable disease protocols	Develop tools to support caregiver carryover of positioning and feeding supports for children at home and training them in their use
Screening and evaluation	Examine the use of specific assessment methods with varying populations	Research commonly used assessments in the skilled nursing facility and development of recommendations for value- and occupation-based assessment choices	Establish tools to support caregiver participation in virtual evaluation Identify screening and assessment tools that can be used in the virtual environment
Intervention	Task analyses on readily available treatment resources and materials in the intensive care unit	Compile a resource binder with information on commonly seen diagnoses, pharmacological issues, and interventions	Develop and implement group programs to address gaps in services Create a video library of occupational therapy interventions for home therapy programs

(continued)

training needs, personal protective equipment) and what a fieldwork experience could look like for one student, never mind five. Not wanting to cancel the placements, using a value-envisioned fieldwork framework, a discourse to reimagine a fieldwork placement in which students would be enmeshed in the occupational therapy process, designing and implementing evaluation and intervention plans, and broadening and deepening their clinical reasoning skills took place. Box 11-3 illustrates the ways in which we approached the challenges and created a school-based value-added fieldwork experience. The outcomes were so impactful, the model has been expanded to school districts throughout the state.

TABLE 11-2 (CONTINUED)
VALUE-ADDED FIELDWORK CONTRIBUTIONS IN ACUTE CARE, SKILLED NURSING, AND OUTPATIENT PEDIATRIC SETTINGS

AREAS OF PERFORMANCE ON THE FIELDWORK PERFORMANCE EVALUATION (AOTA, 2020B)	ACUTE CARE	SKILLED NURSING	OUTPATIENT PEDIATRICS
Management of occupational therapy services	Chart audit to examine the outcomes of acute care interventions	Spend time with discharge planner to deepen understanding of community resources available in the area for effective discharge planning	Develop therapy kits to use in therapy sessions or to share with families for home programs

Compile a database for caregiver handouts and websites for effective dissemination

Establish resources for telehealth provision |
| Communication and professional behaviors | Creation of new patient education materials | Creation of new patient education materials and discharge plans for patients and their caregivers | Create infographics to support therapy services |

Adapted from Virginia Occupational Therapy Education Council. (2020). Setting specific fieldwork innovations: How are they working. https://sites.google.com/view/vaotec/meetings-presentations/past-meetings/november-2020?authuser=0.

Value-added fieldwork experiences provide an important means to strengthen skills in a weakly developed student knowledge or performance area. They can be important tools for challenging the skills of an advanced student as well. They can also serve to support the unique interests of students as they progress through fieldwork and bring their fieldwork experience to a close. Value-added fieldwork experiences provide an opportunity for students to creatively build skills while potentially impacting the capacity of fieldwork and academic educators alike. It is important that value-added experience balance the value between the student and the FWed. If I had a dime for all the times I heard student tell me they did an in service on Parkinson's disease, I'd be rich! That is certainly not to say that a project on this condition is not a value contribution, and, in fact, in some fieldwork situations it may be. Instead, I suggest that as you design value-added fieldwork experience in collaboration with your student; remember the competencies that they bring to the placement and consider the gaps in your practice. Refer to Box 11-4 to guide yosur collaborative generation of ideas of value-added learning activities that benefit you and your practice, as well as your student.

Box 11-3
Case Scenario

To address the challenges of placing students and establishing a fulfilling fieldwork experience in a large school district in Virginia during the COVID-19 pandemic, we began by looking at the ACOTE (2018) standards, the Occupational Therapy Fieldwork Education: Value and Purpose official document (AOTA, 2016), the COE Guidelines for an Occupational Therapy Fieldwork Experience–Level II (2012), the FWPE (AOTA, 2020), the institution's objectives, and the site-specific objectives. We then identified an array of outcomes that we could use to evaluate the students' performance across the component areas of the students' fieldwork placements. A sampling of the outcomes are as follows:

- Fundamentals of practice: Design instructional materials that will enable teachers to help parents with proper positioning of students while they are engaged in remote learning and instruct teachers in their use.
- Screening and evaluation: Examine diagnostic assessments and develop resources to support administration; establish protocols and innovations for remote/virtual evaluation and assessment; develop tools to facilitate the development of an occupational profile in school practice; design clinical reasoning tools on assessment choice and the use of data for collaborative decision making; develop training resources/modules on the tools for the district and state.
- Intervention: Develop vertically aligned learning progressions to align with learning outcomes and identifying the evidence to support occupational therapy's role in high leverage practices; develop tools and strategies to support school/district-wide initiatives in remote learning context for positive behavioral support and mental health; examine intervention research and develop recommendations for home and school; create intervention tools to send home or to be used in remote learning classrooms.
- Communication: Develop caregiver resources (e.g., training, materials, and equipment); establish and provide training for teachers and staff.

We then realigned the site's student learning objectives and pacing guide. We met with the students on their first day and discussed the fieldwork model and the potential outcomes and provided choices for them across the FWPE items. In collaboration with their assigned FWeds, the site clinical coordinator, their AFWCs, and me, the students chose to develop a clinical reasoning resource to support the choice of assessments in school practice. The students evaluated the array of tools available and employed their knowledge of the practice context and their clinical reasoning to identify the clinical scenario for which the assessment would be warranted. They then used the tool later in their fieldwork to choose assessment to evaluate clients in the setting. The tool was distributed to not only the therapists in the school district but to therapists in school practice across the state.

This unique fieldwork model not only enabled the placements to move forward in the pandemic, but it also resulted in a valuable clinical reasoning tool for all. The student evaluations of the placement indicated that not only did the students find the placement valuable, they indicated that their collaborative clinical work on the resource deepened their clinical reasoning and use of the occupational therapy process.

Box 11-4

REFLECTION

Notice nowhere did I suggest the traditional inservice that has become the staple fieldwork project for students on fieldwork. I did not make this suggestion for two reasons. First, value-added learning activities are not, in my mind, projects. It may be nuanced, but value-added learning activities are supplement learning opportunities that enable students to deeply immerse into the occupational therapy process in a way that they might not have the opportunity to do so in the fast-paced therapy setting. When they do so, the learning activities add value to their learning and contribute to their fieldwork site's staff and clients. Second, projects generally add little value. How many times have you sat through an inservice on a topic that either you already know or adds little value to your practice or practice setting?

Take a moment to consider the ways in which you can work collaboratively with the AFWC and your students to design unique learning activities that add value, make your work with students more valuable, and change the course trajectory of your practice and your client outcomes.

Collaboration Is the Key

To effectively design a value-added fieldwork takes the collaborative commitment of students, FWeds, and academic fieldwork coordinators (AFWCs). Working together, each member of the fieldwork education team can shift the experience of fieldwork from volume to value. You will find yourself framing the experience less as a way to give back and more as a way to advance your capacity as a professional and as an occupational therapy practitioner. Table 11-3 outlines just a few of the novel ways that learning might be approached in each area of the FWPE and highlights the contributions that the value-added approach might make to the fieldwork site, student, and academic program. I encourage you to reach out to your academic program and discuss ways in which you might build value in your student programs. It is a fair proposition to ask *"what is it in it for you?"*

TABLE 11-3

CREATING VALUE-ADDED EXPERIENCES IN FIELDWORK

FIELDWORK PERFORMANCE EVALUATION AREAS OF PERFORMANCE (AOTA, 2020B)	HIGHER EDUCATION INSTITUTION FACULTY	FIELDWORK EDUCATOR	OCCUPATIONAL THERAPY STUDENT
Fundamentals of practice	Expand student training opportunities to enhance client safety across the curriculum. Conduct clinical research and knowledge dissemination in alignment with site requirements.	Design high-quality community discharge plans that improve satisfaction and participation and reduce hospital readmissions. Implement evidence-based interventions in behavioral and physical health.	Develop tools and resources for family and staff to eliminate safety hazards and reduce unsafe practices. Design patient resources to enhance safety (e.g., fall prevention, driving safety).
Basic tenets	Enhance understanding and prioritization of research efforts, implementation, and dissemination to address the values, beliefs, and distinct perspectives of the clients and providers served.	Advance skills to lead teams in the development of holistic and individualized client-centered care that improves health outcomes and quality of life. Develop programs to improve health and wellness outcomes by building continuity across the continuum of care. Engage in clinical research.	Access and translate relevant research literature to support practice. Share research evidence with practitioners. Share and develop staff research literacy skills. Use relevant research to advocate for the role of occupational therapy with specific diagnoses and/or interventions. Engage in clinical research.

(continued)

TABLE 11-3 (CONTINUED)

CREATING VALUE-ADDED EXPERIENCES IN FIELDWORK

FIELDWORK PERFORMANCE EVALUATION AREAS OF PERFORMANCE (AOTA, 2020B)	HIGHER EDUCATION INSTITUTION FACULTY	FIELDWORK EDUCATOR	OCCUPATIONAL THERAPY STUDENT
Screening and evaluation	Expand knowledge of available and currently used theory, evaluation practice, and assessment tools.	Expand skill and knowledge in occupation-based evaluation, use of the occupation profile and value and occupation-based assessment tools. Expand the collection of client data to complete the occupation profile and administer related assessments (e.g., Interest Checklist, Canadian Occupational Performance Measure, Depression Scales, Quality of Life Measures).	Explore research on and psychometric properties of assessment tools. Expand the use of outcome measures that address value (e.g., Barthel, Lawton, Functional Reach Test, Get Up and Go Test, clinical observations). Develop recommendations for the use of value and occupation-based assessment tools. Provide training on novel assessment tools.

(continued)

SUMMARY

Innovative value-added learning opportunities in the Level II fieldwork experience offers students as well as fieldwork and academic educators the opportunity to expand knowledge and skills and advance their career trajectories in the field of occupational therapy. Value over volume has been an important construct in the health care market, and it may well serve as an important metric in advancing clinical reasoning and reflective practice in fieldwork education. Value-added fieldwork experiences, built around the collaborative needs and interests of students as well as fieldwork and academic educators, provide a pathway for the enactment of Vision 2025 (AOTA, 2017) by centering learning experiences that build the knowledge, skills, and sustaining leadership capacity of students; strengthen the collaborative, value-focused impact of FWeds; and inform and facilitate the creation and dissemination of knowledge to guide the creation of culturally responsive, occupation-based, and individualized services by academic educators and scholars.

TABLE 11-3 (CONTINUED)

CREATING VALUE-ADDED EXPERIENCES IN FIELDWORK

FIELDWORK PERFORMANCE EVALUATION AREAS OF PERFORMANCE (AOTA, 2020B)	HIGHER EDUCATION INSTITUTION FACULTY	FIELDWORK EDUCATOR	OCCUPATIONAL THERAPY STUDENT
Intervention	Identify knowledge gaps in clinical practice and design clinically relevant research to address practice needs. Design educational opportunities to enhance student knowledge of current best practices. Design learning opportunities for students to critically examine practices currently used in the field.	Critically assess occupational therapy interventions provided.	Engage clients in occupation-based treatment. Provide client education groups to increase health literacy. Develop self-care kits to enhance occupational engagement. Expand opportunities for social and leisure occupations. Expand the array of occupation-based interventions available to practitioners. Collaborate with other disciplines to improve client outcomes. Educate clients on self-advocacy.
Management of occupational therapy services	Collaboratively develop innovative program to meet the needs of clients. Develop community-based programs to educate students and provide needed services. Establish services in nontraditional and role-emerging settings to enhance access.	Examine current program practices, processes, and outcomes. Develop programs to meet the needs of clients.	Establish training resources for appropriate referrals (e.g., providing presentations). Conduct program assessment.

(continued)

TABLE 11-3 (CONTINUED)

CREATING VALUE-ADDED EXPERIENCES IN FIELDWORK

FIELDWORK PERFORMANCE EVALUATION AREAS OF PERFORMANCE (AOTA, 2020B)	HIGHER EDUCATION INSTITUTION FACULTY	FIELDWORK EDUCATOR	OCCUPATIONAL THERAPY STUDENT
Communication and professional behaviors	Disseminate novel practices (e.g., conference presentations, publications).	Disseminate novel practices (e.g., conference presentations, publications).	Create client education handouts and training resources (e.g., chronic disease, depression). Identify and develop handouts on community resources. Attend care conferences and/or meetings with the client and family.

Adapted from Laverdure et al., 2020a, 2020b.

The reciprocity in capacity building through equity partnerships in fieldwork will advance the capacity of occupational therapy professionals to serve as change agents and usher in the value outcomes of evidence-based, client-centered, and cost-effective service delivery. The value proposition for Level II fieldwork lies in its ability to shift the focus of the health care market from volume to value. When academic educators, FWeds, and students collaborate in partnership to prioritize value over volume in learning, they all benefit.

LEARNING ACTIVITIES

1. What are ways academic educators can establish innovative value-added fieldwork experience? Consider the following:

   a. Examining the ACOTE (2018) standards and your program objectives.

   b. Examining course content for student preparation in traditional, nontraditional, and role-emerging practice settings.

   c. Conducting an audit of faculty interest and collaboration.

   d. Examining neighboring institution of higher education, fieldwork site and educators, and students for possible collaboration.

   e. Designing outcome measures that align with the ACOTE (2018) standards and program objectives (may align with the FWPE [AOTA, 2020b] or the performance assessment used at the institution).

   Reflection: The AFWCs of VOTEC meet regularly to discuss the promotion of collaboratively developed learning activities to implement across the state. We have established innovative fieldwork opportunities in traditional settings such as acute care, skilled nursing, inpatient and outpatient, and educational settings, but have also collaborated on experiences in novel areas, such as community-based settings such as homeless shelters and club houses.

2. What are ways FWeds can establish innovative value-added fieldwork experiences? Consider the following:

   a. Examining your practice and your practice setting.

   b. Identifying areas of need and practice/programmatic interest (e.g., client care, research, administration, education, advocacy).

   c. Reaching out to institutions of higher education to develop or expand your fieldwork program.

   d. Developing site-specific and student learning objectives to support the learning outcomes.

   e. Monitoring student progress through the fieldwork experience.

   Reflection: Value-added learning activities are only limited by our imaginations. Imagine the ways that you really go a hold on clinical reasoning or the *Occupational Therapy Practice Framework* (AOTA, 2020d). Where are your gaps in translating knowledge in your practice setting? Spend a few moments jotting down the ways that you might engage your student in learning activities that not only enable them to immerse and engage in reflection in the occupational therapy process and expand their clinical reasoning but add value to you, your practice, and your clients.

3. What are ways occupational therapy students can establish innovative value-added fieldwork experience? Consider the following:

   a. Carefully examining the site description and its site-specific objectives.

   b. Conducting a thorough audit of your learning interest and objectives.

   c. Discussing your interests and objectives with your fieldwork and academic educators.

   d. Designing specific learning outcomes to monitor your learning progress and outcomes. (include the specific measurable outcome, how you will measure it, and when you want to accomplish it).

   e. While you conduct your innovative value-added fieldwork experience, make explicit connections to occupational therapy's philosophical core, values, beliefs (e.g., client centered, occupation based, theory driven, and evidence informed), and the development of your skills in clinical reasoning and reflective practice.

   Reflection: Consider not only your learning needs but also the needs of your FWed, the site, and the clients you collaboratively serve. How might you deepen your clinical reasoning skills through a learning activity that provides value to the fieldwork site? Share your ideas with your FWed and your AFWC. Be open to the ideas of others as you develop your learning activity plans.

REFERENCES

Accreditation Council for Occupational Therapy Education. (2018). 2018 Accreditation Council for Occupational Therapy Education (ACOTE®) Standards and Interpretive Guide. https://www.aota.org/~/media/Corporate/Files/EducationCareers/Accredit/StandardsReview/2018-ACOTE-Standards-Interpretive-Guide.pdf

American Occupational Therapy Association. (n.d.). AOTA's Commitment Statement to the Action Collaborative on Clinician Well-Being and Resilience. https://nam.edu/wp-content/uploads/2020/04/AOTA-Commitment-Statement.pdf

American Occupational Therapy Association. (2012). COE Guidelines for an Occupational Therapy Fieldwork Experience - Level II. https://www.aota.org/~/media/Corporate/Files/EducationCareers/Educators/Fieldwork/LevelII/COE%20Guidelines%20for%20an%20Occupational%20Therapy%20Fieldwork%20Experience%20--%20Level%20II--Final.pdf

American Occupational Therapy Association. (2015). Articulating the distinct value of occupational therapy. https://www.aota.org/Publications-News/AOTANews/2015/distinct-value-of-occupational-therapy.aspx

American Occupational Therapy Association. (2016). Occupational therapy fieldwork education: Value and purpose. *American Journal of Occupational Therapy, 70*(Suppl. 2), 7012410060. http://dx.doi.org/10.5014/ajot.2016.706S06

American Occupational Therapy Association. (2017). Vision 2025. *American Journal of Occupational Therapy, 71*, 7103420010. https://doi.org/10.5014/ajot.2017.713002

American Occupational Therapy Association. (2018a). Fieldwork Level II and occupational therapy students. *American Journal of Occupational Therapy, 72*(Suppl. 2), 7212410020. https://doi.org/10.5014/ajot.2018.72S205

American Occupational Therapy Association. (2018b). Philosophy of occupational therapy education. *American Journal of Occupational Therapy, 72*(Suppl. 2), 7212410070. https://doi.org/10.5014/ajot.2018.72S201

American Occupational Therapy Association. (2020a). AOTA decision guides: Practitioner well-being. https://www.aota.org/-/media/Corporate/Files/Practice/Health/Addressing-Acute-Stress-Anxiety.pdf

American Occupational Therapy Association. (2020b). New Fieldwork Performance Evaluation Tool. https://www.aota.org/Education-Careers/Fieldwork/performance-evaluations.aspx

American Occupational Therapy Association. (2020c). Occupational therapy code of ethics 2020. *American Journal of Occupational Therapy, 74*(Suppl. 3).

American Occupational Therapy Association. (2020d). Occupational therapy practice framework: Domain and process (4th ed.). *American Journal of Occupational Therapy, 74*(Suppl. 2), 7412410010. https://doi.org/10.5014/ajot.2020.74S2001

Brown, M., Brown, G. C., & Sharma, S. (2005). *Evidence-based medicine to value based medicine.* American Medical Association Press.

Canty, G., Roberts, M. J., & Molineux, M. (2020). Characteristics of occupation-based education within entry-level occupational therapy programs: Professional leaders' perspectives. *Journal of Occupational Therapy Education, 4*(2). https://doi.org/10.26681/jote.2020.040202

Centers for Medicare & Medicaid Services. (2017). National Health Expenditures 2017 Highlights. https://www.cms.gov/Research-Statistics-Data-and-Systems/Statistics-Trends-and-Reports/NationalHealthExpendData/Downloads/highlights.pdf

Centers for Medicare & Medicaid Services. (2019a). Overview of the Patient Driven Payment Model (PDGM). https://www.cms.gov/Outreach-and-Education/Outreach/NPC/Downloads/2019-02-12-PDGM-Presentation.pdf

Centers for Medicare & Medicaid Services. (2019b). Patient Driven Payment Model. https://www.cms.gov/medicare/medicare-fee-for-service-payment/snfpps/pdpm

Centers for Medicare & Medicaid Services. (2019c). What are value based programs? https://www.cms.gov/Medicare/Quality-Initiatives-Patient-Assessment-Instruments/Value-Based-Programs/Value-Based-Programs

Cohn, E. S. (2019). Asserting our competence and affirming the value of occupation with confidence. *American Journal of Occupational Therapy, 73*, 7306150010. https://doi.org/10.5014/ajot.2019.736002

Crump, J., & Sugarman, J. (2008). Ethical considerations for short term experiences by trainees in global health. *Journal of the American Medical Association, 300*(12), 1456-1458. https://doi.org/10.1001/jama.300.12.1456

Department of Health. (2015). Accountability headline measures: Technical guide for changes in 2016. [cited 2015 Sept 28]. https://www.gov.uk/government/uploads/system/uploads/attachment_data/file/359909/Technical_Guide_final_for_publication

Drobac, P., & Morse, M. (2016). Medical education and global health equity. *AMA Journal of Ethics, 18*(7), 702-709. https://doi.org/10.1001/journalofethics.2016.18.7.medu1-1607.

Evenson, M. E., Roberts, M., Kaldenberg, J., Barnes, M. A., & Ozelie, R. (2015). Brief report—National survey of fieldwork educators: Implications for occupational therapy education. *American Journal of Occupational Therapy, 69*(Suppl.2), 6912350020. http://dx.doi.org/10.5014/ajot.2015.019265

Feldman, M. D. (2017). Altruism in medical practice. *Journal of General Internal Medicine, 32*(7), 719-720. https://doi.org/10.1007/s11606-017-4067-1

Frenk, J., Chen, L., Bhutta, Z., Cohen, J., Crisp, N., Evans, Timothy, . . . Zurayk, Huda. (2010). Health professionals for a new century: Transforming education to strengthen health systems in an interdependent world. *The Lancet, 376*(9756), 1923-1958. https://doi.org/10.1016/S0140-6736(10)61854-5

Greenhalgh, T., Howick, J., & Maskrey, N. (2014). Evidence based medicine renaissance group: A movement in crisis? *British Medical Journal, 348*, g3725. https://doi.org/10.1136/bmj.g3725

Harris, J. (2017). Altruism: Should it be included as an attribute of medical professionalism? *Health Professions Education, 4*, 3-8. https://doi.org/10.1016/j.hpe.2017.02.005

Jones, R. (2002). Declining altruism in medicine. *British Medical Journal, 324*(7338), 624-625. https://doi.org/10.1136/bmj.324.7338.624

Lamb, A., & McCarley, S. (2019). Practitioners as change agents in PDPM: Maximizing health, well-being, and quality of life. https://www.aota.org/Conference-Events/member-appreciation/webinar-library/Documentation-Coding.aspx

Laverdure, P., Smiley, J., Stoltz, N., & Varland, J. (2020a, June). How fieldwork students can help us address the challenges of client care during COVID – 19 [Paper Presentation]. American Occupational Therapy Association's 2020 Virtual Conference Series. Ideas and Connections. Redefined.

Laverdure, P., Smiley, J., Stotz, N., & Varland, J. (2020b). Student value MVPs: Leveraging fieldwork and capstones to support the volume-to-value reimbursement value shift. *OT Practice, 25*(6), 20-23.

Marzorati, C., & Pravettoni, G. (2017). Value as the key concept in the health care system: How it has influenced medical practice and clinical decision-making processes. *Journal of Multidisciplinary Healthcare, 10*, 101-106. https://doi.org/10.1146/annurev.psych.52.1.397

Maslach, C., Schaufeli, W. B., & Leiter, M. P. (2001). Job burnout. *Annual Review of Psychology, 52*, 397–422.

Miller, C. (2018). Health policy perspectives—Accountable care organizations and occupational therapy. *American Journal of Occupational Therapy, 72*, 7205090010. https://doi.org/10.5014/ajot.2018.725003

Monroe-Wise, A., Kibore, M., Kiarie, J., Nduati, R., Mburu, J., Drake, F.T., Bremner, W., Holmes, K., & Farquhar, C. (2014). The clinical education partnership initiative: An innovative approach to global health education. *BMC Medical Education, 14*(1043). https://doi.org/10.1186/s12909-014-0246-5

Porter, M. E. (2009). A strategy for health care reform – toward a value-based system. *New England Journal of Medicine, 361*(2), 109–112. https://doi.org/10.1001/jama.297.10.1103.

Porter, M. E. (2010). What is value in health care? *New England Journal of Medicine, 363*(26), 2477-2481. https://doi.org/10.1056/NEJMp1011024

Porter, M. E., & Teisberg, E. O. (2006). *Redefining health care: Creating value-based competition on results.* Harvard Business School Press.

Porter, M. E., & Teisberg, E. O. (2007). How physicians can change the future of health care. *Journal of the American Medical Association, 297*(10), 1103–1111. https://doi.org/10.1001/jama.297.10.1103

Rabin, T., Mayanja-Kizza, S., & Rastegar, A. (2016). Medical education capacity-building partnerships for health care systems development. *AMA Journal of Ethics, 18*(7), 710-717. https://doi.org/10.1001/journalofethics.2016.18.7.medu2-1607.

Rogers, J., & Dodson, S. (1988). Burnout in occupational therapists. *American Journal of Occupational Therapy, 42*, 787–792. https://doi.org/10.5014/ajot.42.12.787

Scott, B., & Eminger, T. (2016). Bundled payments: Value-based care - Implications for providers, payers, and patients. *American Health and Drug Benefits, 9*(9), 493-496. PMCID: PMC5394559 PMID: 28465776

Tickle-Degnen, L. (2020). Client-centered practice, therapeutic relationship, and the use of research evidence. *American Journal of Occupational Therapy, 46*, 460-474. https://doi.org/10.5014/ajot.56.4.470

Virginia Occupational Therapy Education Council. (2020). Setting specific fieldwork innovations: How are they working. https://sites.google.com/view/vaotec/meetings-presentations/past-meetings/november-2020?authuser=0

Wilkinson, T., Wade, W., & Knock, L. (2009). A blueprint to assess professionalism: Results of a systematic review. *Academic Medicine, 84*(5), 551-558. https://doi.org/10.1097/ACM.0b013e31819fbaa2.

Zeman, E., & Harvison, N. (2017). Burnout, stress, and compassion fatigue in occupational therapy practice and education: A call for mindful, selfcare protocols. *NAM Perspectives. Commentary, National Academy of Medicine.* https://doi.org/10.31478/201703g

12

Summative Assessment of Student Learning

Jayson Zeigler, DHSc, MS, OTR

Evaluation of student performance is an essential component in experiential learning. Not only is an evaluation mechanism a requirement set by the Accreditation Council for Occupational Therapy Education (ACOTE) in the United States, but evaluation provides the student and fieldwork educator (FWed) the opportunity for reflection and feedback, which promotes personal and professional growth. Evaluation can occur informally or formally, be focused on the process or the outcome, and might also include a self-assessment, which helps students to reflect and become more self-aware. FWeds should be mindful that the evaluation process for Level II differs from Level I. Level II fieldwork summative and formative assessment differs from Level I because the student is usually expected to meet more standardized competencies such as those within the American Occupational Therapy Association (AOTA) Fieldwork Performance Evaluation (FWPE) for the Occupational Therapy Student, which was created in 2002 and was recently updated in 2020.

Understanding how to be an effective evaluator to support your fieldwork student's growth and development is a professional responsibility. Not only does this involve being knowledgeable about the mechanism that the occupational therapy program uses to evaluate Level II fieldwork but also to understand characteristics of being an effective evaluator and common pitfalls to avoid. This chapter will dive deeper into the evaluation process, provide an overview and comparison between the prior AOTA FWPE and the current version of the tool, discuss common scenarios where bias or stigma can influence the evaluation process, and suggest resources for effective evaluation.

DeIuliis, E. D., & Hanson, D. (Eds.).
Fieldwork Educator's Guide to Level II Fieldwork (pp. 345-370).
© 2023 Taylor & Francis Group.

KEY WORDS

- **Evaluation:** A means by which to collect information about student performance related to their didactic knowledge, clinical skill, and professional behavior skill acquisition (University of Michigan Center for Research on Teach and Learning, 2021).

- **Formal evaluation:** The utilization of a data-based measure for gathering information on an occupational therapy student's learning and demonstration of knowledge in systematic competencies predetermined as imperative to enter the profession.

- **Formative evaluation:** Information collected about a student to improve curriculum design of an academic institution, or the educator is collecting information on teaching a particular skill set to a student with immediate evaluation of performance conducted to assess instruction efficacy (University of Michigan Center for Research on Teach and Learning, 2021; Wiggins, 1998).

- **Informal evaluation:** The actions conducted by FWeds that are embedded in the day-to-day clinical environment learning activities and that gather information on student performance and progress.

- **Summative evaluation:** Information collected on the student's demonstration and competence for translation of knowledge from classroom to clinic at various points of time in a student's curriculum (University of Michigan Center for Research on Teach and Learning, 2021; Wiggins, 1998).

LEARNING OBJECTIVES

By the end of reading this chapter and completing the learning activities, the reader should be able to:

1. Identify the importance of evaluation within Level II fieldwork education.
2. Differentiate between informal and formal evaluation of Level II fieldwork student performance.
3. Understand the developmental history of the AOTA FWPE tool.
4. Analyze student performance based on FWPE competencies and apply appropriate scores.
5. Avoid common pitfalls when evaluating Level II fieldwork student performance.
6. Identify strategies and resources to support an objective evaluation process.

THE IMPORTANCE OF EVALUATION DURING LEVEL II FIELDWORK

Occupational therapy programs (across all degree levels and in all countries) are required to have some sort of mechanism in place to evaluate Level II fieldwork. Evaluation mechanisms are recognized as an important tool to ensure quality clinical education and contribute to providing the student best clinical education structure, processes, and outcomes (Jette et al., 2014). Likewise, to the construct of supervision, which has been discussed throughout this book, evaluation is a mutual process and experience. In the United States, ACOTE (2018) Standard C.1.12 stipulates a requirement that there is an evaluation of the effectiveness of the supervision of the FWed (a process led by the fieldwork student), and Standard C.1.15 requires that there is a formal evaluation of the student's performance (a process led by the FWed). Outside of accreditors outlining an expectation and requirement for evaluation, the AOTA also identifies evaluation as a key component of fieldwork. For example, evaluation is identified as an essential performance skill competency within the role of the FWed (Dickerson, 2006).

Evaluation is a needed and expected aspect of any experiential learning experience. It is a means by which to collect information about student performance related to their didactic knowledge, clinical skill, and professional behavior skill acquisition (University of Michigan Center for Research on Teach and Learning, 2021). An important mindset to have as a FWed is to not view evaluation as a critical or punitive concept. Embodying a more strength-based mindset will allow the FWed, and ultimately the fieldwork student, to view the evaluation process as an essential step in their growth and development toward entry-level practice. There are different approaches and forms of evaluation. For instance, evaluation can be informal or formal, or summative or formative.

Formal Evaluation

Formal evaluation is the utilization of a data-based measure to gather information on an occupational therapy student's learning and the student's demonstration of knowledge in systematic competencies predetermined as imperative to enter the profession. Examples of formal evaluation include a standardized midterm and final evaluation (such as the AOTA FWPE, 2020a) or structured weekly feedback forms. Examples of a structured weekly feedback form can be found in Appendix A. Weekly feedback forms provide the fieldwork student with more frequent opportunities to receive critical or constructive feedback (Costa, 2015). Weekly feedback forms, such as those found in the Appendix, can be integrated into weekly feedback sessions with your fieldwork student or at set intervals throughout the fieldwork experience. Weekly feedback forms provide the educator with the opportunity to identify problem areas that may have clinical consequences and communicate solutions to solve these problems for the student (Costa, 2015). The weekly feedback forms also provide a mechanism for the FWed to document student progress and performance throughout the fieldwork experience, which can be helpful to guide ratings and comments during formal evaluation at midterm and final. While formal evaluations occur at set intervals, it is important to understand that evaluation is not just a two-time phenomenon (midterm/final) in Level II fieldwork. Effective FWeds should complete evaluation of their students' performance and progress throughout the fieldwork experience. These can be referred to as informal evaluations.

Informal Evaluation

Informal evaluation are actions conducted by FWeds that are embedded in the day-to-day fieldwork learning activities and that gather information on student performance and progress.

Examples of informal evaluation are:

- Comparative evaluation using a site-specific learning objective (SSLO) checklist
- Observation
- Recorded time samplings
- Facilitated critical reflections after significant clinical situations and scenarios (see example prompts to foster reflection within Chapters 7 and 8).

Comparative Evaluation Using a Site-Specific Learning Objective Checklist

Here is an example of how a site-specific learning objective checklist can be used to evaluate student progress and performance. As you already know, creating SSLOs is a best practice approach of a FWed. SSLOs can be used to provide a clear picture of expected performance, and to create benchmarks to guide and measure progress toward the end-goal. In other words, the expected level of performance at week 8 or 12 (which should be aligned with entry-level practice) can be downgraded to reasonable performance levels at midterm, or even other intervals such as week 3 or week 9, appropriate for the practice setting and complexity of caseload. See Table 12-1, which provides an example using Section I: Fundamentals of Practice, which has three items that evaluate a student's competency in areas of ethics, safety, and judgment (AOTA, 2020a). It is important to denote that occupational therapy programs in the United States are not required to utilize the AOTA FWPE tool. FWeds should seek out the evaluation mechanism utilized by the occupational therapy program and familiarize themselves with the tool and process prior to the onset of the experience.

As part of regular feedback sessions, the FWed can use the checklist to document student progress for each SSLO at set intervals. Documentation in the checklist can then be used to provide objective feedback and distinct examples to the student during more formal reviews at midterm and final.

Observation

Observation can be considered a method of informative evaluation to provide critical or constructive feedback frequently as mentioned previously when discussing weekly feedback forms. However, to provide more frequent feedback the FWed can observe student behaviors on a day-to-day basis and provide the student with real-time critical feedback to offer solutions and strategies for areas of growth (Costa, 2015). For example, the FWed observes that the Level II fieldwork student is demonstrating difficulty with remembering to don non-skid socks on patients prior to a functional sit to stand transfer at the bedside. The FWed communicates these observations to the student prior to the midterm Level II fieldwork evaluation and discusses how safety and judgment are critical competencies to meet in order to reach entry-level practice. The FWed can then accurately document and communicate areas of growth at midterm and identify any further action items related to this performance problem.

Recorded Time Samplings

Time sampling is a data collection strategy that also involves direct observation and can also include audio or video recording to assess whether student performance (or a specific action or behavior) occurs or does not occur during specific time periods. If using audio or video recording, the FWed should obtain the student's permission first and explain in advance how the recordings will be used to identify skill performance and growth. For example, a fieldwork program might have a SSLO that a Level II fieldwork student is responsible for leading the hospital's preoperative total joint group program each week. After observing their FWed complete the group session two times, the student is expected to lead the weekly group sessions. The FWed might observe and/or record the student performance each week to foster discussion on strengths and areas of growth. The FWed and the student can watch the recordings on a weekly basis to discuss progress made and improve the student's skill progression week to week.

While informal assessment approaches can be a good approach to evaluate progress, it should not completely replace formal evaluation. We need both, as one complements the other, in depicting accurate pictures of our students. We can use either type (depending on the intended purpose) to improve teaching and learning.

TABLE 12-1

EXAMPLE OF SITE OBJECTIVE CHECKLIST

AOTA FWPE—OT AREA	WEEK 1 STUDENT PROGRESS AND EXAMPLE	WEEK 3 STUDENT PROGRESS AND EXAMPLE	SSLO—INDICATOR OF SUCCESS AT MIDTERM	WEEK 8 STUDENT PROGRESS AND EXAMPLE	WEEK 10 STUDENT PROGRESS AND EXAMPLE	SSLO—INDICATOR OF SUCCESS AT FINAL
1. Adheres to ethics			Verbalizes importance of HIPAA regulations and department HIPAA procedures			Maintains patient confidentiality by consistently locking computer, shredding printed documents at the end of the day 100% of the time
2. Adheres to safety regulations			Adheres to department "hold and reorder polices" by utilizing the printed reference guide			Demonstrates safe adherence to the reorder and hold polices without the use of printed reference guide
3. Uses judgment and safety			Demonstrates safe moving and handling techniques during patient care with no more than two verbal cues from FWed per day			Maintains and demonstrates safe moving and handling techniques 100% of the time and articulates to caregivers the importance of body mechanics

---

BOX 12-1

Examples of summative assessment include:

- Assessment of evaluation skills within occupational therapy specialty settings (e.g., oncology, pediatric specialty clinics, psychosocial settings)
- Assessment of student performance for advanced intervention skills such as serial casting to facilitate constraint induced movement therapy or wound care within a burn unit after the student's participation in an elective occupational therapy graduate course
- Assessment of acquired intrinsic and extrinsic qualities of professionalism throughout a curriculum
- Assessment of interprofessional collaboration skills within an intensive care unit after student participates in advance acute care best practices graduate course

---

BOX 12-2

Examples of formative assessment during Level II fieldwork assessing student performance include:

- The student is taught how to coban wrap upper extremity digits within a burn unit and provided ample practice time to understand and demonstrate skill for which they are later assessed for the performance to initiate and complete the skill
- The student learns from the educator the proper steps for interprofessional communication related to patient handoffs and provided opportunity to practice the skill to be later assessed for competency in this skill
- The student learns and practices how to perform screening a patient and completing a chart review using the site's electronic medical record platform to be later assessed for competency in this skill

---

Summative and Formative Assessment

Summative and formative assessments are also both needed to enhance the educator's teaching and the student's learning during Level II fieldwork. The type of assessment we should use should match the intended purpose of the assessment. Box 12-1 provides examples of summative assessment that would occur after the student acquires knowledge and skill acquisition for the occupational therapy process within a certain practice setting and population, while Box 12-2 provides examples of formative assessment for the Level II student who learns a skill and acquires knowledge, practices the skills, and is provided feedback on performance.

Regardless of what type of assessment, the FWed should consider understanding what actions they can take to effectively gather information on student progress and provide feedback on the student's performance. First, the educator should attempt to provide objective feedback that is based on **direct observations** using methods previously mentioned in this chapter. Second, the objective feedback should provide the student with information or **actionable data that facilitate reflection** internally within the student. In order to observe the student's response to feedback and how they internalize the feedback, **provide opportunity for deliberate practice for skill development** within the identified problem areas of their performance. If the FWed finds the student is having difficulty reflecting on problem areas previously identified by the FWed, consider the use of audio or video recordings to provide the student the opportunity to observe themselves in action. An overview of best practice tips to facilitate effective evaluation during Level II fieldwork can be found in Box 12-3.

BOX 12-3

Tips for Level II FWeds to facilitate an effective evaluation and quality Level II fieldwork clinical education experiences adopted from clinical and general education models for evaluation of performance (Jette et al., 2014; Moody, 2018):

1. Provide *objective feedback* that facilitates student reflection.
2. Gather *actionable data* that will better facilitate an observable student response to feedback from FWed.
3. Ensure that information gathered will provide opportunity for *deliberate practice* in which the student can demonstrate response to feedback on evaluation. This would typically be implemented by a FWed during the midterm formal evaluation tool use or informal tool use such as a critical reflection facilitated after one clinical session and practice provided to correct performance in the next session.
4. If able, *utilize technology* (video) to help students gain a better understanding for subjective skill demonstration using objective measures that will facilitate deeper critical reflection on how to improve performance. While video is not always permitted in the clinical environment, role-playing with you as their educator or with another work colleague could be considered as an alternative to help with this trait of effective evaluation.
5. Know your organization's or site's *structures* which include settings, available staff, and clinical education funding.
6. Provide adequate and efficient supervision, evaluation mechanisms, and administrative *processes* must work in harmony with a site's structures for an effective clinical education experience that include evaluation processes of student performance to be perceived as successful completion for all participants (fieldwork stakeholders).
7. Communicate your site's expected *outcomes* that parallel the expected competencies for the student during a clinical experience and be aware of the resources needed to help achieve these outcomes for all stakeholders.

HISTORY ON THE AOTA FIELDWORK PERFORMANCE EVALUATION

In the early 2000s, the AOTA (2002) published the *Fieldwork Performance Evaluation* as a 42-item assessment instrument designed to measure an occupational therapy student's performance for applying the occupational therapy process within Level II fieldwork. There was a separate form for the occupational therapy student and the occupational therapy assistant student. Each item was scored by the FWed using a four-point Likert-like scale with 1 = unsatisfactory, 2 = needs improvement, 3 = meets standards, and 4 = exceeds standards (AOTA, 2002). While the general purpose of the tool was to have a formal mechanism to evaluate student fieldwork performance as "entry-level," some occupational therapy programs also might have used the final score received on the AOTA FWPE tool to correlate to a final grade to award the student in the fieldwork course that they were enrolled in. An interesting aspect of the older version of the AOTA FWPE was how a Rasch analysis revealed an ordering continuum based upon level of difficulty (Atler, 2002). In other words, this type of analysis can provide a framework for evaluators to understand a hierarchy of simple to complex or more difficult items. For example, certain competencies such as positive interpersonal skills are known to be easier to observe and evaluate because of an observable action and behavior. You know it when you see it. Whereas other competencies such as understanding occupational therapy philosophy are noted to be more challenging items to measure by a FWed.

> ### Box 12-4
>
> *Why are the psychometrics of the new FWPE important to me as a FWed?*
>
> Having a psychometrically sound evaluation tool provides the opportunity for the occupational therapy profession and pedagogy of fieldwork to be more science-driven. Collecting data at the national level allows AFWCs and other academic researchers to investigate key constructs of fieldwork and enhance the profession's social responsibility to train and educate optimally future practitioners. Psychometrics provides the opportunity to produce evidence that our fieldwork education aligns with the signature pedagogies of the occupational therapy education.

Although the AOTA FWPE (2002) tool was a widely used tool across numerous academic programs, validity and reliability for this instrument were never established in the literature. In 2015, AOTA began an intensive process to develop a psychometrically established Level II fieldwork performance evaluation to assess student performance in preparation for entry-level practice (Preissner et al., 2020). This process has focused on establishing content validity (stage one) and evaluation of internal structure, response processes, fairness in testing, and item precision on the AOTA FWPE (Preissner et al., 2020, p. 2).

In 2020, AOTA unveiled the new *Fieldwork Performance Evaluation for the Occupational Therapy Student* (AOTA, 2020a). Due to copyright laws, use of the prior form (whether hard copy or electronic format) is not permitted by AOTA. In comparison to the previous version of the AOTA FWPE (2002), the new and revised AOTA *Fieldwork Performance Evaluation for the Occupational Therapy Student* (2020a) is a 37-item assessment instrument designed to measure an occupational therapy student's performance in preparation for entry-level practice. Table 12-2 outlines the construct items that FWeds should understand to assess and score for Level II fieldwork student performance on the AOTA *Fieldwork Performance Evaluation for the Occupational Therapy Student* (2020a). Each item is scored by the FWed using a four-point Likert-like scale with 1 = unsatisfactory performance, 2 = emerging performance, 3 = proficient performance, and 4 = exemplary performance (AOTA, 2020a). In comparison to the AOTA FWPE (2002) tool, this tool has and is undergoing intense psychometric property establishment regarding content validity and reliability. See Box 12-4

Another significant change with the new tool is that it is only available in an online format, which is currently housed in the FormStack platform. The FWed should expect to work with the student's academic program (usually via the AFWC) to gain access to the FormStack portal. It is in this portal that the FWed will be provided an emailed link to access the midterm and final AOTA FWPE form. FWeds do have the ability to save the form and return to the link at a later time to complete the evaluation. Once the final evaluation is complete and submitted in Formstack, academic programs can set up the "fieldwork recognition certificate," often used to formally recognize the amount of supervision provided to a practitioner to satisfy professional development units, to be automatically emailed to the supervising FWed.

Although resources and training materials are provided by AOTA, there are some complexities that exist within this new tool related to a FWed's interpretation of competency items. Therefore, future work is underway to better understand the complexities within FWeds' interpretations of items within this tool (Preissner et al., 2020). FWeds should feel more confident in using the updated tool because of the psychometric property establishment and know that future literature

TABLE 12-2

COMPARISON OF AOTA FWPE TOOLS

	AOTA FWPE (2002)	AOTA FWPE (2020A)
Number of Items	42	37
Format	Hardcopy or online format available	Online format only
Likert Scoring Scale	1 – Unsatisfactory 2 – Needs improvement 3 – Meets standards 4 – Exceeds standards	1 – Unsatisfactory performance 2 – Emerging performance 3 – Proficient performance 4 – Exemplary performance
Passing Score	Midterm • Satisfactory performance = 90 and above Final • Pass = 122 points and above • Scores for the ethics and safety items must be scored at 3 or above to receive a pass	Midterm • **There is not a passing score identified** Final • Pass = 111 points and above • Scores of 3 or higher required on AOTA's *Code of Ethics* (AOTA, 2020b) and safety items • **Scores of 1 on any of the items is not allowed to receive a pass**
Expected Student Competencies	1. Fundamentals of practice 2. Basic tenets of occupational therapy 3. Screening and evaluation 4. Intervention 5. Management of services 6. Communication 7. Professional behaviors	1. Fundamentals of practice 2. Basic tenets 3. Screening and evaluation 4. Intervention 5. Management of occupational therapy services 6. Communication and professional behaviors

will identify preliminary evidence that enhances how students are educated and evaluated for entry-level practice. In summary, Table 12-2 provides a visual picture for FWeds to compare FWPE tools (most recent version vs. older version). Then, Table 12-3 provides a comparison of rating scale definitions between the two AOTA FWPE tools for FWeds to familiarize themselves with prior to assessing Level II fieldwork student performance formatively and in summation.

TABLE 12-3

COMPARISON OF RATING SCALE DEFINITIONS FOR AOTA FWPE TOOL

AOTA FWPE TOOLS	RATING SCALE	PERFORMANCE DESCRIPTION
AOTA FWPE (2002)	4 – Exceeds standards	Performance is highly skilled
	3 – Meet standards	Consistent with entry-level practice
	2 – Needs improvement	Performance is progressing but still needs improvement to entry-level practice
	1 – Unsatisfactory	Performance is below standard and requires development to entry-level practice
AOTA FWPE (2020a)	4 – Exemplary performance	Demonstrates satisfactory competence in specific skills consistently; demonstrates substantial breadth and depth in understanding and/or skillful application of fundamental knowledge and skills
	3 – Proficient performance	Demonstrates satisfactory competence in specific skills; demonstrates adequate understanding and/or application of fundamental knowledge and skills
	2 – Emerging performance	Demonstrates limited competence in specific skills (inconsistencies may be evident); demonstrates limited understanding and/or application of fundamental knowledge and skills (displays some gaps and/or inaccuracies)
	1 – Unsatisfactory performance	Fails to demonstrate competence in specific skills; performs in an inappropriate manner; demonstrates inadequate understanding and/or application of fundamental knowledge and skills (demonstrates significant gaps and/or inaccuracies)

FIELDWORK PERFORMANCE EVALUATION COMPETENCIES

As outlined in the AOTA FWPE (2020a), the Level II fieldwork student is expected to demonstrate competency in fundamentals of practice, basic tenets, screening and evaluation, intervention, management of occupational therapy services, and communication and professional behaviors. As you further review the competency items, reflect on the language used in the rating scale to think about what exemplar, proficient, emerging, and unsatisfactory performance might look like at your setting.

Box 12-5

CLINICAL VIGNETTE ONE

A FWed is supervising a Level II fieldwork student in an acute care setting. Specifically, the FWed is working with the student within an intensive care unit in which patients are ventilator dependent. The site's policy and procedure related to ventilator settings to sit a patient at the edge of bed on this unit is that a respiratory therapist must be present before this action is completed by a therapist. The supervising occupational therapist has exclusively practiced on this unit for over 15 years and is overly confident in working with this population and changes the ventilator settings on their own prior to the student completing the functional transfer. As the weeks progress, the student follows and demonstrates this practice observed from their FWed.

At midterm, the FWed rates the student a "1"—unsatisfactory performance—for items #2 and #3 on the AOTA FWPE (2020a) noting the occurrence of several unsafe behaviors observed during functional transfers and transitions within the intensive care unit due to a respiratory therapist not being present during these attempts.

Safety actions demonstrated by the student during the first half of the Level II fieldwork rotation are learned behaviors modeled by the FWed. Therefore, the FWed should reconsider the student's summative and formative learning up to this point in the rotation and objectively teach and demonstrate the site's policy and procedure for transition patients who are ventilator dependent to the site of the bed. The student should then be provided the opportunity to practice (formative evaluation) and demonstrate summative learning skills at the final Level II fieldwork evaluation that is not dependent on tacit knowledge demonstrated by the educator.

Fundamentals of Practice

In Section 1: Fundamentals of Practice, the student is expected to demonstrate fundamental knowledge in the ability to adhere to the AOTA (2020b) *Code of Ethics*, adherence to safety policies and procedures at their site, and the ability facilitate safety in all fieldwork tasks by utilizing a proactive approach to all clinical situations (AOTA, 2020a). The FWed, when scoring the Level II fieldwork student, should avoid applying their own interpretation of the site's safety regulations, policies, and procedures and strictly hold the student accountable to demonstrate this competency to those safety policies and procedures that are site specific and in writing. This action will avoid conflict when providing feedback to the student in a constructive manner. See Box 12-5 for an example.

Basic Tenets

In the Basic Tenants section of the AOTA FWPE tool, the Level II fieldwork student must demonstrate the ability to articulate the meaning of the occupational therapy profession to society, the value of the profession, and the role of the profession (AOTA, 2020a). Scoring this section for student performance is subjective to your patient population that the student is providing services to and the diverse interactions that they will engage with many different individuals at the site. See Box 12-6 for an example of a scenario

---

Box 12-6

Clinical Vignette Two

An occupational therapist in a rehab hospital is supervising a Level II fieldwork student in their second rotation. The student must participate in many interactions with several different disciplines. The rehab hospital hosts a new group of medical student residents every 3 months. The occupational therapy fieldwork student is given the responsibility to communicate the meaning of occupational therapy, the value of occupational therapy services to this patient population, and the role of discipline on the rehab team. The fieldwork student claims that they did a similar task at their first Level II fieldwork site, which was in a community-based early intervention pediatrics program (role-emerging site). Prior to midterm assessment of student performance, when observing the student's performance during their first meeting with residents, the educator provides feedback to the student that they seem to have difficulty utilizing professional medical terminology to communicate the meaning and value of the occupational therapy profession in this setting. Further feedback is provided to the student that their examples from a community-based setting to better define occupational therapy and the role of the profession did not make a clear connection with the intended audience of medical residents.

Is a rating of 2 (emerging performance) out of 4 at midterm an accurate score for student performance on the AOTA FWPE (2020a) in this situation?

Screening and Evaluation

In the Screening and Evaluation section of the AOTA FWPE, students are evaluated on performance-based skills related to the student's ability to perform a chart review, communicate their rationale for evaluation decisions, select relevant assessment tools for clinical decision-making initiation, develop an occupational profile, and demonstrate fidelity of measurement to reveal best patient outcomes in a manner that is clearly and concisely documented (AOTA, 2020a).

Intervention

Closely related, the FWed will need to evaluate the student's performance for selecting relevant interventions based on evaluation findings, facilitating client-centered and occupation-based interventions, implementing appropriate clinical reasoning skills during interventions, and documents the client's response to intervention in a manner that justifies goal-directed interventions (AOTA, 2020a).

Management of Occupational Therapy Services

Next, the FWed assesses the student's performance for management of occupational therapy services. Scoring this competency is based on the FWed's interprofessional environment and subjective organizational standards that the student will be exposed to during the Level II fieldwork experiences. This competency is also where the FWed will evaluate the student's ability to manage occupational therapy assistants and aides as well as meet productivity standards that are site

---

Box 12-7

CLINICAL VIGNETTE THREE

A FWed meets with their site's clinical education coordinator to prepare for supervising a Level II fieldwork student. The clinical education coordinator has communicated to the FWed that the student will be held to the same productivity standards as a staff occupational therapist by week 6 of a 12-week Level II fieldwork rotation. The occupational therapist reflects on this request and recognizes internally that the site productivity standard is often difficult for themself to meet this expectation and worries that this is unrealistic for a student. The student starts the rotation and by week 6 is only capable of meeting 75% of the site's productivity standard with no noted performance weaknesses in managing documentation or preparation for implementing clinical services. How should the FWed have implemented this request by the clinical education coordinator, and how should the educator fairly score the student in the competency area for managing occupational therapy services?

---

specific. The FWed should approach the scoring of this competency with caution. It is advised that prior to the student starting the Level II fieldwork experience, the FWed should collaboratively or independently work to establish weekly expectations for productivity for the student. See Box 12-7.

As you reflect on the vignette in Box 12-7, refer back to Chapters 4 and 5, which provide guidelines of how to structure a learning plan and orientation schedule. Having a clear learning plan will provide a benchmark for student progress that will aid in providing clear and unbiased feedback on a weekly basis to the student. The use of an orientation schedule will help you to track when and where the student was introduced to the competencies expected at your site and the supports that were available to support proficiency. The student should also be directed to these documents to support ownership for learning.

Communication and Professional Behaviors

Finally, the student's intrinsic and extrinsic qualities of professionalism (DeIuliis, 2017; verbal and nonverbal communication skills, interpersonal skills, time management skills, cultural and generational sensitivity, etc.) will be evaluated during the Level II fieldwork experience in the Communication and Professional Behavior section (AOTA, 2020a). It is recommended that the FWed utilize a type of feedback form, such as those found in the chapter appendices, to record objective findings of this competency daily. This also aids in the development of a paper trail, which can be useful evidence to have if the student's performance does not improve. As discussed in Chapter 10, having a paper trail is critical to provide effective support to an underperforming student. See Box 12-8.

In summary, a brief overview of the expected AOTA FWPE (2020a) competencies was provided, highlighting skills that the student is responsible to demonstrate competency as an emerging entry-level occupational therapy practitioner. The FWed is responsible for administratively organizing their objective findings of student performance on a weekly basis and providing feedback to the student in a manner that facilitates skills acquisition for the student to develop into an entry-level practitioner.

> **BOX 12-8**
> ## CLINICAL VIGNETTE FOUR
>
> A FWed meets with their student each morning in order to stay informed of the daily patient load schedule in a timely manner. The Level II FWed observes that the student deviates away from the schedule daily without communicating schedules changes and reasoning to the educator. The FWed fails to document the student's behaviors related to the extrinsic quality of professionalism and time management skills (Deluliis, 2017). Due to the lack of a paper trail, at midterm, the educator is forced to rate the student's professionalism in communication and time management as proficient vs. emerging or unsatisfactory due to a lack of evidence related to the observed student performance in these competency areas.

COMMON PITFALLS DURING THE EVALUATION PROCESS

Despite having a psychometrically sound evaluation tool and specific competencies identified to evaluate, a FWed can experience some challenges. At times, there might be some snags in the evaluation process, or some difficulties experienced by the FWed that might have some unintentional consequences related to assessment bias. These pitfalls include (1) management of conflicting qualities of professionalism between student and FWed, (2) failure to fail a student, and (3) the FWed not understanding, from a metacognitive standpoint, their own self-efficacy as an educator. Figure 12-1 represents the cyclical nature of these internal and external pitfalls occurring during the collaborative process of the FWed facilitating summative assessment of student performance.

Management of Conflicting Qualities of Professionalism

First, FWeds should understand internally what their own intrinsic and extrinsic qualities of professionalism are before assessing these qualities in their Level II fieldwork students. Intrinsic qualities of professionalism include self-management, clinical reasoning skills, integrity, dependability, and generational as well as cultural sensitivity (Deluliis, 2017). Extrinsic qualities of professionalism are professional image, time management skills, interpersonal skills or emotional intelligence, teamwork (interprofessionalism), conflict management, and e-professionalism (Deluliis, 2017). Managing and balancing these qualities can be difficult for a FWed during the summative assessment process for student performance. If one or more qualities of professionalism becomes imbalanced or disjointed, the summative assessment for student performance can become biased, leading to the common pitfall of a FWed rating competencies for students with inaccurate scale scores that compromise the fidelity of the measurement tool. See Box 12-9.

Figure 12-2 represents how the FWed should view the collaborative process of the student and educator managing these qualities of professionalism during the summative assessment process to ensure that fidelity of measurement is not compromised.

Next, look at a case scenario (Box 12-10) related to the balance of intrinsic and extrinsic qualities within both the FWed and student.

Thus far, the examples are primarily examples of imbalanced qualities of professionalism that show up in summative assessment of student performance. However, this imbalance also occurs in formative assessment. For example, a FWed might be attempting to improve a student's interactional clinical reasoning skills with a focus on improving eye contact with patients. After providing critical feedback, the FWed is hoping to see an improvement in the student's active listening and clinical observation skills. The FWed models the expected behavior during the next intervention

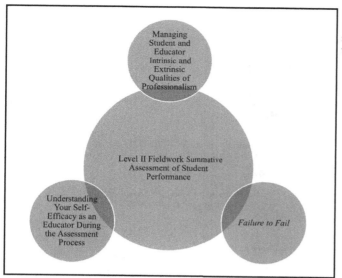

Figure 12-1. Cyclical process of common pitfalls for FWeds during Level II fieldwork summative assessment for student performance.

CLINICAL VIGNETTE FIVE

A FWed (from the Baby Boomer generation) is expected to host a Level II fieldwork (from Generation Z). The FWed identified this based on demographic information reviewed on the student personal data form, provided by the school prior to the onset of the experience. The FWed knows that this generation can be known to have associated-stereotypes and therefore a bias is created towards the student prior to their arrival on site (Deluliis, 2017; Deluliis & Saylor, 2021). The student arrives on day one of the Level II fieldwork experience demonstrating an abundance of confidence and claims to be an over-achiever. The FWed now starts to have biased thoughts about expectations of scoring this student with inaccurate scale scores within the FWPE (2020) competencies. This could have been avoided by the FWed recognizing the generational differences but not allowing their qualities of professionalism become disjointed from the students thus creating a bias of the student. The student's scores for the FWPE (2020) competencies are inaccurate representations of the student performance based on the educator's bias and imbalance of the of FWed's intrinsic qualities of professionalism.

---

session, but it is observed by the student that the educator frequently alternates between brief eye contact with the patient and attention to their note pad and laptop for documentation. The student internally questions the interactional clinical reasoning skills of the educator who is attempting to teach such skills. The student is advised to practice better eye contact with patients to facilitate improved clinical reasoning skills but also models the educator's behavior previously described. The educator then further provides the student with critical feedback about demonstrating more eye contact with the patient and less eye contact on their note pad without recognition of how the modeled behavior has influenced the student's performance. The antidote for this type of situation is practitioner self-reflection and self-awareness as well as open communication between the student and FWed as to expectations.

At the end of this chapter, you will have the opportunity to reflect on your own intrinsic and extrinsic qualities of professionalism to better facilitate the harmonic balance that occurs when collaborating with a fieldwork student during the formative and summative assessment process of their performance during Level II fieldwork.

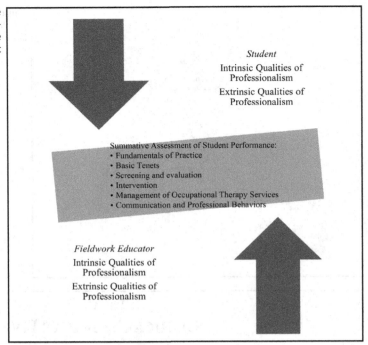

Figure 12-2. The harmonic balance of qualities of professionalism during the Level II fieldwork summative assessment process for both student and FWed.

Student
Intrinsic Qualities of
Professionalism

Extrinsic Qualities of
Professionalism

Summative Assessment of Student Performance:
• Fundamentals of Practice
• Basic Tenets
• Screening and evaluation
• Intervention
• Management of Occupational Therapy Services
• Communication and Professional Behaviors

Fieldwork Educator
Intrinsic Qualities of
Professionalism

Extrinsic Qualities of
Professionalism

Failing to Fail

The next common pitfall for the FWed is the phenomena of "failure to fail" (Cardell et al., 2017, p. 1). This phenomenon is defined by the ability of a student to enter a field despite observed poor academic and fieldwork performance (Cardell et al., 2017). Or in other words, the FWed provides high ratings during the final evaluation despite the student not displaying satisfactory nor entry-level performance. This might involve an emotional or ethical dilemma for the FWed. See Box 12-11.

Lack of measurable proof on fieldwork performance tools, vague terminology (procedural guidelines for failing) on student performance assessment tools, and lack of confidence were revealed by Cardell et al. (2017) as reasoning for false positive student performance scores on fieldwork. Lack of measurable proof may include:

- Lack of time management skills—student displays excessive tardiness

- Portrayal of unprofessional self-image—lack of adherence to the site's dress code policy, which might include clinically appropriate apparel and coverage of tattoos and piercings

However, what if there is no tangible evidence to justify these performance problems? No paper trail created by the FWed? Or no indication that direct feedback was provided by the FWed to the student regarding this performance problem? Even though the FWed has judged the student's performance to be unsatisfactory or poor, the FWed might realize that they in turn have failed to address these issues and take the blame.

With the new AOTA FWPE (2020a), terminology in the rating scale, including cut scores, have been clarified. However, the FWed should be aware that their interpretation of failing guidelines may vary and complicate their reasoning for failing or not failing a Level II fieldwork student. For example, a Level II FWed is supervising an occupational therapy student during their last week of a 12-week rotation. The student is observed to make a mental error by not donning the gait belt prior to standing a patient to ambulate to the sink in the hospital room to complete grooming. The patient falls as the student is ambulating with the patient to the sink. The patient is not injured, and

---

BOX 12-10

QUALITIES OF PROFESSIONALISM CASE SCENARIO

Jill is serving as a Level II FWed for the first time within an acute care setting. After week 6 of a 12-week Level II fieldwork experience, she observes that her student is not proactively remembering to the don the gait belt prior to completing a functional transfer of a patient from sitting to standing to complete activities of daily living within their room. However, after reflection, Jill remembers during weeks 1 to 6 that she did not consistently model this behavior for her student when the student was observing the typical routine for evaluation and interventions sessions within the acute setting.

Reflection Questions:

- What should she do to provide an accurate score for the student's competencies in the Fundamentals of Practice section on the AOTA FWPE (2020a) summative assessment tool?
- What qualities of professionalism could Jill reflect on and improve as a FWed to avoid this common pitfall in the future related to the summative assessment process for a Level II fieldwork student?

BOX 12-11

DID YOU KNOW ... ?

In the role of evaluator, 26% of occupational therapy FWeds had provided false positive performance scores on fieldwork, which compromises the assumption and expectation that health care students will be knowledgeable and competent when they graduate and enter the professional workforce (Cardell et al., 2017).

---

the student is able to safely position the patient in the bedside chair to recover from the fall. The educator is now contemplating failing the student due to lack of safety and judgment. However, the student has demonstrated understanding and competence for the fundamentals of practice such as adherence to safety procedures and policies on site during the previous 11 weeks of the experience. The FWed is aware if the student receives a score of 2 within the safety section of the AOTA FWPE (2020a), despite earning a 3 or higher on the rest of the items, the student will fail the experience. Does the educator evaluate and synthesize the student's overall performance during the entire 12-week experience, or focus on this one event where the student demonstrated a lack of safety and judgment? It is these types of scenarios that make being a Level II FWed difficult and complicates the evaluation of student performance process. In this situation, if accurate weekly feedback forms are kept, it should be visible that this situation is not representative of the student's performance during the entire rotation. Further, it should be seen by the educator as an opportunity to teach the student about complacency in practice and to facilitate reflective learning in the student as a future practitioner. Therefore, their initial interpretation of the event could be seen as a concrete failure of the student, but upon further reflection the student could be provided with the score of 3 (proficient performance) on the AOTA FWPE (2020a) with additional time spent with the student to ensure learning and reflection of consequences, for such practices are fundamental to a practitioner's knowledge and skill acquisition. Moreover, the educator could consider the event representative of the student's entire preparedness for entry-level practice.

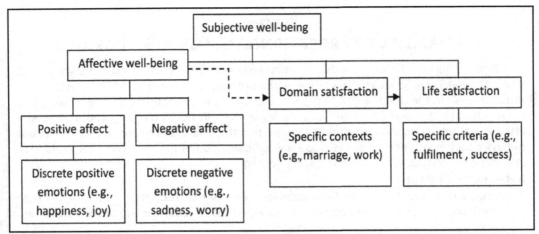

Figure 12-3. Conceptual model for FWeds related to factors influencing the presence of impact bias. (Adapted from Diener, E., Napa Scollon, C., & Lucas, R. E. (2009). The evolving concept of subjective well-being: The multifaceted nature of happiness. In, Assessing well-being: Social indicators research series. Springer, Dordrecht. https://doi. org/10.1007/978-90-481-2354-4_4.)

Understanding Your Own Self-Efficacy as an Educator

Impact bias can play a role in the summative assessment process for your Level II fieldwork student. This type of bias within a FWed is their observed behavior to overestimate the intensity and duration of their emotional reactions to past and present events related to teaching, scoring, and providing feedback for Level II student performance (Grimes et al., 2017). Figure 12-3 provides the FWed a guide to help visualize and reflect on their subjective well-being in preparation to avoid impact bias that will negatively or positively influences summative assessment of Level II fieldwork student performance. Refer to Box 12-12 for an illustration of a scenario.

Ways to Avoid Common Pitfalls During the Evaluation Process

Two methods can be considered by the FWed to avoid these common pitfalls. First, the FWed should consider the completion of the AOTA *Self-Assessment Tool for Fieldwork Educator Competency* (2009). This tool can be used to facilitate an ongoing process of improving a FWed's proficiency in summative assessment and facilitating practice education for the student (AOTA, 2009). Therefore, it provides the opportunity for FWeds to avoid compromising the student's accurate summative assessment of performance by first understanding self-competency as an educator.

Second, weekly and midterm feedback forms (Appendix A) offer the opportunity for continued and ongoing learning to take place using collaborative efforts between the student and FWed. Moreover, use of weekly feedback forms validate and make reliable the feedback provided by the educator at midterm and final, thus avoiding false positive reactions between the educator and student. For example, the FWed scores the student as having unsatisfactory performance during the administration of evaluations. However, the student was not aware of their poor performance in this clinical skills area due to the nonuse of weekly feedback forms.

Finally, FWeds should engage in the role of the reflective practitioner to better understand their strengths and challenges regarding summative assessment. Table 12-4 provides the FWed with traits of ineffective FWeds during the summative assessment process.

BOX 12-12

IMPACT BIAS CASE SCENARIO

Tom is a Level II FWed for an occupational therapy assistant student from a local academic program. The student is approaching midterm of their Level II fieldwork experience. Tom has recently experienced a divorce and is in the process of moving from his permanent residence he has known for 20 years. The student observes that Tom has aggressive responses to her questions and is demonstrating emotional lability. At midterm, Tom provides all scores of "1" in every competency section with no feedback on the reasoning for these score selections.

TABLE 12-4

TRAITS OF INEFFECTIVE FIELDWORK EDUCATORS DURING THE SUMMATIVE ASSESSMENT PROCESS FOR LEVEL II FIELDWORK STUDENT PERFORMANCE

An *ineffective* FWed engaged in the summative assessment process for Level II fieldwork student performance is ...

CHARACTERISTIC	EXAMPLE
Biased	The FWed communicates to the student that "all occupational therapy students from 'your school' struggle in this clinical environment."
Lacks cultural and generational sensitivity	The FWed assumes that a Level II student who has communicated that they are Muslim is comfortable facilitating all basic activities of daily living during evaluation and intervention sessions.
Dependent on static learning and demonstrates native intelligence within their setting and is close-minded to student's suggestions for evidence-based practice	The FWed frequently states, "I know you learned this at your school out of the textbook, but here, we do it this way."
Quick to deviate away from the AOTA FWPE (2020a) competencies expected for the student and is dependent on their own interpretation of the competencies to score the student	The FWed in a skilled nursing facility limits intervention choices for the student and provides few opportunities for the Level II fieldwork student to demonstrate intervention planning and formation of rationale for intervention choices.
Unaware of their own modeling behaviors related to clinical skills and AOTA FWPE (2020a) expected competencies	The FWed is unable to identify evidence for practice when modeling evaluation and intervention skills. For example, the FWed facilitates the assembly of the same puzzle for all four children in an outpatient setting based on reasoning that the children all have the same diagnosis and would all benefit from the same intervention plan.

Box 12-13

EXAMPLES FROM THE STUDENT EVALUATION OF FIELDWORK EXPERIENCE

- How did the student view their orientation and onboarding experience?
- Were the SSLOs helpful?
- How did they evaluate the type and amount of supervision provided?
- Did they perceive they had adequate and timely feedback?
- Were the learning activities or supplemental assignments meaningful to their professional development and growth?
- How did they perceive the role modeling of professionalism?
- Did they experience adequate exposure to the occupational therapy process?
- Were there enough opportunities for interprofessional collaboration?
- How was evidenced-based practice modeled for the student?

Common pitfalls for FWeds engaged in the process for summative assessment for a Level II fieldwork student can be avoided by understanding your own intrinsic qualities of professionalism, valuing the professional responsibility to fail a student, and internalizing your self-efficacy as an educator who is evaluating Level II fieldwork student performance.

Reflecting and Using Feedback From the Student Evaluation of Fieldwork Experience

As mentioned earlier in this chapter, evaluation of Level II fieldwork is an expectation of both the FWed and occupational therapy student. Academic programs are required to ensure that each Level II fieldwork experience is evaluated by the fieldwork student. This is usually an expectation that occurs during the final week of the experience. In 2016 year, AOTA debuted the *Student Evaluation of Fieldwork Experience* (SEFW) tool, which many occupational therapy programs have adopted or adapted as a means to evaluate the effectiveness of supervision provided and provide as means of evaluation to ensure that the fieldwork is performed in settings that provide educational experiences reflecting the curriculum design. The student is usually coached by their AFWC to contribute to the SEFW throughout their Level II fieldwork experience. Once the student completes the form, the student evaluation is typically reviewed by and discussed between the student and FWed at the end of the experience. Outside of acknowledging they reviewed the student evaluation with a signature, Level II FWeds should be empowered to actively use feedback from the student to maximize their own professional growth and development as a FWed. Feedback from the student evaluation might directly correlate to the administration of your fieldwork program; see Box 12-13.

Some student evaluations also ask the student to make suggestions or provide advice for future students who wish to prepare for a fieldwork at your site. These suggestions might bring unique perspectives to integrate into your student onboarding process and FAQ documents that are sent to future students. FWeds should use the SEFW as a measure of quality to guide the fieldwork experience. Read and refer back to the tool often; reflect and integrate on the student's feedback to strengthen your own skill set as a FWed and the overall success of your fieldwork program.

CONSIDERATIONS FOR SUPERVISORY MODELS

As this chapter concludes, let's layer in perspectives of how some of these best practice principles for evaluation of the Level II fieldwork student might be applied within a Level II experience that uses a nontraditional supervision model (such as those covered in Chapter 2 of this book).

Collaborative Model

A collaborative supervision model occurs in Level II fieldwork when there are two or more students supervised by one FWed (Costa, 2015). Evaluation of student performance is a shared responsibility between the student and the educator in this type of model. There is a balance between the student being self-aware and facilitating self-directed learning and the FWed facilitating formal and informal assessment of student performance to provide critical feedback (Costa, 2020). An inherent aspect of the collaborative model is the peer-to-peer relationship. Students might receive insightful feedback from the other students in their cohort. Therefore, the FWed should intentionally create opportunities for the students to provide feedback to one another, which can be used to contribute to formal evaluations.

Shared Supervision

This type of supervision model occurs during Level II fieldwork when two FWeds share the supervision responsibilities and assessment of student performance responsibilities for one student (Costa, 2015). This may occur because of a clinician's schedule restrictions or a FWed who is new to this role is being mentored by another, more experienced FWed. It is important for FWeds using this model to present the student with agreed-upon expectations and outcomes. The educators should consider having weekly meetings to discuss provided critical feedback to the student and share strategies communicated to the student to improve student learning and outcomes. An imbalance of feedback, expectations, and strategies for improved student learning only leads to student frustration and the potential for imbalanced qualities of professionalism demonstrated by the student causing conflict during the rotation. Communication is key in this model for all stakeholders during the assessment of student performance starting at the first week and concluding during the last week of the rotation. Feedback from the educators during midterm and final assessments can be provided individually or facilitated during a conference, face-to-face, with all stakeholders in attendance.

Role-Emerging

During a role-emerging Level II fieldwork experience, the occupational therapy FWed may only be providing direct supervision on a limited basis; a minimum of 8 hours is the requirement. Therefore, the method by which the student is formally and informally assessed looks different when this model is facilitated for assessment of student performance. Meaning, the FWed must be dependent on other stakeholders who are on-site full time or who interact with the student frequently during the experience to provide critical feedback to the student. The FWed should consider the information gathered on their student's performance while on-site and collect information from other stakeholders to fully assess the student's performance on a daily basis, weekly basis, at midterm, and final time periods during this nontraditional placement. The FWed is dependent on the site to provide structure and daily processes to the student as mentioned previously in Box 12-3 in order to best facilitate education outcomes for the student during this type of rotation.

TABLE 12-5

LEVEL II EVALUATION CONSIDERATIONS ACROSS SUPERVISORY MODELS

SUPERVISION MODEL	CONSIDERATIONS FOR THE EVALUATION PROCESS
Collaborative	Although experience occurs in a cohort-model, perform formative student evaluation individually.
	Provide opportunities for the students to provide feedback to one another.
Shared supervision/multiple mentoring	Seek out and consider feedback from all FWeds involved.
	Identify an evaluation plan prior to formal evaluation periods (e.g., are there specific AOTA FWPE competencies each evaluator should consider?).
Role-emerging	Determine how to interpret AOTA FWPE competencies in a role-emerging or nontraditional setting (e.g., screening and evaluation skills might translate to the student's ability to complete a needs assessment to guide program or project development).

Table 12-5 provides an overview of Level II fieldwork evaluation considerations for an educator across supervisory models.

SUMMARY

The evaluation process for both the FWed and student is complex. In some sense, the FWed might consider themselves as gatekeepers for deciding who enters the profession of occupational therapy or responsible for providing a stamp of approval that an occupational therapy student is "entry-level," "graduation-ready," and eligible to sit for the certification exam. This professional responsibility can be difficult for the FWed to process and agree to participate in. However, utilizing the tools in this chapter, engaging in self-reflection and independent study, accessing Level II FWed resources, and attending continuing education to enhance your skills as a Level II FWed can improve your abilities to assess student performance. The efforts that you take promote the fidelity of measurement for clinical education opportunities for occupational therapy students attempting to enter the profession.

LEARNING ACTIVITIES

1. Using the following blank spaces, list your intrinsic and extrinsic qualities of professionalism that should be considered when engaging in the summative assessment process for your Level II fieldwork student. How will these qualities influence your score selection for the AOTA FWPE (2020a) competencies for your student at midterm and final assessments for their performance?

   Intrinsic Qualities:

   Extrinsic Qualities:

2. Using Box 12-3, what is your site's structures, department processes, and expected Level II fieldwork student outcomes that can be listed to ensure a quality clinical education experience and accurate evaluation of student performance?

3. What traits should you possess and avoid as a FWed who is participating in the summative assessment process for your Level II fieldwork student?

REFERENCES

Accreditation Council for Occupational Therapy Education. (2018). Standards and interpretative guide [PDF]. https://www.aota.org/~/media/Corporate/Files/EducationCareers/Accredit/StandardsReview/2018-ACOTE-Standards-Interpretive-Guide.pdf

American Occupational Therapy Association. (2002). Fieldwork performance evaluation for the occupational therapy student. AOTA Press.

American Occupational Therapy Association. (2009). Self-assessment tool for fieldwork educator competency. https://www.aota.org/-/media/Corporate/Files/EducationCareers/Educators/Fieldwork/Supervisor/Forms/Self-Assessment%20Tool%20FW%20Ed%20Competency%20(2009).pdf

American Occupational Therapy Association. (2020a). Fieldwork performance evaluation for the occupational therapy student. AOTA Press. https://www.aota.org/-/media/Corporate/Files/EducationCareers/Fieldwork/Fieldwork-Performance-Evaluation-Occupational-Therapy-Student.pdf

American Occupational Therapy Association. (2020b). AOTA 2020 code of ethics. *American Journal Occupational Therapy, 74*(Supplement 3), 1-13.

Atler, K. (2002). *The complete guide: Using the fieldwork performance evaluation forms.* AOTA Press.

Cardell, B., Koski, J., Wahl, J., Rock, W., & Kirby, A. (2017). Underperforming students: Factors and decision-making in occupational therapy programs. *Journal of Occupational Therapy Education, 1*(3), 1-13. https://doi.org/10.26681/jote.2017. 010301

Costa, D. M. (2015). *The essential guide to occupational therapy fieldwork education: Resources for educators and practitioners.* AOTA Press.

DeIuliis, E. D. (2017). Professionalism and fieldwork education. In E. DeIuliis (Ed.), *Professionalism across occupational therapy practice* (pp. 201-222). SLACK Incorporated.

DeIuliis, E. D., & Saylor, E. (2021). Bridging the gap: Three strategies to optimize professional relationships with generation Y and Z. *The Open Journal of Occupational Therapy, 9*(1), 1-13. https://doi.org/10.15453/2168-6408.1748

Dickerson, A. E. (2006). Role competencies for a fieldwork educator. *American Journal of Occupational Therapy, 60*(6), 1-2. https://doi.org/10.5014/ajot.60.6.650

Diener, E., Napa Scollon, C., & Lucas, R. E. (2009). The evolving concept of subjective well-being: The multifaceted nature of happiness. In, Assessing well-being: Social indicators research series. Springer, Dordrecht. https://doi.org/10.1007/978-90-481-2354-4_4

Grimes, A., Medway, D., Foos, A., & Goatman, A. (2017). Impact bias in student evaluations of higher education. *Studies of Higher Education, 42*(6), 1-19.

Jette, D., Nelson, L., Palaima, M., & Weatersbee, E. (2014). How do we improve quality in clinical education? Examination of structures, processes, and outcomes. *Journal of Physical Therapy Education, 28*(10), 1-7. https://doi.org/10.1097/00001416-201400001-00004

Preissner, K., Duke, K. B., Killian, C., Luangdilok Ouyang, R., Jarek, E. D., & Kottorp, A. (2020). The revised american occupational therapy association fieldwork performance evaluations: Evaluation of content validity – Part 1. *American Journal of Occupational Therapy, 74*(6), 1-13.

University of Michigan Center for Research on Learning and Teaching. (2021). Summative and formative evaluation. https://crlt.umich.edu/tstrategies/tsfse

Wiggins, G. P. (1998). Educative assessment: Designing assessments to inform and improve student performance. (Volume 1). Jossey-Bass.

APPENDIX A
Program Developed Weekly Feedback Forms

University of North Dakota
Occupational Therapy Student Weekly Review Form

Student Name _____

Fieldwork Educator Name _____

Date _____ Week # _____

FUNDAMENTAL BASIC TENETS OF PRACTICE	
Areas of Strength	**Areas of Need**
EVALUATION AND SCREENING	
Areas of Strength	**Areas of Need**
INTERVENTION	
Areas of Strength	**Areas of Need**
MANAGEMENT OF OCCUPATIONAL THERAPY SERVICES	
Areas of Strength	**Areas of Need**
COMMUNICATION/PROFESSIONAL BEHAVIORS	
Areas of Strength	**Areas of Need**

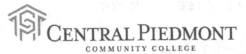

Fieldwork Weekly Feedback Form

Occupational Therapy Assistant Program – Level II Fieldwork

Student and FWE both complete a form prior to weekly feedback meetings. Use the results to promote dialogue and collaborate on goals for the following week(s).

Student Name	Week #	Date

Strengths and Successes this Week:

Areas for Growth:

Goals:

Signatures

Student Signature:	
FWE Signature:	

Central Piedmont Community College | P.O. Box 35009, Charlotte, NC 28235-5009 | cpcc.edu

13

Level II Fieldwork as a Gateway to the Doctoral Capstone Experience

Understanding the Role and Responsibilities of the Site Mentor

Ann B. Cook EdD., OTD, OTR/L, CPAM

As fieldwork education has been a formal, required part of occupational therapy education for more than 100 years, it is expected that the roles, responsibilities, and structure are relatively well-known to most practitioners across practice settings. Although the dialogue at the professional level about entry-level degree pathways for occupational therapy has been a hot topic over the past decade, it may be surprising to learn that the entry-level occupational therapy doctorate degree has existed for more than 20 years (American Occupational Therapy Association [AOTA], 2014). With this, and the exponential growth of new doctoral programs and master's-level programs transitioning to the doctoral level, there remains a lot of misconception among the profession, particularly related to the relationship between fieldwork education and the doctoral capstone (Cook, 2019).

Occupational therapy practitioners may be more familiar with their responsibilities in the role of a fieldwork educator (FWed) than they are in the role of a site mentor to a doctoral capstone student. As of the end of 2021, there are more than 50 fully accredited entry-level occupational therapy doctoral (OTD) programs across the United States, and more than 100 occupational therapy programs in process to transition to the doctorate or within candidacy/pre-accreditation status to develop an OTD program. This number is expected to increase by almost 400% in the next decade (Accreditation Council for Occupational Therapy Education [ACOTE], 2018a). With increasing numbers of occupational therapy programs across the nation transitioning to offer the entry-level doctoral degree, the number of individuals needed to serve as doctoral capstone site mentors will increase (Kemp et al., 2020). Simultaneous to the growth of doctoral programs in

DeIuliis, E. D., & Hanson, D. (Eds.).
Fieldwork Educator's Guide to Level II Fieldwork (pp. 371-413).

occupational therapy, there continues to be a shortage of fieldwork sites (Evenson et al., 2015), as well as a traumatic impact to the sustainability of fieldwork placement models due to the global COVID-19 pandemic. Because of these contextual factors, it is reasonable for occupational therapy practitioners to be prepared to be asked to serve the profession, both as a FWed and a doctoral capstone site mentor. While this may seem daunting, there are clear benefits of serving in both roles. Prior to accepting an opportunity to mentor a doctoral capstone student, the occupational therapy practitioner should understand how the role, responsibilities, and skill sets of the FWed compare and contrast with those of the site mentor.

This chapter will provide an overview of the doctoral capstone, which includes a mentored experience and a capstone project. Practitioners who are more familiar with the model and structure of fieldwork education will learn about the importance of mentorship that is required within the doctoral capstone and how to enhance known skill sets that support fieldwork to align with the objectives of the doctoral capstone. Benefits of serving as a site mentor and benefits of the capstone project to the practice setting will also be discussed.

KEY WORDS

- **ACOTE focus areas**: "Clinical practice skills, research skills, administration, leadership, program and policy development, advocacy, education, and theory development" (ACOTE, 2018b, p. 52).

- **Capstone chair**: Faculty member in the occupational therapy program who collaborates with the student and with the capstone coordinator throughout the capstone process to ensure the capstone aligns with the curriculum design and meets ACOTE standards.

- **Capstone coordinator**: "Faculty member who is specifically responsible for the program's compliance with the capstone requirements of Standards Section D.1.0 and is assigned to the occupational therapy educational program as a full-time core faculty member as defined by ACOTE" (ACOTE, 2018b, p. 55).

- **Doctoral capstone**: "An in-depth exposure to a concentrated area, which is an integral part of the program's curriculum design. This in-depth exposure may be in one or more of the following areas: clinical practice skills, research skills, scholarship, administration, leadership, program and policy development, advocacy, education, and theory development. The doctoral capstone consists of two parts: the capstone experience and the capstone project" (ACOTE, 2018b, p. 57).

  - **Capstone experience**: "A 14-week full-time in-depth exposure in a concentrated area that may include on-site and off-site activities that meets developed goals/objectives of the doctoral capstone" (ACOTE, 2018b, p. 55).

  - **Capstone project**: "A project that is completed by a doctoral-level student that demonstrates the student's ability to relate theory to practice and to synthesize in-depth knowledge in a practice area that relates to the capstone experience" (ACOTE, 2018b, p. 56).

- **Mentoring**: "A relationship between two people in which one person (the mentor) is dedicated to the personal and professional growth of the other (the mentee). A mentor has more experience and knowledge than the mentee" (ACOTE, 2018b, p. 59).

- **Site mentor**: An individual with expertise consistent with the student's area of focus for the doctoral capstone experience. "The site mentor does not have to be an occupational therapist" (ACOTE, 2018b, p. 58).

- **Supervising**: To "direct and inspect the performance of workers or work" (ACOTE, 2018b, p. 54).

LEARNING OBJECTIVES

By the end of reading this chapter and completing the learning activities, the reader should be able to:

1. Define the key differences between Level II fieldwork and the doctoral capstone.

2. Compare and contrast the role, responsibilities, and skill sets of the Level II FWed and the doctoral capstone site mentor.

3. Understand how to encourage students' critical thinking, problem-solving, and self-directed learning as they transition from fieldwork to the doctoral capstone.

4. Explore alternative mentorship models and the benefits of the mentorship role.

5. Articulate the process for becoming a doctoral capstone mentor.

COMPARING AND CONTRASTING LEVEL II FIELDWORK AND THE DOCTORAL CAPSTONE

As discussed in prior chapters of this book, the goal of Level II fieldwork is to "develop competent, entry-level, generalist occupational therapists" (ACOTE, 2018b, p. 42). Fieldwork students are expected to be able to evaluate clients with a variety of diagnoses, deliver appropriate and effective interventions, and assess the outcomes of such interventions. In addition, Level II fieldwork students should demonstrate competence in the administration and management of occupational therapy services (e.g., documentation, interprofessional collaboration, discharge planning). The emphasis on Level II fieldwork is on solidifying skills for direct practice. The individual who provides supervision, evaluation, clinical instruction, and guidance to the fieldwork student is referred to as the FWed. While fieldwork is required for both the entry-level master's and entry-level doctoral degrees, a signature difference between the two degrees is the requirement of the doctoral capstone.

A capstone is not an uncommon requirement for doctoral-level education in health professions (Krusen et al., 2020). The purpose of the capstone is quite variable across and even within health profession degrees. In occupational therapy, the doctoral capstone has evolved over time, both in the terminology used to describe the capstone and in the requirements of the capstone itself. For instance, in the 2011 ACOTE standards, the language used was a 16-week doctoral experiential component that was to "develop occupational therapists with advanced skills (those that are beyond a generalist level)" (ACOTE, 2011, p. 37). The doctoral experiential component was to include an in-depth experience in one or more of the following: clinical practice skills, research skills, administration, leadership, program and policy development, advocacy, education, or theory development. The experience was to align with the student's individualized specific objectives, and the doctoral student was required to complete a culminating project which aligned with their chosen focus area(s) (ACOTE, 2011).

While current accreditation standards are similar in some ways, there are also some notable changes in terminology and content required. The 2018 ACOTE standards coined a broader term to describe this educational requirement, the doctoral capstone. The interpretative language in the accreditation standards further unpacks the description of the doctoral capstone to include two main components: an experience and a project (ACOTE, 2018b). The doctoral capstone experience (DCE) is at minimum a 14-week experience (560 hours). This shortened time frame fits a little more neatly within a traditional college semester; however, each OTD program may situate

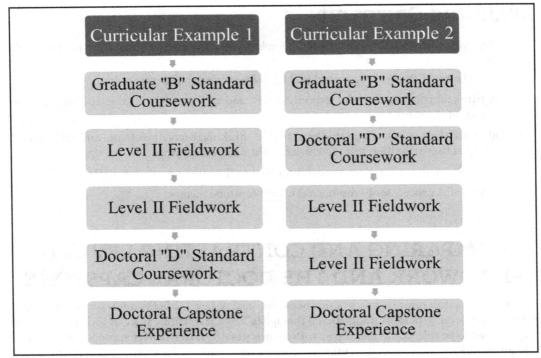

Figure 13-1. Examples of the DCE situated within curricula.

the DCE differently within their curriculum. For example, some occupational therapy programs might complete all the prerequisite coursework for the capstone even before Level II fieldwork, and a doctoral student then moves right from completing Level II fieldwork to the DCE. Other programs might situate the required preparatory coursework (which requires the student to develop a literature review, complete a needs assessment, create goals and objectives for the project, and an evaluation plan) after Level II fieldwork, and therefore there is another didactic semester that occurs between Level II fieldwork and the DCE. See Figure 13-1 for two different examples of curricular designs surrounding the DCE. Similar to the previous accreditation standards, the student's capstone project is to demonstrate the ability to synthesize in-depth knowledge in the chosen focus area(s) (ACOTE, 2018b). This next section will further describe the make-up of a doctoral capstone.

The Doctoral Capstone Experience

While Level II fieldwork is meant to prepare students for generalist practice, the goal of the DCE is "to provide in-depth exposure to one or more of the following: clinical practice skills, research skills, administration, leadership, program and policy development, advocacy, education, and theory development" (ACOTE, 2018b, p. 44). It is through the mentored DCE that an occupational therapy student can develop in-depth skills in their chosen focus area(s). A national survey determined that advanced clinical skills was the most selected focus area followed by program and policy development (Kemp et al., 2020).

TABLE 13-1

DOCTORAL CAPSTONE EXPERIENCE FOCUS AREAS

FOCUS AREA	DESCRIPTION
Clinical practice skills	The OTD student gains in-depth clinical skills by working with a specific population or within a specialized practice setting, as overseen by an expert mentor. Examples: advancing skills in hand therapy, work hardening, or in the neonatal intensive care unit
Research skills	The OTD student collaborates with researchers on a particular research project, including leading various portions of the study. Example: leading a research project regarding the effectiveness of fall prevention education for rehab staff
Administration	The OTD student collaborates with distinguished occupational therapists who manage private practices, therapy departments, or specialized sites. Examples: gaining in-depth skills related to billing, insurance, quality care outcomes, and entrepreneurship
Leadership	The OTD student develops skills to lead and represent the profession at the national and/or international level or within the organization. Examples: serving on the board of an organization within the practice setting or developing clinical best practice information and presenting at a conference
Program development	The OTD student completes a needs assessment, program planning, proposal writing, implementation, and measurement of program outcomes in a clinical or community setting. Examples: identifying the need for occupational therapy in an underrepresented setting (such as prenatal care for mothers in a homeless shelter) and implementing a sustainable program at the site

(continued)

As students may choose to gain in-depth skills in more than one focus area, their time could be spent in a variety of ways, working toward their learning objectives and honing particular skills. It is not uncommon for students to choose to develop skills in both program development and clinical practice (e.g., both administration and leadership, or in both policy development and advocacy). Stephenson et al. (2020) shared that the majority of the doctoral students do choose two or more focus areas and in agreement with Kemp et al. (2020), that the most chosen combination was advanced clinical skills and program development. Table 13-1 provides a description and examples of each of the focus areas. These are just a few of the numerous ways in which a doctoral capstone student can not only further their own learning and professional development but also make a direct impact on the site and clients. Site mentors should not be afraid to think outside of the box!

TABLE 13-1 (CONTINUED)
DOCTORAL CAPSTONE EXPERIENCE FOCUS AREAS

FOCUS AREA	DESCRIPTION
Policy development	The OTD student analyzes a site-specific, state, or national health care policy and proposes a change in the policy.
	Example: meeting with stakeholders impacted by the policy and collaborating with recognized individuals to lobby for change related to the policy
Advocacy	The OTD student advocates for the profession at the local, state, or federal level.
	Examples: advocating for occupational therapy services in the neonatal intensive care unit at a local hospital, representing the profession at legislative meetings regarding current issues
Education	The OTD student gains knowledge related to the role of the educator, whether formally in academia or in practice in the clinic.
	Examples: contributing to a course as a guest speaker with a local university, developing and delivering a series of continuing education courses for clinicians regarding best practice techniques
Theory development	The OTD student actively works with individuals to test models related to occupational therapy in regard to specific types of intervention.
	Examples: analyzing neurodevelopment treatment techniques and outcomes of interest, conducting research as it pertains to evidence-based practice

The Doctoral Capstone Project

In addition to the capstone experience, doctoral students are required to complete a capstone project to "demonstrate synthesis and application of knowledge gained during the experience" (ACOTE, 2018b, p. 46). Ensuring that the capstone project aligns with the student's chosen focus area(s) is important, as is ensuring that it aligns with the site's mission, vision, and values. It is critical that the site mentor understands that the capstone project is not the same as the experience. Depending on the program's requirements, a completed capstone project could be a written manuscript or report, practice guidelines, portfolio, or another tangible product that relates to the DCE and demonstrates synthesis of in-depth knowledge (ACOTE, 2018b; Cook, 2019; Wasmuth & Polo, 2019). While the DCE is more evident as a 14-week experience, the project is demonstrative of the culmination of their learning and should be related to the student's chosen learning objectives and focus areas.

There are no specifics regarding the amount of time that should be spent on the project, but it really should be the focal point of the student's whole experience. Certainly, doctoral students can spend time during their DCE on other tasks that increase their knowledge and skills, but creation and implementation of the culminating project should also be occurring. Students may spend the initial weeks of their DCE orienting themselves to the site and finalizing plans for the project based on the feedback of the site mentor. From there, the project may be carried out over the course of several weeks, perhaps 8 to 10, depending on the scope of the project, with the final weeks of the DCE spent on finalizing deliverables and educating the site and site mentor regarding

---

Box 13-1

CASE SCENARIO

A doctoral student is completing their capstone at an inpatient rehabilitation facility, specifically on a spinal cord injury unit. The student's focus areas are clinical practice and program development. The student's capstone project is focused around creating a more structured patient-education program that occurs within the unit's discharge process. One of the student's individualized learning objectives is to gain in-depth knowledge in bowel and bladder management.

In collaboration with their site mentor, the student initiates communication with various professionals, including the lead nurse on the unit that teaches bowel and bladder training. The student and the nurse set a schedule that allows the student the opportunity to engage in direct observation of individualized training and group therapy sessions that occur on the unit. The site mentor also provides support and guidance to the doctoral student to work alongside other professionals on the unit such as a registered respiratory therapist who specializes in working with individuals who have new quadriplegia.

Over the course of 14 weeks, the student is simultaneously working to achieve the individualized learning objectives as well as complete the capstone project. Action steps for the capstone project might include refining the needs assessment, become familiar with related literature, building a problem statement and gap analysis, collecting data or feedback from stakeholders, analyzing outcomes and/or evaluating the effectiveness of the program, etc. As the DCE comes to an end, the student presents the revamped patient-education discharge program to the site staff and administration, as well as participates in a formal dissemination at the occupational therapy program, such as a poster session or symposium event.

---

the outcomes of the project and any continuation that should occur after the student finishes. It is critical that the site mentor keep the student's learning objectives in mind when considering additional learning experiences to offer outside of the capstone project. See Box 13-1 for an example.

Another important consideration for the DCE is the time requirement, which differs from Level II fieldwork. Whereas the expectation for occupational therapy fieldwork students is that they spend their time on-site, usually engaged in direct practice for 24 weeks, the DCE does allow for some flexibility in time spent on-site vs. off. Eighty percent of the DCE must occur on-site, while 20% of the experience may occur off-site. This off-site time can be spent engaged in learning opportunities unavailable to the capstone student at the site itself or spent creating deliverables related to the project. Using the example in Box 13-1, where the DCE is occurring on an inpatient spinal cord injury unit, the doctoral student might plan to use off-site time to attend relevant trainings to enhance content knowledge captured in the individualized student learning objectives. In addition, there might be a weekly or monthly educational event offered by the local chapter of the National Spinal Cord Injury Association. Another example is that the capstone student might plan to regularly attend a support group in the area to learn more about the lived experience of the population. Alternatively, the student might plan for a recurring weekly or monthly day to shadow other health care practitioners who work with this population in different settings, such as outpatient, or even a driver's rehabilitation program. See Appendix A for examples of tasks appropriate for time spent both on- and off-site. It is the capstone student's responsibility to communicate with their site mentor regarding how they plan to spend their hours and obtain approval as needed from the site mentor for hours spent off-site. See Box 13-2 for some examples of beneficial learning opportunities for the doctoral student.

Box 13-2

CONSIDER BENEFICIAL LEARNING OPPORTUNITIES

Clinicians, consider what makes the most sense for the doctoral capstone student's time on site. Keep in mind their chosen focus area(s) and learning objectives. Consider the following questions:

- Are there particular days when opportunities are available that would be valuable learning experiences for the capstone student? For example, do team "rounds" occur on a particular day of the week?
- For advancing their clinical skills, are there particular days when new patients are admitted and evaluated?
- For leadership, are there recurring meetings in which their participation would be beneficial?

TRUTH OR MYTH ABOUT SERVING AS A SITE MENTOR?

Although entry-level occupational therapy doctoral programs have existed for more than 20 years, the purpose and expectations have continued to shift. Practitioners might have outdated knowledge, assumptions, or misconceptions that impact their willingness to serve as a site mentor. This next section will highlight a few scenarios that might raise questions regarding the requirements of the doctoral capstone. Are they truth or are they myth? See Table 13-2 for common assumptions and misconceptions.

THE SITE MENTOR

An essential difference between fieldwork and the doctoral capstone is the critical role of a mentor and the concept of mentorship. Clinicians serving as Level II FWeds are responsible for providing supervision of and direct instruction to fieldwork students. Clinicians must provide frequent assessment of student progress toward their learning objectives (ACOTE, 2018b). During Level II fieldwork, supervision should be direct and progress to less direct as the student becomes more competent (ACOTE, 2018b). Instead of a FWed serving as a role model and teacher for entry-level generalist practice skills, the capstone requires the doctoral student to be mentored. This individual is referred to as the site mentor. As the purpose and goal of the doctoral capstone differs from fieldwork, it is critical for individuals who are interested in serving as a site mentor to understand how their role and responsibilities will shift. See Box 13-3 for a list of responsibilities of the site mentor.

According to ACOTE (2018b), the site mentor is responsible for mentoring the doctoral student in their focus area(s). The capstone coordinator, who is an academic faculty member, is required to ensure that there is a valid memorandum of understanding (MOU) in place, which shares the roles and responsibilities of the doctoral student, site mentor, and possibly the faculty member who serves as a capstone chair to the student's project.

TABLE 13-2

FREQUENT ASSUMPTIONS OR MISCONCEPTIONS ABOUT THE DOCTORAL CAPSTONE

SCENARIO	TRUTH OR MYTH
A doctoral student is torn between advancing their clinical skills with clients with dementia and developing a program for caregivers. The student cannot address both and must choose one focus area for the doctoral capstone experience.	**Myth**. The student may choose more than one focus area, such as a combination of advanced clinical skills and program development skills.
A doctoral student has chosen to focus on advancing clinical practice skills during the DCE at an acute care hospital. Because of their chosen focus area, the student is required to maintain a full caseload of clients.	**Myth**. There are no guidelines requiring a doctoral capstone student to maintain a full caseload. While this could occur, it may make more sense for the student to evaluate and treat some of the more complex clients while spending a portion of the DCE gaining knowledge in another area (e.g., learning the roles of other professionals on the care team) and completing their capstone project.
A doctoral student proposes their schedule at their DCE to be four, 10-hour days; however, the student's mentor works a traditional 5 days per week schedule. The student must maintain the same schedule as their site mentor.	**Myth**. The student is to be mentored, not supervised, during the capstone. The site mentor and doctoral student do not need to work the same hours as long as the mentor is comfortable with the student's ability to work independently.
A doctoral student would like to telecommute or work remotely on Mondays, preparing materials for their project implementation throughout the week. They will then be present at the site Tuesday through Friday. This is permissible based on accreditation standards.	**Truth**. ACOTE (2018b) standards require that the student spend 80% of their time on-site, and the student may spend up to 20% of their time off-site. This could be similar to four, 8-hour days on-site and one, 8-hour day off-site each week, or it could be more variable, depending on the site's needs and the student's project.

(continued)

Memorandum of Understanding

The MOU is the agreement in which the student and the site mentor officially document the student's individualized learning objectives, plans for supervision and mentorship, and an agreement regarding the responsibilities of all parties involved (ACOTE, 2018b). Each program's MOU will look a little different but should include verbiage similar to a contract in which the clinician is agreeing to mentor the doctoral student, evaluate their progress, collaborate on scholarly products (perhaps as a contributing author), and provide evidence of their expertise. Evidence of expertise in the student's chosen focus area(s) could include an updated résumé or curriculum vitae, a job description, a copy of a relevant advanced certification received, or evidence of continued education beyond the generalist level in a particular area of practice. See Appendix B for an example of one program's MOU.

TABLE 13-2 (CONTINUED)

FREQUENT ASSUMPTIONS OR MISCONCEPTIONS ABOUT THE DOCTORAL CAPSTONE

SCENARIO	TRUTH OR MYTH
A doctoral student is completing the doctoral capstone at a community site at which no occupational therapists are employed. The student is creating and implementing vocational skills groups for young adults. The student must find an occupational therapist who is willing to be present during the group sessions.	**Myth**. The doctoral student does not need to be supervised by an occupational therapist. They are to be supervised by someone with expertise in their focus area.
A doctoral student who is evaluating and/or treating clients and billing for occupational therapy services must be supervised by an occupational therapist.	**Truth**. While the student's site mentor does not have to be an occupational therapist, for any billable services, an occupational therapist must supervise the student as the student does not have a license or certification according to their State Practice Act, or guidelines stipulated by the third-party payer, such as Centers for Medicare & Medicaid Services.
A doctoral student would like to be mentored by a clinician with expertise in traumatic brain injury practice. The clinician earned their master's degree and has practiced for the last 10 years with the population; however, because they do not have a doctoral degree, they cannot serve as a site mentor to an occupational therapy doctoral student.	**Myth**. ACOTE (2018b) standards do not stipulate the degree level of individuals who can serve as site mentors. In fact, a site mentor does not even have to be an occupational therapist. Professionals who have mentored doctoral students have included physical therapists, teachers, social workers, and even graphic designers (Kemp et al., 2020). Site mentors must have documented expertise aligned with the student's focus area.

Individualized Learning Objectives and Evaluation

Similar to responsibilities of the FWed, the site mentor is also responsible for evaluating the doctoral student's performance during the capstone experience. For fieldwork, students might be evaluated based upon their ability to meet site-specific objectives or achieve certain performance competencies such as within the AOTA FWPE (2020) tool. Within the DCE, achievement of the in-depth knowledge and skill should coincide with the individualized student learning objectives stipulated in the MOU. Occupational therapy doctoral programs might have their own established learning objectives that align with the program's curriculum (ACOTE, 2018a); thus, it is important that the site mentor familiarize themselves with the learning objectives early in the process, in order to be on the lookout for student progress toward these objectives. Alongside these general

> **BOX 13-3**
> # RESPONSIBILITIES OF THE SITE MENTOR
>
> The DCE site mentor should understand their role in providing appropriate mentorship to the capstone student. The site mentor should:
>
> - Have expertise in the student's focus area(s). The site mentor may be asked by the OTD program to provide evidence of expertise, such as a résumé or curriculum vitae for the program's accreditation records.
> - Meet with the student regarding the needs assessment and connect them with other key stakeholders for this process. The timing and length of the needs assessment will vary by program.
> - Collaborate with the student regarding creating individualized learning objectives for the DCE.
> - Provide an initial orientation to the site, overview of important processes, and introduce other key staff members.
> - Provide mentorship to the capstone student during the 14-week experience.
> - Provide support when necessary while allowing the student the autonomy to make decisions and problem solve challenges.
> - Collaborate with and guide the capstone student as they seek feedback.
> - Complete an evaluation of student progress toward the DCE learning objectives (this may vary by program, yet it may occur around the midterm [week 7] and final [week 14]).
> - Communicate with program's capstone coordinator, especially regarding any questions or issues that may arise.
> - Consider contributing to and being listed as a contributing author on any disseminated work related to the DCE by the capstone student.

objectives, the doctoral student would then also be expected to initiate and maintain collaboration with their site mentor to create individualized learning objectives. These individualized learning objectives should clearly relate to the in-depth skills the student wants to gain during their experience and will also most likely relate to their capstone project.

A clinician who is mentoring a doctoral capstone student for the first time may be interested in learning how to ensure that the experience is increasing the student's knowledge and skills beyond that of a generalist. Creating the "just-right challenge" for the student to gain in-depth knowledge does not need to be difficult. Many site-specific fieldwork objectives can be used as a starting point for considering how to facilitate the student's growth. Things to consider include the setting and population that the student will address during the DCE, the student's chosen focus area(s), and the objectives that they have already achieved during their fieldwork experiences. The site mentor should ask themselves, *What is the next step?* Figure 13-2 depicts a formula to convert traditional Level II fieldwork site-specific objectives across various settings into DCE learning objectives that align with ACOTE focus areas. It is important that these focus areas, as well as the setting and population, are considered to create realistic learning objectives.

While this seems like a simple equation, it may be helpful to view various examples based on each of the focus areas and with a variety of practice settings in mind. Table 13-3 includes examples of Level II fieldwork objectives with a graded challenge specific to the student's area of focus in order to become appropriate DCE objectives.

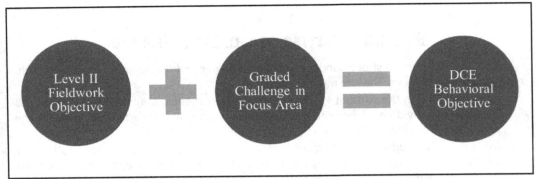

Figure 13-2. Process for creating DCE objectives from Level II fieldwork objectives.

It is important to keep in mind that these are examples of how to create DCE objectives from existing Level II fieldwork objectives; however, this is not a hard-and-fast rule. Although it is best practice, a site may not have site-specific objectives. The site mentor could consider asking the program for examples of their objectives. There are also resources available online to use as a starting point (AOTA, n.d.). In other cases, students may have very particular or unique interests, therefore, being creative with DCE objectives may be necessary. Some questions that the site mentor should consider asking themselves are, *"Is this an objective that a student would typically meet upon completing Level II fieldwork?"* or *"Is this a competency area that is aligned with entry-level occupational therapy practice?"* If the answer is yes, then the site mentor should guide the doctoral student to think about how to elevate the objective into a measurable statement that leads to more in-depth knowledge and skills. Following are a few more examples of creative learning objectives that aim for in-depth skills beyond that achieved upon completion of Level II fieldwork:

- Focus area—Clinical skills: Student will be able to demonstrate proficient ergonomic consultations for health care workers in a hospital setting.

- Focus area—Research: Student will evaluate the outcomes of animal-assisted therapy vs. Neurodevelopmental Treatment on postural control for children with decreased tone.

- Focus area—Program development: Student will increase clinical practice skills in relation to group therapy by creating a therapeutic leisure group for residents based on the outcomes of the Leisure Interest Checklist.

See Box 13-4 for a tip for creating objectives.

The authorship of the learning objectives requires the doctoral student to be self-directed and take ownership of their learning. One way to encourage the doctoral student to be self-directed early on, even before the DCE starts, is to ask them to create action steps and a timeline to meet their individualized learning objectives. Doing so will allow them to create very clear criteria for themselves regarding what it would mean to successfully meet each of their learning objectives. Appendix C includes two charts that can be used as examples. The first chart is completed as the student writes individualized learning objectives, the actions or steps they will take to meet the objectives, a proposed timeline for completion of each objective, the skills they possess and the resources available to them to support their success, and objective evidence to confirm accomplishment. The second chart requires the student to plan a 14-week timeline for their DCE.

TABLE 13-3

EXAMPLES OF CONVERTING LEVEL II FIELDWORK OBJECTIVES INTO DOCTORAL CAPSTONE EXPERIENCE OBJECTIVES

SETTING	LEVEL II FIELDWORK OBJECTIVE	DCE OBJECTIVE
Inpatient rehabilitation	Student will demonstrate competency in evaluation procedures, including the administration, scoring, and interpretation of assessments appropriate for inpatient rehabilitation.	*Focus Area: Research* Student will demonstrate the ability to statistically analyze client outcomes from initial assessment to discharge based on change measured with selected assessment tools after receiving chosen intervention.
Outpatient hand therapy	Student will demonstrate proficiency in the application of therapeutic activities, including grading, adapting, and modifying, for patients referred for outpatient services.	*Focus Area: Advanced Clinical Skills* Student will demonstrate advanced knowledge and proficiency with orthotic fabrication including the creation of dynamic and static progressive orthoses.
Home health	Student will demonstrate effective oral and written communication skills as demonstrated by their documentation of service provision and interactions with patients and staff.	*Focus Area: Leadership* Student will lead home health clinicians on best practices for completing communication logs for the patient and caregiver for increased adherence to home programs.
Long-term acute care	Student will demonstrate the ability to establish and sustain therapeutic relationships.	*Focus Area: Theory Development* Student will explore the therapeutic use of self as a motivating factor for clients when evaluating and treating clients through the lens of the Model of Human Occupation.

(continued)

Similar to Level II fieldwork, doctoral programs must have an evaluation mechanism in place for the DCE. As there is not a formal tool endorsed by the profession (Kemp et al., 2020), most doctoral programs create their own evaluation approach for the site mentor to provide feedback on the student's performance. Doctoral programs might require the student to be evaluated around midterm (7 weeks into the experience) and final (14 weeks), though that is not necessarily the rule. See Appendix D as an example of an evaluation.

TABLE 13-3 (CONTINUED)
EXAMPLES OF CONVERTING LEVEL II FIELDWORK OBJECTIVES INTO DOCTORAL CAPSTONE EXPERIENCE OBJECTIVES

SETTING	LEVEL II FIELDWORK OBJECTIVE	DCE OBJECTIVE
Inpatient acute care	Student will demonstrate the ability to work as a member of a treatment team.	*Focus Area: Administration* Student will establish decision trees for all members of the therapy team to screen patients upon initial evaluation to determine if a need for other services is warranted.
Inpatient psychiatric unit	Student will appropriately consider and address psychosocial factors related to client's occupational performance.	*Focus Area: Program Development* Student will create and implement a support group for patients to explore appropriate use of free time through meaningful leisure activities and healthy social interactions.
Skilled nursing facility	Student will demonstrate respect for patient confidentiality and autonomy.	*Focus Area: Advocacy* Student will advocate for the patient's rights by promoting through their state association and local policies a definition of medical necessity that fully encompasses their patient's needs.
School-based	Student will demonstrate the ability to integrate evidence into the selection of appropriate interventions for treatment of the child.	*Focus Area: Education* Student will create an evidence-based weekly module for families to educate them on the benefits of and techniques to engage in therapeutic play with their child.

UNDERSTANDING SUPERVISION VERSUS MENTORSHIP

It is critical to understand that being a mentor to a doctoral student is a different role than being a FWed who provides supervision to a fieldwork student. The two learning experiences are different, and thus the expectations and roles of the student and clinician are different. It may be helpful for the site mentor to consider Dr. Paula Kramer's description of the capstone in relation to AOTA's (2017) Vision 2025. Kramer stated,

I think both the experience and the capstone project can do exactly what the vision projects for the future. That is, provided that the experiences and the capstone are truly at a higher level, and involve careful research and/or program development related to

---

Box 13-4

ADVICE FOR CREATING DCE LEARNING OBJECTIVES

Although the DCE learning objectives should be derived from a collaboration between the doctoral student and the site mentor... when in doubt, reach out to the program's capstone coordinator. They are well versed in the programs' curriculum design and expectations as well as the student's interests. They can help to create appropriate learning objectives.

---

occupations, and are not simply seen as an extension of the Level II fieldwork experience or just a project to be completed without deeper meaning and insight. (Whitney & McCormack, 2020, p. 2)

The emphasis on "higher level" is key. To compare, the DCE differs from Level II fieldwork in several ways. First, with Level II fieldwork in traditional settings, the student is usually supervised by an occupational therapist. Standard C.1.13 states that Level II fieldwork supervision is required to be "direct and then decreases to less direct supervision as appropriate for the setting, the severity of the client's condition, and the ability of the student to support progression toward entry-level competence" (ACOTE, 2018b, p. 43). In contrast, with the DCE, the student is to be mentored by an individual with expertise in their in-depth area of focus (ACOTE, 2018b). This person may or may not be an occupational therapist. In fact, students may choose to complete their experience and project at a role-emerging site at which there is no employed occupational therapist on staff or, depending on the nature of their focus area or objectives, a student's mentor might be another health or administrative professional such as a dietician or quality improvement coordinator within a health system.

Models of Supervision

A quality fieldwork experience is expected to include detailed and clear expectations of the student, quality feedback from the supervisor, and a structured learning environment (Rodger et al., 2011). Often, FWeds are very hands-on at the beginning of the experience and only in the final weeks may they feel comfortable allowing the student to direct the occupational therapy process. Interestingly, this type of one-to-one supervision can impede students from developing critical thinking and problem solving due to reliance on their fieldwork supervisor for direction (Copley & Nelson, 2012), and this model is certainly not ideal for the DCE. However, other models for fieldwork supervision can be useful for facilitating students' self-directedness in preparation for the DCE.

As covered in Chapter 2 of this book, the collaborative model of fieldwork supervision is one such model. In this model, a FWed supervises two or more students at the same time, and the students are able to collaborate to problem solve and learn together (Hanson & DeIuliis, 2015). Students can share their ideas with one another, feel empowered to share ideas with the supervisor, and learn that there is often more than one way to approach a clinical problem. Students who experience this type of fieldwork supervision are more team oriented, self-directed, and learn to give and receive feedback as a professional, skills that are essential for a successful DCE.

An additional model that supports the self-directedness and autonomy of the student is one in which the student is supervised in a role-emerging setting. Within this type of fieldwork setting, the role of the occupational therapist is not yet clearly defined. Whereas in more traditional settings, students may easily model or follow the lead of the supervising therapist, a role-emerging setting requires creativity, the establishment of new processes, and the distinct value of occupational therapy to be asserted. Mattila et al. (2018) shared that students who completed fieldwork in

Box 13-5

Building Skills on Fieldwork for the Doctoral Capstone Experience

Provide the fieldwork student with the opportunity to develop their professional identity in a variety of ways. Allow them to introduce themselves and the role of occupational therapy in interprofessional team meetings; have them explain the role of occupational therapy to patients, family members, and caregivers; and allow them to observe other professionals and learn how the two professions collaborate for quality patient care. Provide opportunity for the student to visit area facilities that provide related services to your clients in the community and rehearse with them how they might explain the role of occupational therapy to professionals outside of the health care arena. After the visit, discuss what went well and how they might improve their explanations in future field trips.

Seek out opportunities for the student to collaborate with other students. Perhaps a Level II student could explain to a Level I student the rationale behind their intervention choices. Ask the fieldwork student to lead a co-treatment with a physical therapy student and then analyze with the student factors that impacted the success of the intervention. Give and receive feedback from one another as to professional strengths and areas of challenge; make a collaborative plan for professional development and future treatment sessions.

Know when to provide guidance and when to allow the fieldwork student the autonomy to make choices, even if that means they will need to experience a challenge in order to grow. For example, rather than reviewing with them the needs of a target population, challenge them to conduct a needs assessment process and use the results to identify an intervention plan. Remember, providing the "just-right challenge" applies to supervising and mentoring students as well as treating clients!

a role-emerging setting were able to provisionally try new roles in an interprofessional setting and increase their self-awareness of their skills as a future clinician. The autonomy required in role-emerging fieldwork settings prepares the student to have confidence in their professional identity, an essential attribute for the DCE.

Of course, the FWed may not work in a role-emerging setting, and they may not have the opportunity to supervise two fieldwork students using the collaborative model. However, there are experiences that can be offered to the student to mimic these models and thus create similar learning opportunities. While supervising a fieldwork student who plans to complete a DCE, the mentor can create opportunities in which the student can collaborate with other students, assert the value of occupational therapy to build their professional identity, and challenge them in ways that will foster autonomy. See Box 13-5 for advice on preparing fieldwork students with the skills needed for the DCE.

Models of Mentorship

Because the process and product of the doctoral capstone differs from fieldwork, it is necessary for all stakeholders to adopt a different mindset and way of thinking. Human-centered design has been pinpointed as one framework to help guide thinking about the doctoral capstone for occupational therapy students, faculty, and site mentors (DeIuliis & Bednarski, 2019). Human-centered design is one type of design thinking that showcases an iterative process to help a "designer," a doctoral student, to move through phases of discovery, brainstorming possibilities, and implementing their ideas (Brenner et al., 2016; IDEO, n.d.). Similar to the occupational therapy process, design thinking is iterative. It is not linear. Therefore, during the development and planning for the doctoral capstone a student might revisit various phases of the process, and growth is experienced when they get feedback from their site mentor, learn from mistakes or failures, or experience success. Preparing for and educating a doctoral student and site mentor about the differences in the process and outcome is important. While students are often afraid to take risks and make mistakes, allowing them to make decisions and experience the consequences (positive or negative) will help them to learn and grow. Of course, safety is of utmost importance, so any unsafe situations need to be avoided. But to promote divergent thinking, it is okay for the mentor to allow the doctoral student to attempt a task and fail, reflect on the process, and make changes to be successful in the future.

Another framework that the mentor might consider is the Systems and Experiential Learning Framework (S.E.L.F.) approach. This framework has been utilized for the creation of fieldwork and capstone handbooks to clearly articulate the policies, purpose, and intended outcomes of these learning experiences. The capstone site mentor might also use the framework for designing individualized learning objectives for the doctoral student. S.E.L.F. uses a structured evidence-based theoretical approach and includes the process of planning, designing, developing, writing, and evaluating fieldwork and capstone education with an accompanying manual (Delbert et al., 2020). The S.E.L.F. approach is grounded in systems and learning theories with core development strategies of plan, design, develop, write, and evaluate (Delbert et al., 2020). A site mentor can utilize these strategies with the doctoral student to consider factors impacting the learning experience and to ensure that student learning is prioritized.

Preparing Students for the Shift From Supervision to Mentorship

While the supervisory expectations are relatively clear for the FWed, the expectations of the site mentor are not as straightforward for the DCE, due to the individualized nature of the capstone experience and project, as well as the variation in pre-existing knowledge and comfort level of the capstone student in their focus area(s). Whereas the Level II fieldwork student is expected to be supervised, the doctoral capstone student is to be self-directed and take charge of their learning. In cases where the student is providing billable occupational therapy services, they should receive supervision, as they have not yet earned an entry-level occupational therapy degree nor their license and certification; however, in other aspects of the experience, the supervision should shift to mentorship, with the capstone student seeking feedback as needed from their site mentor. See Table 13-4 for a comparison of fieldwork supervision and doctoral capstone mentorship responsibilities.

For undergraduate students, Crisp (2009) suggested that mentoring is:

Support provided to college students that entails emotional and psychological guidance and support, help succeeding in academic coursework, assistance examining and selecting degree and career options, and the presence of a role model by which the student can learn from and copy their behaviors. (p. 189)

By the time students are enrolled in the DCE, they most likely have already completed most of their didactic coursework, but here the focus is on role modeling and guidance. It is vital that the mentor understand the student's pre-existing knowledge and professional goals to provide opportunities for growth (Johnson et al., 2001). Over time, the mentor's confidence in the student's abilities should foster trust and increased autonomy of the student. But one might ask, how does a mentor demonstrate confidence in the student?

Freeman et al. (2017) suggested that **regular and focused meetings** between the mentor and mentee can help to develop a student's confidence. It may be helpful to have a recurring meeting

TABLE 13-4

FIELDWORK SUPERVISION AND DOCTORAL CAPSTONE MENTORSHIP RESPONSIBILITIES

FIELDWORK SUPERVISION	DOCTORAL CAPSTONE MENTORSHIP
Start as direct, progressing to less direct supervision as the student gains entry-level skills	Initial onboarding may require more frequent mentorship but shortly thereafter should shift to regularly scheduled meetings and as-needed mentorship
Explain and demonstrate the policies, procedures, and daily operations to be modeled by the student	Provide the policies and procedures and immerse the student in the daily implementation early on
Foster development of entry-level, generalist skills	Foster development of in-depth knowledge in the student's chosen focus area(s)
Provide constructive criticism regarding the evaluation, intervention, and discharge planning processes led by the student	Collaborate with the student regarding their ideas, support creativity, and respect their foundational knowledge of the profession
Structure the fieldwork experience so that the student gradually builds to evaluating and treating a caseload of clients	Ensure that the student completes a culminating capstone project that demonstrates application and synthesis of knowledge gained
Complete a formal evaluation of the student's performance and progress toward entry-level generalist skills	Complete a formal evaluation of the student's performance and progress toward individualized learning objectives

at the same time each week to ensure consistent communication between the student and mentor, as with the busyness of clinical practice, time can pass without the mentor realizing it. The site mentor should **set clear expectations** at the start of the experience, so the student knows how and when to best communicate with the site mentor. One way to encourage the doctoral student to be self-directed is to require them to send a meeting agenda ahead of time. This will allow them to direct the conversation and ask questions or address areas of concern that they have. Since the agenda is written and shared, they should feel empowered to address each agenda item without feeling that they are "bothering" the site mentor. See Box 13-6 for communication expectations.

An additional way to build self-directed thinking is to **promote divergent thinking** discussed earlier. Divergent thinking is a specific type of thought process used for idea and solution genera-tion (Bednarski & DeIuliis, 2021). This differs from convergent thinking, which is the ability to give the "correct answer" to basic questions that do not require much creativity or problem solv-ing (Bednarski & DeIuliis, 2021). For Level II fieldwork, students might utilize more convergent thinking. They may need to recall information on-the-spot, such as developmental milestones, understand and respond to safety contraindications, and visualize anatomical landmarks during upper extremity examination, etc. Level II fieldwork is a much more linear process in competency development. The doctoral capstone requires that the student develops and uses divergent think-ing. The doctoral capstone requires the occupational therapy student to be comfortable with the exploration of multiple solutions and multiple idea formations, and the student often needs to go back to the drawing board to iterate (again) and shift their plan. See Table 13-5 for examples of convergent and divergent thinking.

Box 13-6

COMMUNICATION EXPECTATIONS

Following are questions that the site mentor should consider and discuss with the capstone student regarding their communication expectations. The site mentor should discuss these with the capstone student at the beginning of the experience:

What is the best way for the student to make contact—email, call, text, face to face? Are there any times that are off-limits? How much notice is needed in order to schedule a meeting—1 day or week? How much time is needed for the mentor to be able to review and provide feedback on any materials or products created by the capstone student?

Ensure that the student understands that it would be helpful if they saved non-urgent questions for regularly scheduled meetings, while more immediate needs can be discussed in the agreed-upon fashion (i.e., email, call, text) as needed.

TABLE 13-5

CONVERGENT VERSUS DIVERGENT THINKING

CONVERGENT	DIVERGENT
"I have a challenge …"	"How can I approach this …?"
"I learned something new …"	"What else can you tell me about this …?"
"I have an idea …"	"How do I build it …?"

Divergent thinking encourages the student to be curious, engage in brainstorming, generate ideas, think through problems, take risks, and to be creative, which are arguably essential components for a successful doctoral capstone. A site mentor's communication and interactions with the doctoral student should promote this type of thinking. Mattila et al. (2020) shared that students undergo a transformation during their doctoral capstone learning experiences. The student is presented with a new experience that is often disorienting, perhaps confusing, and presents a challenge. This "disorienting dilemma" is an opportunity for the student to reflect, examine their own knowledge, and seek available resources to support their ability to address the dilemma (Mattila et al., 2020). During this phase of the process, it is important for the mentor to encourage self-directedness. For instance, if a doctoral student comes to the mentor with a problem and asks for advice on what they should do, the site mentor should prompt them to think of creative solutions. A way to role model this type of thinking is to use the prompt, *"How might we …?"* The goal is for the student to have a free flow of thinking and more spontaneous idea generation rather than having their educator or mentor provide the answer.

Embracing and learning from failures is also important for the site mentor to role model. Due to the iterative process of the doctoral capstone, the student needs to be aware that their initial plan for the capstone project might shift, change, or even get scrapped all together. When the student successfully overcomes a challenge, asking the student what they learned and how it can be applied in the future will help them to take new skills and generalize them. The process of "becoming" an occupational therapy practitioner is fostered through this process of experiencing a problem, brainstorming creative solutions, implementing them, and learning from the results (Mattila et al., 2020). See Box 13-7 for a case scenario.

> **Box 13-7**
> ## CASE SCENARIO
>
> A doctoral student is completing their capstone experience at an inpatient rehabilitation hospital for military veterans. The student's project focuses on creating an education program for patients with new limb amputations. After spending a week at the site, the student has realized that many of the veterans who have amputations are not in rehab because of a new amputation but for other complications, some related to their amputation and some not related. The student is unsure of how to implement a project that is now less applicable to the patient population. The student approaches their site mentor, saying, "My project idea isn't going to work. The patients don't have new amputations. I don't think they need the information I'm creating for this program."
>
> The site mentor thinks about the student's dilemma and has several suggestions. But instead of sharing them, the site mentor asks the following questions:
> - *How might we utilize the information you've already created? Is there a way to build off of this foundation?*
> - *Are all of the patients well-versed in the information you've created?*
> - *Let's think about why the patients have been re-admitted in relation to their amputation. What are some of the recurring issues?*
>
> After hearing these questions and brainstorming with the mentor, the student can come up with creative solutions to the problem and redirect the project focus. The student can use some of the original materials as intended and adds others where appropriate.

BEST PRACTICE QUALITIES OF A SITE MENTOR

To be effective as a site mentor, the practitioner needs the ability to communicate effectively, to collaborate with the doctoral student, and should genuinely care for the student's learning. While these seem like the characteristics of any good clinical educator, there are some differences in application between fieldwork and the capstone.

There are five standards that are attributed to being a competent FWed: knowledge, critical reasoning, performance skills, interpersonal skills, and ethical reasoning (AOTA, 2006). DeIuliis (2017) further outlined attributes of a successful FWed, and these are starting points for considering the attributes of an effective doctoral capstone site mentor. While there is not an official paper within the profession to emulate role competencies of the site mentor, Table 13-6 outlines how these FWed competencies can be shifted to reflect an effective site mentor.

CREATIVE SCENARIOS FOR THE SITE MENTOR

Given the increased demand for FWeds, clinicians may be asked to supervise one or more fieldwork students at the same time. Now, with entry-level doctoral programs on the rise across the country, a clinician may be more likely to be asked to mentor a doctoral student. So, what exactly is the most ideal scenario for mentoring a doctoral student? The truth is that a clinician can mentor a doctoral student in many different scenarios. Just like there are numerous models to supervise fieldwork students, there are different ways to mentor doctoral capstone students.

TABLE 13-6
ROLE COMPETENCIES OF A FIELDWORK EDUCATOR AND ATTRIBUTES OF AN EFFECTIVE SITE MENTOR

ROLE COMPETENCIES OF A FIELDWORK EDUCATOR	ATTRIBUTES OF AN EFFECTIVE SITE MENTOR
Developing and maintaining proficiency through formal education, continuing education, and self-study	Demonstrating expertise in particular focus area(s) and maintaining expertise through formal education, continuing education, and self-study
Maintaining knowledge of current standards, rules, and regulations	Making improvements to processes based on current standards, rules, and regulations
Evaluating interpersonal dynamics	Utilizing effective interpersonal skills with clients, students, and colleagues to improve situational outcomes
Projecting a positive self-image	Mentoring the student to recognize their strengths and to draw on such strengths to overcome challenges
Demonstrating a positive attitude toward practice and supervision	Enthusiastically collaborating with the student in a partnership to draw upon each other's knowledge and creating experiences to help the student grow
Planning fieldwork experiences that prepare ethical practitioners	Facilitating divergent thinking by sharing realistic challenges faced in the practice setting and supporting the student in problem-solving ethical dilemmas
Acting as a role model	Acting as a role model and helping the student to identify characteristics and skills in themselves that will help them to model the same behaviors

Same-Site Model (for Fieldwork and Doctoral Capstone Experience)

Consider this: A clinician is supervising a student during their Level II fieldwork. The fieldwork student is professional and hard-working, and the clinician very much enjoys supervising them as a FWed. The student mentions during conversation that following Level II fieldwork, they will be continuing in their studies to receive an entry-level doctoral degree. The student will need to complete a DCE as part of their degree. Wouldn't it be great if the clinician could choose to work with this student on their DCE? They probably can! The clinician should reach out to the program's doctoral capstone coordinator. If the student plans to live in the same area for their doctoral education and their focus area aligns with the site's needs, it may be a welcome suggestion for the student to work at the same site on a capstone project to meet a current need at the site. The clinician should discuss it with the student while they are completing their fieldwork. See Box 13-8 for an example of a same-site model.

Box 13-8
EXAMPLE OF A SAME-SITE MODEL

A Level II fieldwork student is midway through her second Level II fieldwork at a large inpatient rehabilitation hospital. She and her FWed have a good working relationship, and the student has shared that she is continuing her education and will be completing her DCE and project, though she is unsure of where she will be located. The student hopes to complete her experience in a hospital setting but is open to ideas for her capstone project.

One day, the FWed and student are attending the bi-weekly staff meeting where the director of rehab shares results of the post-discharge patient satisfaction surveys. Unfortunately, patients have been sharing that they do not feel involved in setting their own goals for therapy, and therefore they are not motivated to participate. The FWed is concerned by this and wants to know how to best address the problem. After thinking about it, the FWed approaches the student with an idea to improve patient experiences at the hospital. The student agrees that she, too, is interested in this project and wonders if it could be feasible for her doctoral capstone. Together, they approach the program's capstone coordinator about the possibility of future collaborations.

The capstone coordinator is happy to hear of the great working relationship between the supervisor and student and agrees that the project would help the student gain in-depth skills in clinical practice and theory development. The student returns to the hospital to complete her DCE and project. Using the Cognitive Orientation to Daily Occupational Performance approach, patients participated in goal setting and driving the therapeutic process. Because of the successful outcomes of the project, a system-wide initiative was implemented to utilize the approach with all rehabilitation patients.

Dual Duty: Supervision and Mentorship Model

How about this scenario? A clinician is slated to have a Level II fieldwork student and is asked to mentor a doctoral student at the same time. Is that possible? Yes! Given that the doctoral student is to be much more self-directed than the Level II fieldwork student, a clinician can supervise a fieldwork student, continue to treat a caseload of clients, and mentor a doctoral student. It is important that the clinician sets clear guidelines regarding the best methods for communication given this scenario. For example, if the clinician is only free during a scheduled lunch break, that may be a good time for the doctoral student to check in. As the fieldwork student becomes more independent, meeting with the doctoral student may become easier on an as-needed basis, such as when the fieldwork student is documenting. See Box 13-9 for an example of dual duty.

Collaborative Mentorship Model

Consider one last scenario—a clinician mentoring two doctoral students at a time. The students could be working on two related capstone projects that contribute to a larger initiative or two completely different projects that meet current needs at the site. The students may enjoy feeling the support of a peer and can be encouraged to use one another as sounding boards before approaching their site mentor for advice. They will be able to critique one another, provide feedback, and share their knowledge of the site's processes rather than having to approach the mentor for this information. Refresh your memory about the best practices associated with collaborative supervision models in Chapter 2. See Box 13-10 for an example of the collaborative mentorship model.

BOX 13-9

EXAMPLE OF DUAL DUTY

A clinician who works in an outpatient clinic is supervising a Level II fieldwork student from one program while mentoring a doctoral student from another. The clinician sees a large caseload of clients with upper extremity injuries and also completes wheelchair fittings. The Level II fieldwork student focuses on gaining entry-level practice skills by evaluating and treating the clients with upper extremity issues. The doctoral student is completing a project focusing on the creation of a wheelchair skills training clinic for new wheelchair users. While the clinician provides direct supervision to the fieldwork student, the clinician is also able to provide feedback and input on the creation of the wheelchair clinic as needed.

BOX 13-10

EXAMPLE OF THE COLLABORATIVE MENTORSHIP MODEL

Two students are completing their capstones at a school for children with autism spectrum disorder. The site mentor expressed that there is a need for carryover of sensory diets implemented with the students by the therapists. Both staff at the school and families of the students have difficulty understanding and implementing the diets in the classroom and in home life. One student decides to complete a project that focuses on staff education on sensory diets while the other decides to complete a project that focuses on family understanding and implementation. While their projects are different, the hope is that together projects will lead to increased carryover of sensory diet implementation to the benefit of the students.

While no two scenarios of mentorship will be the same, it is possible to mentor doctoral capstone students in addition to the clinician's current responsibilities. Projects that the clinician has been considering or needs that the site has had for some time but that have not been addressed could be tackled with the right doctoral student. Think of mentorship as a win-win situation for both the site/clinician and the student. See Box 13-11 for some strategies to brainstorm how a doctoral capstone student or capstone project might serve a specific need at your work setting.

BENEFITS OF SERVING AS A SITE MENTOR

Similarly, as to what was discussed in Chapter 1 of this book, there are both intrinsic and extrinsic benefits to serving as a mentor to a doctoral student. First, this section will discuss the tangible, more objective benefits. Then, the internally motivating factors will be discussed.

A clinician can earn professional development units (PDUs) for mentoring a doctoral student. Each week of mentorship is the equivalent of earning one PDU. Up to 18 PDUs can be earned per each National Board for Certification in Occupational Therapy renewal period (2019). The occupational therapy program will usually provide a certificate or formal letter which outlines the name of the doctoral student and the number of weeks that the student was mentored for. Site mentors might also be able to use mentorship of a doctoral student to satisfy state licensure continuing competence requirements. Reviewing your state board regulations in advance is important.

BOX 13-11

BRAINSTORMING CAPSTONE PROJECTS

The variety of focus areas for the DCE translates to endless possibilities for capstone projects. But a capstone project should really be a win-win for the practitioner/site and the student. A savvy practitioner will have brainstormed a variety of projects that would both interest a doctoral student but also benefit the site.

Consider your workplace. Are there current quality improvement initiatives being pushed by administration? Or are there programs that have been in consideration but have not been executed due to limited time? Consider the list below to generate ideas of projects that could benefit your workplace.

- Is your workplace working toward an accreditation or certification? Is this something a student could organize?
- Does your site have ongoing or new quality improvement initiatives such as preventative measures, increased client satisfaction, or compliance goals?
- Does your site have a need for increased education for staff or volunteers?
- Are there established best-practices guidelines for treating the population(s) at your workplace?
- Does your facility provide niche interventions that could benefit from further validation?

Do not be afraid to get creative. Consider the many capstone focus areas and the roles that occupational therapists do and could play at your workplace. You will likely come up with some very interesting and needed projects.

Second, a doctoral student's project should be designed to help to meet a need at the site. If the clinician or site has certain projects that have been placed on hold, whether due to lack of time or uncertainty about the best way to approach the project, it is likely that a doctoral student has the time and resources to tackle the project (or a portion of it). For example, consider quality initiatives at the site such as improving fall prevention measures. Or consider whether the site is seeking or renewing an accreditation (like The Joint Commission or Commission of Accreditation for Rehabilitation Facilities) of some sort. These are great opportunities for students whose focus area(s) include administration and/or program development.

Mentoring a student who is interested in research would be a great way for a site mentor to collaborate on a research project with outcomes being disseminated at the state or national level. A site mentor could be listed as a co-author or contributor on a conference poster or session, depending on their level of input. This increased scholarship could be included on the clinician's annual performance review or help support mobility up a clinical ladder.

In addition to the more objective benefits, clinicians who serve as site mentors will benefit for subjective reasons. Taking pride in helping a student learn and grow in their skills as an occupational therapist is often motivation enough for clinicians. In addition, collaborating with a student can challenge the mentor to also learn, grow, and stay up to date with the latest evidence-based practices. Clinicians who regularly supervise and mentor students can be some of the most informed clinicians. Serving as a site mentor is a practical way to help occupational therapy achieve AOTA's (2016) Vision 2025 by helping to shape future clinicians and the sites and clients they serve.

HOW TO BECOME A SITE MENTOR

At this point, one might be thinking, *"This all sounds great! But how does one actually become a site mentor to a doctoral student?"* Following are several steps to consider taking to become a mentor.

First, a clinician should brainstorm on their own and with their colleagues about potential project ideas or current needs at the site. The clinician should consider using the ACOTE (2018b) focus areas as a starting point. It is also important to consider current initiatives at the site, such as accreditation or compliance standards, certifications, or quality improvement projects. If unfamiliar with these areas, the clinician should seek out administration for their input.

A smart second step is to talk with the site's student clinical coordinator and the education or quality improvement department. It is important to know if there is a particular process for accepting and placing students at the site as well as for implementing projects. One should follow the student coordinator's lead regarding onboarding students as well as the quality improvement department's guidelines for gaining permission to execute a future project.

Once permission is granted from the student coordinator or any other necessary parties, the clinician should reach out to local occupational therapy doctoral programs' capstone coordinators. A list of local OTD programs can be found on ACOTE's website: https://acoteonline.org/schools/ot-doctorate/. Call the occupational therapy department or email them, with attention to the capstone coordinator.

The clinician may want to ask for resources related to the program's requirements for the DCE, the specific timeframe for the DCE, as it will differ from program to program, and be prepared to share information about their own area(s) of expertise and current needs of the site. The capstone coordinator will likely be happy to hear about the clinician's interest. From there, the capstone coordinator should take the initiative to create an affiliation agreement between the OTD program and the site if one does not already exist. Similar to fieldwork, occupational therapy programs will want to formalize the experience with a formal contract with the site/organization, which also will usually include a certificate of insurance for liability purposes.

SUMMARY

Given the growing number of occupational therapy programs offering the entry-level doctoral degree, it is likely that clinicians will have the opportunity to (or be expected to) mentor a doctoral capstone student. This can be a rewarding experience, for both the clinician and the student, as mutual learning, collaboration, and growth occurs. In addition, the student's capstone project can benefit the site by meeting a current need.

It is important that the clinician understand that fieldwork is to prepare generalist practitioners whereas the capstone experience and project are to advance the student's skills in one or more focus areas. Supervisors can help to prepare students who are on fieldwork for the capstone experience by providing opportunities for decision making and by promoting divergent thinking. Clinicians who provide effective mentorship are not only role models who communicate and collaborate with the doctoral student but also allow the doctoral student to self-direct their learning while promoting divergent thinking. The tools included in this chapter should empower the clinician to prepare fieldwork students for the transition to the DCE as well as provide effective mentorship to the student during the doctoral capstone.

LEARNING ACTIVITIES

1. If your workplace has site-specific learning objectives, use those as a starting point to create DCE objectives. If your workplace does not have them, refer to AOTA's Site-Specific Objectives (AOTA, n.d.) for a starting point. Consider the examples provided in Table 13-3. and write a few DCE objectives that would be pertinent for your site.

2. Do you have ideas for doctoral capstone projects? Consider your site's program development and quality improvement initiatives as well as their accreditation standards and certifications. Create a list of current needs that projects could meet in each of these areas. Share this with your local occupational therapy programs to increase student interest.

3. Consider the professionals with whom you work. Do any of them have particular expertise that could benefit a doctoral capstone student's learning in their chosen area(s) of focus? Create a chart of the focus areas and the professionals who might contribute to a doctoral capstone student's learning in those areas. Gauge their interest in providing learning experiences to a doctoral student.

4. Consider the skills that are required of the student during the DCE. How can you provide exposure for skill development during a Level II fieldwork experience? Refer to the examples of learning objectives that are listed in Table 13-3 for skills that might be required in each focus area.

REFERENCES

Accreditation Council for Occupational Therapy Education. (2018a). Schools. https://acoteonline.org/all-schools/

Accreditation Council for Occupational Therapy Education. (2018b). Standards and interpretive guide (effective July 31, 2020). https://www.aota.org/~/media/Corporate/Files/EducationCareers/Accredit/StandardsReview/2018-ACOTE-Standards-Interpretive-Guide.pdf

American Occupational Therapy Association. (n.d.). Site-specific objectives. https://www.aota.org/Education-Careers/Fieldwork/SiteObj.aspx

American Occupational Therapy Association. (2006). Role competencies for a fieldwork educator. *American Journal of Occupational Therapy, 60*(6), 650–651. https://doi.org/10.5014/ajot.60.6.650

American Occupational Therapy Association. (2011). Accreditation Council for Occupational Therapy Education (ACOTE) standards. *American Journal of Occupational Therapy, 66*(6), S6–S74. https://doi.org/10.5014/ajot.2012.66s6

American Occupational Therapy Association. (2014). AOTA Board of Directors position statement on entry-level degree for the occupational therapist [OTD statement]. https://www.aota.org/AboutAOTA/GetInvolved/BOD/OTD-Statement.aspx.

American Occupational Therapy Association. (2017). Vision 2025. *American Journal of Occupational Therapy, 71,* 7103420010. https://doi.org/10.5014/ajot.2017.713002

American Occupational Therapy Association. (2020). Fieldwork performance evaluation for the occupational therapy student. AOTA Press. https://www.aota.org/-/media/Corporate/Files/EducationCareers/Fieldwork/Fieldwork-Performance-Evaluation-Occupational-Therapy-Student.pdf

Bednarski, J., & DeIuliis, E.D. (2021, April 9). Facilitate innovative entry-level doctorate capstones to align with the AOTA Vision 2025 using human centered design framework [short course]. American Occupational Therapy Association Annual Conference.

Brenner, W., Uebernickel, F., & Abrell, T. (2016). Design thinking as a mindset, process, and toolbox. Experiences from research and teaching at the University of St. Gallen. Design Thinking for Innovation. https://doi.org/10.1007/978-3-319-26100-3_1

Cook, A. B. (2019). Suggested components of the final capstone report. In E. DeIuliis & J. Bednarski (Eds.), *The entry level occupational therapy doctorate capstone: A framework for the experience and project* (pp. 195-214). SLACK Incorporated.

Copley, J., & Nelson, A. (2012). Practice educator perspectives of multiple mentoring in diverse clinical settings. *British Journal of Occupational Therapy, 75*(10), 456-462. https://dx.doi.org.10/4276/030802212X13496921049662

Crisp, G. (2009). Conceptualization and initial validation of the College Student Mentoring Scale (CSMS). *Journal of College Student Development, 50*(2), 177–194. https://doi.org/10.1353/csd.0.0061

DeIuliis, E. D. (2017). What is fieldwork education? In E. D. DeIuliis (Ed.), *Professionalism across occupational therapy practice* (pp. 163-199). SLACK Incorporated.

DeIuliis, E.D., & Bednarski, J. (2019). *The entry level occupational therapy doctorate capstone: A framework for the experience and project*. SLACK Incorporated.

Delbert, T., Stepansky, K., & Lekas, T. (2020). The S.E.L.F. approach: Systems and experiential learning framework for fieldwork and capstone education development. *The Open Journal of Occupational Therapy, 8*(3), 1-11. https://doi.org/10.15453/2168-6408.1710

Evenson, M. E., Roberts, M., Kaldenberg, J., Barnes, M.A., & Ozelie, R. (2015). National survey of fieldwork educators: Implications for occupational therapy education. *American Journal of Occupational Therapy, 69*(Suppl. 2) 6912350020p1-5. https://doi.org/10.5014/ajot.2015.019265

Freeman, J. C., & All, A. (2017). Academic support of programs utilized for nursing students at risk of academic failure: A review of the literature. *Nursing Education Perspectives, 38*(2), 69–74. https://doi.org/10.1097/01.NEP.0000000000000089

Hanson, D. J., & DeIuliis, E. D. (2015). The collaborative model of fieldwork education: A blueprint for group supervision of students. *Occupational Therapy in Health Care, 29*(2), 223-239. https://doi.org/10.3109/07380577.2015.1011297

IDEO.org. https://www.designkit.org/resources/1?utm_medium=ApproachPage&utm_source=www.ideo.org&utm_campaign=FGButton

Johnson, T. R. B., Settimi, P. D., & Rogers, J. L. (2001). Mentoring for the health professions. *New Directions for Teaching and Learning*, (85), 25–34. https://doi.org/10.1002/tl.3

Kemp, E., Domina, A., Delbert, T., Rivera, A., & Navarro-Walker, L. (2020). Development, implementation and evaluation of entry-level occupational therapy doctoral capstones: A national survey. *Journal of Occupational Therapy Education, 4*(4). https://doi.org/10.26681/jote.2020.040411

Krusen, N. E., Murphy-Hagan, A., & Foidel, S. (2020). The purpose of capstone in an entry-level clinical doctorate: A scoping review. *Journal of Occupational Therapy Education, 4*(4). https://doi.org/10.26681/jote.2020.040404

Mattila, A., DeIuliis, E. D., & Cook, A. B. (2018). Increasing self-efficacy through role emerging placements: Implications for occupational therapy experiential learning. *Journal of Occupational Therapy Education, 2*(3). https://doi.org/10.26681/jote.2018.020303

Mattila, A., DeIuliis, E. D., & Cook, A. B. (2020). Evaluating the professional transformation from a doctoral capstone experience. *Journal of Transformative Learning, 7*(2), 34-44.

National Board for Certification in Occupational Therapy. (2019). NBCOT certification renewal activities chart. https://www.nbcot.org/-/media/NBCOT/PDFs/Renewal_Activity_Chart.ashx?la=en&hash=1B1765963E596B6BF27064B05197B2DA48157E8A

Rodger, S., Fitzgerald, C., Davila, W., Millar, F., & Allison, H. (2011). What makes a quality occupational therapy practice placement? Students' and practice educators' perspectives. *Australian Occupational Therapy Journal, 58*(3), 195–202. https://doi.org/10.1111/j.1440-1630.2010.00903.x

Stephenson, S., Rogers, O., Ivy, C., Barron, R., & Burke, J. (2020). Designing effective capstone experiences and projects for entry-level doctoral students in occupational therapy: One program's approaches and lessons learned. *The Open Journal of Occupational Therapy, 8*(3), 1-12. https://doi.org/10.15453/ 2168-6408.1727

Wasmuth, S. & Polo, K. M. (2019). Scholarly deliverables and impact of the capstone. In E. DeIuliis & J. Bednarski (Eds.), *The entry level occupational therapy doctorate capstone: A framework for the experience and project* (pp. 215-226). SLACK Incorporated.

Whitney, R. V., & McCormack, G. (2020). They said: Perspectives on capstone experience and projects in occupational therapy. *The Open Journal of Occupational Therapy, 8*(3), 1-5. https://doi.org/10.15453/2168-6408.1778

APPENDIX A

80/20 Rule Examples

FOCUS AREA	TIME SPENT ON-SITE	TIME SPENT OFF-SITE
Clinical practice skills	Evaluating clients with specific or complex diagnoses and providing intervention; attending team meetings, attending on-site trainings; engaging in interprofessional collaboration and learning from other disciplines their role in client care	Creating a best practices guideline for newly hired therapists; participating in continued education to benefit clinical practice skills; reading evidence-based practice articles to inform client care
Research skills	Measuring client outcomes; comparing medical charts; reviewing research protocols; gaining informed consent; interviewing	Using statistical software to run analyses; transcribing interviews; coding; updating literature review
Administration	Learning directly alongside administrators; attending managerial level meetings; preparing reports for accreditors	Reviewing Medicare guidelines, Joint Commission accreditation guidelines, and employee handbook
Leadership	Attending meetings, events, and forums; interviewing leaders to learn what makes an effective leader	Taking an online leadership course; reflecting on one's own leadership style
Program and policy development	Meeting with stakeholders necessary to implement a program or policy; delivering a program; implementing a policy; documenting reactions or outcomes	Designing the logistics of the program or policy; evaluating outcomes
Advocacy	Attending meetings with stakeholders; engaging in advocacy events; attending forums; meeting with legislators	Reading about the current policies; writing a letter to a legislator; creating an advocacy pamphlet
Education	Directly delivering a lecture; administering a learning activity; instructing a hands-on lab	Designing an exam; pre-recording a webinar or lecture; creating a learning activity
Theory development	Applying the theory in on-site interactions with clients, family, or staff	Reading literature about the theory; attending trainings on how to apply theory to the practice setting and population

APPENDIX B
Memorandum of Understanding

Doctoral Capstone Memorandum of Understanding

OTD Student Name: _____

Area of Primary Focus:

☐ Research	☐ Administration	☐ Teaching
☐ Adv Clinical Practice	☐ Leadership	☐ Theory Development
☐ Adv Community Practice	☐ Advocacy	☐ Other - Describe: _____

Area of Secondary Focus (if applicable):

☐ Research	☐ Administration	☐ Teaching
☐ Adv Clinical Practice	☐ Leadership	☐ Theory Development
☐ Adv Community Practice	☐ Advocacy	☐ Other - Describe: _____

Name of DCE Site: _____

DCE Setting: _____

Primary Site Mentor Name, Title and Credentials: _____

Site Mentor Preferred Email Address: _____

Site Mentor Preferred Phone: _____

Description of Qualifications of Site Mentor Aligned With the Focus Area:

Please also attach evidence via a résumé, curriculum vitae or other qualification that shows expertise aligned with focus area.

General Overview of Doctorate Capstone Experience and Project (100 words or less):*

This may be subject to change based on the completion of the needs assessment but is meant to ensure the site mentor and OTD student are considering the capstone project in similar ways.

*Page 1 should be completed by the OTD student

Relationship to Duquesne Curriculum Design Acknowledgement of Duquesne OTD Behavioral Objectives

Below are the OTD DCE learning objectives aligned with the curriculum design at Duquesne University (https://www.duq.edu/academics/schools/health-sciences/academic-programs/occupational-therapy/resources-for-students/doctoral-capstone-experience). You will see that there is space provided for the OTD student and you, the site mentor, to mutually decide upon three student-specific objectives that would be achievable within the 14-week experience. These should align with the student's chosen area of focus. Once the three objectives are agreed to, students should continue to collaborate with you to outline action steps, activities, or strategies to help achieve their goals (see action plan and weekly schedule template provided).

1. Demonstrate effective communication skills and work interprofessionally with those who receive and provide care/services.

2. Display positive interpersonal skills and insight into one's professional behaviors to accurately appraise one's professional disposition strengths and areas for improvement.

3. Exhibit the ability to practice educative roles for consumers, peers, students, interprofessionals, and others.

4. Develop essential knowledge and skills to contribute to the advancement of occupational therapy through scholarly activities.

5. Apply a critical foundation of evidence based professional knowledge, skills, and attitudes.

6. Apply principles and constructs of ethics to individual, institutional, and societal issues and articulate justifiable resolutions to these issues and act in an ethical manner.

7. Perform tasks in a safe and ethical manner and adhere to the site's policies and procedures, including those related to human participant research when relevant.

8. Demonstrate competence in following program methods, quality improvement, and/or research procedures utilized at the site.

9. Learn, practice, and apply knowledge from the classroom and practice settings at a higher level than prior fieldwork experiences with simultaneous guidance from site mentor and DU OT faculty.

10. Relate theory to practice and demonstrate synthesis of advanced knowledge in a specialized practice area through completion of a doctoral field experience and scholarly project.

11. Acquire in-depth experience in one or more of the following areas: clinical practice skills, research skills, administration, leadership, program and policy development, advocacy, education, and theory development.

12. Student identified objective

13. Student identified objective

14. Student identified objective

Site Mentor Signature: _____   Date: _____

OTD Student Signature: _____   Date: _____

Site Mentor Acknowledgment of Supervision/Mentorship

I, _____ , agree to:

(site mentor name)

1. Serve as a site mentor to _____ during a 14-week DCE placement, which includes regular (at least weekly) communication. (insert student name above)

2. Collaborate with the OTD Student to create three individualized student learning objectives to customize this capstone experience.

3. Provide guidance and mentorship to the student's action plan to support accomplishment of the student learning objectives over the 14-week placement.

4. Complete a midterm and final evaluation of the OTD student using the DCE Evaluation of the OTD student.

5. Communicate with the Capstone Coordinator regarding any concerns or needs during the experience.

6. Collaborate with the OTD Student and be listed as a contributing author (as appropriate) regarding scholarly products, including but not limited to manuscripts, presentations, and posters.

7. Provide documentation of expertise in the OTD Student's chosen focus area(s) by submitting a copy of a résumé, CV, or continued education in the area(s).

8. Watch the Site Mentor webinar found at: https://www.duq.edu/academics/schools/health-sciences/academic-programs/occupational-therapy/resources-for-fw-educators (Under **Educator Development Resources**, then **DCE Site Mentor Guide**).

Site Mentor Signature: _____ Date: _____

OTD Student Acknowledgment of Supervision/Mentorship

I, _____ , agree to:

(OTD Student name)

1. Initiate a discussion with the Site Mentor to create three individualized student learning objectives to customize this capstone experience using the DCE Behavioral Objectives Form.

2. Collaborate with the Site Mentor on an action plan designed to accomplish the individualized student learning objectives.

3. Work together with Site Mentor to create a schedule that will consist of at least 80% on-site and no more than 20% off-site.

4. Create and implement a capstone project informed by evidenced and based upon a Needs Assessment at the DCE site.

5. Complete the Student Evaluation of the DCE Site form at completion of the DCE.

6. Proactively communicate with the Site Mentor regarding any questions during the experience.

7. Proactively communicate with the capstone coordinator regarding any concerns or needs during the experience.

8. Collaborate with and include my Site Mentor, Faculty Capstone Chair, and any other appropriate parties as contributing authors on scholarly products, including but not limited to, manuscripts, presentations, and posters.

9. Demonstrate respectful interaction and communication with the student cohort, faculty, mentors, doctoral capstone coordinator, and other individuals who may be a part of the capstone.

10. Utilize constructive feedback from faculty, site mentor, and capstone coordinator for personal and professional growth.

11. Take responsibility for their own skills and professional development. (This can include professional writing skills, knowledge of IRB application process, etc.)

12. Complete and disseminate a culminating capstone project in a format and forum, within the timeframe determined by the academic program.

OTD Student Signature: _____ Date: _____

Mail/fax/email this form and supporting documentation to the Capstone Coordinator within 2 weeks after completion of the Needs Assessment.

APPENDIX C
Doctoral Capstone Experience Action Plan to Achieve In-Depth Skills

Outline how you will achieve your self-authored goals (designed in collaboration with your site mentor) below by indicating your learning objectives, activities to achieve your objectives, and proposed evidence of achievement of your learning objectives (add rows to the table as needed).

Individualized Learning Objectives	Activities, Strategies and Actions to Achieve Learning Objectives	Proposed Timeline for Each Learning Objective	The Skills You Possess and the Resources You Can Access to Support Success	Proposed Evidence of Achievement of Each Learning Objective
Example: I will gain in-depth clinical skills related to infant handling and positioning in the NICU	Shadow the NICU OT	Weeks 1 to 2	Foundational knowledge of infant development, sensory processing Quick learner who learns by seeing and doing Ability to seek and integrate feedback	Treat at least one infant on caseload each day during weeks 4 to 12 Create educational materials on proper positioning and handling for families
	Learn about other professionals' roles in NICU	Weeks 1 to 14		
	Work under supervision of OT	Weeks 3 to 12		
	Educate families on proper handling of infants	Weeks 6 to 12		

Signatures below signify acceptance of the above proposal and approval to move forward with implementation. It is the student's responsibility to access resources, carry out these and/or other strategies to increase their knowledge and skill, aligned with their chosen focus area.

Student Signature: _____   Date: _____

Site Mentor Signature: _____   Date: _____

Proposed Timeline for the 14-Week Doctoral Capstone Experience (Please Include Doctoral Capstone Project Components)

Please complete the following schedule as a tentative plan of how you foresee your time spent during the 14-week doctoral experience. This plan may be general at this point and subject to change. This is a tool to help you consider how you will spend time to meet your learning objectives as well as complete your culminating capstone project. Experiences, actions, and steps that you will take should align with your chosen focus area(s). Please share this with your entire capstone team.

WEEK	EXPERIENCES, ACTIONS, STEPS	NOTES/MISCELLANEOUS
Week 1		
Week 2		
Week 3		
Week 4		
Week 5		
Week 6		
Week 7 Midterm Evaluation Due		
Week 8		
Week 9		
Week 10		
Week 11		
Week 12		
Week 13		
Week 14 Final Evaluation Due		

APPENDIX D

Duquesne University
Doctoral Capstone Experience Evaluation of the OTD Student

Site Mentor Form

Student Name: _____   Site Mentor Name: _____

Placement Dates: _____   Site/Setting: _____

Date of Midterm Review: _____   Date of Final Review: _____

Select the focus of the residency:

☐ Research   ☐ Administration   ☐ Teaching
☐ Adv Clinical Practice   ☐ Leadership   ☐ Theory Development
☐ Adv Community Practice   ☐ Advocacy   ☐ Other - Describe: _____

Instructions

The site mentor will complete this evaluation form at midterm (7 weeks) and final (14 weeks). The site mentor and the OTD student will review the evaluation collectively and sign that they agree on the evaluation. The OTD student is encouraged to complete a self-assessment to guide discussion and the learning process. The self-reflection is to be completed by the student separate from and prior to meeting with the site mentor. This is used to foster self-reflection on the student's performance including areas of growth and areas for improvement related to the learning objectives and student-specific objectives.

Learning objectives 1 through 11 are derived from the DU OTD Doctoral Capstone Experience Behavioral Objectives.

Note that there is space provided (potential objectives 12 to 14) for both the OTD student and the site mentor to add three student-specific objectives, mutually decided upon by the OTD student and site mentor based on what the student wants/needs to know and what skills the student needs to develop. All objectives must be: (1) relevant to the fieldwork experience setting; (2) understandable to the student, site mentor, and Doctoral Capstone Coordinator AFWC; (3) measurable; (4) behavioral/observable; and (5) achievable within the specified time frame.

Please use this scale to rate the objectives below:

5= Exceeding, 4= Met, 3= Making Progress, 2= Not Making Progress, 1= Needs Attention

Provide comments to indicate evidence, as indicated.

DU OTD Objective #1: Student will demonstrate effective communication skills and work inter-professionally with those who receive and provide care.

Evidence of Accomplishment, to be completed by Student and Site Mentor:

_____

_____

Midterm   ☐ 5   ☐ 4   ☐ 3   ☐ 2   ☐ 1

Comments:

_____

Final   ☐ 5   ☐ 4   ☐ 3   ☐ 2   ☐ 1

Comments:

_____

_____

DU OTD Objective #2: Student will demonstrate positive interpersonal skills and insight into one's professional behaviors to accurately appraise one's professional disposition, strengths, and areas for improvement.

Evidence of Accomplishment, to be completed by Student and Site Mentor:

_____

_____

Midterm   ☐ 5   ☐ 4   ☐ 3   ☐ 2   ☐ 1

Comments:

_____

Final   ☐ 5   ☐ 4   ☐ 3   ☐ 2   ☐ 1

Comments:

_____

_____

DU OTD Objective #3: Student will demonstrate the ability to practice educative roles for clients, peers, students, interprofessionals, and others.

Evidence of Accomplishment, to be completed by Student and Site Mentor:

_____

_____

Midterm   ☐ 5   ☐ 4   ☐ 3   ☐ 2   ☐ 1

Comments:

_____

_____

Final   ☐ 5   ☐ 4   ☐ 3   ☐ 2   ☐ 1

Comments:

_____

_____

DU OTD Objective #4: Student will develop essential knowledge and skills to contribute to the advancement of occupational therapy through scholarly activities.

Evidence of Accomplishment, to be completed by Student and Site Mentor:

_____

_____

Midterm   ☐ 5   ☐ 4   ☐ 3   ☐ 2   ☐ 1

Comments:

_____

_____

Final   ☐ 5   ☐ 4   ☐ 3   ☐ 2   ☐ 1

Comments:

_____

_____

DU OTD Objective #5: Student will apply a critical foundation of evidence-based professional knowledge, skills, and attitudes.

Evidence of Accomplishment, to be completed by Student and Site Mentor:

_____

_____

Midterm   ☐ 5   ☐ 4   ☐ 3   ☐ 2   ☐ 1

Comments:

_____

_____

Final   ☐ 5   ☐ 4   ☐ 3   ☐ 2   ☐ 1

Comments:

_____

_____

DU OTD Objective #6: Student will apply principles and constructs of ethics to individual, institutional, and societal issues and articulate justifiable resolutions to these issues and act in an ethical manner.

Evidence of Accomplishment, to be completed by Student and Site Mentor:

_____

_____

Midterm   ☐ 5   ☐ 4   ☐ 3   ☐ 2   ☐ 1

Comments:

_____

_____

Final   ☐ 5   ☐ 4   ☐ 3   ☐ 2   ☐ 1

Comments:

_____

_____

DU OTD Objective #7: Student will perform tasks in a safe and ethical manner and adhere to the site's policies and procedures, including those related to human participant research, when relevant.

Evidence of Accomplishment, to be completed by Student and Site Mentor:

_____

_____

Midterm   ☐ 5   ☐ 4   ☐ 3   ☐ 2   ☐ 1

Comments:

_____

_____

Final   ☐ 5   ☐ 4   ☐ 3   ☐ 2   ☐ 1

Comments:

_____

_____

DU OTD Objective #8: Student will demonstrate competence in following program methods, quality improvement, and/or research procedures utilized at the site.

Evidence of Accomplishment, to be completed by Student and Site Mentor:

_____

_____

Midterm   ☐ 5   ☐ 4   ☐ 3   ☐ 2   ☐ 1

Comments:

_____

_____

Final   ☐ 5   ☐ 4   ☐ 3   ☐ 2   ☐ 1

Comments:

_____

_____

DU OTD Objective #9: Student will learn, practice, and apply knowledge from the classroom and practice settings at a higher level than prior fieldwork experiences, with simultaneous guidance from Site Mentor and DU OT Faculty.

Evidence of Accomplishment, to be completed by Student and Site Mentor:

_____

_____

Midterm   ☐ 5   ☐ 4   ☐ 3   ☐ 2   ☐ 1

Comments:

_____

_____

Final   ☐ 5   ☐ 4   ☐ 3   ☐ 2   ☐ 1

Comments:

_____

_____

DU OTD Objective #10: Student will relate theory to practice and demonstrate synthesis of advanced knowledge in a specialized practice area through completion of a doctoral capstone component and scholarly project.

Evidence of Accomplishment, to be completed by Student and Site Mentor:

_____

_____

Midterm   ☐ 5   ☐ 4   ☐ 3   ☐ 2   ☐ 1

Comments:

_____

_____

Final   ☐ 5   ☐ 4   ☐ 3   ☐ 2   ☐ 1

Comments:

_____

_____

DU OTD Objective #11: Acquire in-depth experience in one or more of the following areas: clinical practice skills, research skills, administration, leadership, program and policy development, advocacy, education, and theory development.

Evidence of Accomplishment, to be completed by Student and Site Mentor:

_____

_____

Midterm   ☐ 5   ☐ 4   ☐ 3   ☐ 2   ☐ 1

Comments:

_____

_____

Final   ☐ 5   ☐ 4   ☐ 3   ☐ 2   ☐ 1

Comments:

_____

_____

OTD Student-Selected Objective #1:

Evidence of Accomplishment, to be completed by Student and Site Mentor:

_____

_____

Midterm   ☐ 5   ☐ 4   ☐ 3   ☐ 2   ☐ 1

Comments:

_____

_____

Final   ☐ 5   ☐ 4   ☐ 3   ☐ 2   ☐ 1

Comments:

_____

_____

OTD Student-Selected Objective #2:

Evidence of Accomplishment, to be completed by Student and Site Mentor:

_____

_____

Midterm   ☐ 5   ☐ 4   ☐ 3   ☐ 2   ☐ 1

Comments:

_____

_____

Final   ☐ 5   ☐ 4   ☐ 3   ☐ 2   ☐ 1

Comments:

_____

_____

OTD Student-Selected Objective #3:

Evidence of Accomplishment, to be completed by Student and Site Mentor:

_____

_____

Midterm   ☐ 5   ☐ 4   ☐ 3   ☐ 2   ☐ 1

Comments:

_____

_____

Final   ☐ 5   ☐ 4   ☐ 3   ☐ 2   ☐ 1

Comments:

_____

_____

We are interested in obtaining an accurate profile of the OTD student's capacity for the profession. We would appreciate your additional comments regarding the areas in which you rated the student on the previous pages.

Overall Strengths:

Areas for Growth:

Student Signature: _____   Date: _____

Site Mentor Name (Print): _____

Phone: _____

Email Address: _____

Site Mentor Signature: _____   Date: _____

FINANCIAL DISCLOSURES

Dr. Julie A. Bednarski reported no financial or proprietary interest in the materials presented herein.

Dr. Ann B. Cook reported no financial or proprietary interest in the materials presented herein.

Dr. Elizabeth D. DeIuliis reported no financial or proprietary interest in the materials presented herein.

Dr. Anna Domina reported no financial or proprietary interest in the materials presented herein.

Dr. Cherie Graves reported no financial or proprietary interest in the materials presented herein.

Dr. Debra Hanson reported no financial or proprietary interest in the materials presented herein.

Dr. Caryn Reichlin Johnson reported no financial or proprietary interest in the materials presented herein.

Dr. Angela Lampe reported no financial or proprietary interest in the materials presented herein.

Dr. Patricia Laverdure reported no financial or proprietary interest in the materials presented herein.

Dr. Elizabeth LeQuieu reported no financial or proprietary interest in the materials presented herein.

Dr. Amy Mattila reported no financial or proprietary interest in the materials presented herein.

Dr. Ranelle Nissen reported no financial or proprietary interest in the materials presented herein.

Dr. Hannah Oldenburg reported no financial or proprietary interest in the materials presented herein.

Dr. Rebecca Ozelie reported no financial or proprietary interest in the materials presented herein.

Dr. Alexandria Raymond reported no financial or proprietary interest in the materials presented herein.

Dr. Michael Roberts reported no financial or proprietary interest in the materials presented herein.

Dr. Rebecca L. Simon reported no financial or proprietary interest in the materials presented herein.

Dr. Bridget Trivinia reported no financial or proprietary interest in the materials presented herein.

Dr. Jayson Ziegler reported no financial or proprietary interest in the materials presented herein.

INDEX

Printed in the United States
by Baker & Taylor Publisher Services